Vascular Technology
Examination PREP

Vascular Technology Examination PREP

Second Edition

Raymond Gaiser, MS, RDMS, RVT
Director of Radiology
Pennsylvania Hospital
Clinical Instructor, Vascular Sonography
Department of Medical Imaging & Radiation Sciences
Jefferson College of Health Professions
Thomas Jefferson University
Philadelphia, Pennsylvania

Traci B. Fox, EdD, RT(R), RDMS, RVT
Associate Professor, Diagnostic Medical Sonography
Department of Medical Imaging & Radiation Sciences
Jefferson College of Health Professions
Thomas Jefferson University
Philadelphia, Pennsylvania

New York   Chicago   San Francisco   Athens   London   Madrid   Mexico City
Milan   New Delhi   Singapore   Sydney   Toronto

3 4 5 6 7 8 9   DSS   26 25 24 23

ISBN 978-1-260-46761-1
MHID 1-260-46761-9

This book was set in Minion Pro by KnowledgeWorks Global Ltd.
The editors were Susan Oldenburg and Kim J. Davis.
The production supervisor was Richard Ruzycka.
Project management was provided by Revathi Viswanathan, KnowledgeWorks Global Ltd.
The cover design was W2 Design.

This book is printed on acid-free paper.

Library of Congress Cataloging-in-Publication Data

Names: Gaiser, Ray, author. | Fox, Traci B, author.
Title: Vascular technology examination PREP / Raymond Gaiser, Traci B. Fox.
Description: Second edition. | New York: McGraw Hill, [2021] | Includes bibliographical references and index. | Summary: "The purpose of this book is to provide a comprehensive yet concise review of all aspects of vascular disease and testing for sonographers at any level of their career"—Provided by publisher.
Identifiers: LCCN 2020038868 (print) | LCCN 2020038869 (ebook) | ISBN 9781260467611 (paperback: alk. paper) | ISBN 9781260467628 (ebook)
Subjects: MESH: Vascular Diseases—diagnostic imaging | Cerebrovascular Disorders—diagnostic imaging | Diagnostic Techniques, Cardiovascular | Ultrasonography | Examination Questions
Classification: LCC RC388.5 (print) | LCC RC388.5 (ebook) | NLM WG 18.2 | DDC 616.8/1075—dc23
LC record available at https://lccn.loc.gov/2020038868
LC ebook record available at https://lccn.loc.gov/2020038869

McGraw Hill books are available at special quantity discounts to use as premiums and sales promotions or for use in corporate training programs. To contact a representative, please visit the Contact Us pages at www.mhprofessional.com.

Contents

Preface

One of the greatest gifts for an educator is when someone comes up to you and says, "I passed my boards because of you." We are proud that our first edition helped so many people pass their vascular technology exams. This second edition expands on the first by adding more images, newer procedures, and updated normal/abnormal values. In addition, it includes recently published (at the time of publication) consensus group recommendations on arterial and venous waveforms. We hope that this second edition continues to help a new generation with lasting vascular learning.

Through the many years we've spent educating inspiring vascular technologists, we have answered a very simple question numerous times: "What is a good resource to use to help me pass the vascular technology boards?" Our answer would always jokingly be, "Just study my notes from class and you should pass with no problem." Of course, we would always follow with some of our favorite review materials that have previously been published. It wasn't until a couple of years ago that we decided that our initial answer to that repeated question was not that far-fetched. Traci Fox and I share the same passion for educating, and it was at that time we decided to take our combined years of clinical and teaching experience and create a comprehensive review for vascular technologists and students.

The purpose of this book is to provide a comprehensive yet concise review of all aspects of vascular disease and testing for sonographers at any level of their career. It can serve as a point of reference for practicing technologists in any laboratory as well as a systematic, well-organized review for new technologists preparing for the ARDMS (VT) or CCI (RVS) examinations. It can also be used by interpreting physicians, residents, and fellows as a reference as well as a resource of review material for the RPVI examination.

With over 40 images per chapter, this text offers an extensive review of vascular testing presented in a clear and thorough manner that is easy to read and understand. Each chapter outline follows the outline for the ARDMS vascular technology examination which covers hemodynamics and vascular anatomy, pathology, patient assessment and integration of data, protocols, interpretation of results, treatments, and other related testing for each of the vascular systems in the body. Each section is explained in a way that can be understood and applied to every aspect of a vascular technologist's duties. For the novice sonographer, this book provides the knowledge necessary to practice as well as to become a registered vascular technologist.

The key feature of this text is that it is an all-encompassing, comprehensive review book focused on vascular principles that includes both the content as well as review questions for each chapter. When studying, knowing what you do not know is an important part of studying. Therefore, each chapter has the relevant content for each vascular topic as well as a complete list of questions followed by the answers and explanations. In addition to the review questions at the end of each chapter, there is a full practice examination with an additional 120 questions also followed by answers and explanations designed to mimic the ARDMS national registry examination for vascular technology.

We are very pleased to be able to share this text with you. We wrote this text with the intent to help expand the knowledge of vascular technology for those currently practicing while providing the foundation of knowledge for others just getting started. We really enjoyed writing this text and hope that you and it to be a valuable resource throughout your career.

Raymond Gaiser, MS, RDMS, RVT
Traci B. Fox, EdD, RT(R), RDMS, RVT

Acknowledgments

I would like to dedicate this book to my real-life hero, my father Raymond Gaiser, Jr. Even though he is no longer with us, I will always remember the lessons he taught me. Without the traits he instilled in me throughout my life none of this would be possible. I would like to thank to the most important women in my life who are my Mother Joan, wife Diana, and our three beautiful daughters Ava, Mia, and Alina. You make me prouder with each passing year. They keep me grounded and provide unconditional support always. I would also like to thank many colleagues and friends who made all this possible. Their contributions to this book are what make it so great. Special thanks to Adam Olsen, Rita Brooks, Rachel Lucchese, Katie Nahill, Doreen Kuestner, and Clara Lombardi. I would also like to make my gratitude known to all the vascular technologists at Capital Health Medical Center and Pennsylvania Hospital for their commitment to quality and skill level which made it possible for us to provide you with such amazing images. Finally, but certainly not least, I would like to personally thank my esteemed partner in crime on this project, Traci Fox, for her dedication to this project. Without her knowledge, expertise, and drive, this would not have been possible.

Raymond Gaiser, MS, RDMS, RVT

I would like to thank Thresa for her continued unbelievable patience and understanding. To her, I'm just the weird noise coming from the first-floor office. Special shoutout to my friends and family for their everlasting support, and sending much love to my "Aunt Sukey," who left us since the first edition. I would also like to thank all my colleagues who offered images as well as their own anatomy for this project. Extra special thanks to the following people who helped expand my knowledge and, through their contributions, made my work easier: Laurence Needleman, MD; Flemming Forsberg, PhD; Roger Lown, BS, RVT, RDMS, RMSKS; Lauren Lown, BS, RVT, RDMS, RMSKS; JoAnne Aichroth, BS, RDMS, RVT, RMSKS; Renee McKinney, BS, RVT, RDMS; Ayaz Anaan BS, RDCS; Dallas Peyton, BS, RDMS, RVT; Doreen Kuestner, MS, RDMS, RVT; George Berdejo, BA, RVT, FSVU; Patrick Washko, BS, RDMS, RVT, FSVU; Adam Olsen, BS, RVT; Renee T. Kinney, BS, RVT, RDMS; Melanie Kinkler, BS, RVT; Patricia McGinnis, BS, RDMS, RVT, and probably many others. I would especially like to thank my colleague and co-author Ray Gaiser, for his knowledge, experience, and dedication to this project (again). Ray and I both experienced extreme challenges during this project, but our combined strength kept this project moving forward. Lastly, I just want to say fight cancer and fight Alzheimer's and dementia.

Traci B. Fox, EdD, RT(R), RDMS, RVT

We are grateful to be surrounded by so many talented and intelligent people who all made this possible. We hope you enjoy reading the text as much as we enjoyed writing it.

Vascular Technology
Examination PREP

Instrumentation, Hemodynamics, and Doppler

INSTRUMENTATION

Transducers

Ultrasound (US) is a technology that is constantly evolving. Although this chapter will review common technologies in use today to make diagnoses with ultrasound, there is a new era on the near horizon that is changing the way sound is generated, received, and processed. Modern US transducer arrays use a row of piezoelectric elements made of a lead zirconate titanate (PZT) ceramic to create sound waves. Sound waves are generated by the transducer and sent into the patient when the piezoelectric elements are shocked by electricity. The sound waves are reflected by reflectors in the body, and the sound returns to the piezoelectric elements, which generate electricity. The electrical signals produced by the piezoelectric elements are sent to the US machine for processing, and an image is produced. Doppler is possible because red blood cells (RBCs) reflect sound. RBCs are a type of nonspecular reflector called a Rayleigh scatterer, which is a type of scattering that occurs from reflectors that are very small compared to the wavelength of the beam.

Transducers can operate in pulsed-wave (PW) or continuous-wave (CW) operation, depending on their design (Fig. 1–1). In vascular sonography, CW transducers most commonly resemble a pencil probe with two separate piezoelectric elements (Fig. 1–2). The CW pencil probe is commonly used to insonate the distal arteries during noninvasive peripheral arterial examinations. CW transducers need to have two piezoelectric elements: one to continuously transmit sound waves and one to continuously receive sound waves. The constant transmission of the sound means the machine is not able to measure the travel time of the sound, which is only possible with PW ultrasound. Therefore, CW ultrasound transducers do not produce an image, only a spectral Doppler waveform, and the operator cannot select a specific vessel to insonate.

The curvilinear, linear, and sector transducers are PW transducers used for different purposes. The curvilinear (aka convex or curved) array is commonly used for abdominal work or for venous examinations on patients with a large body habitus. The linear array, which produces a rectangular-shaped image, is used for most peripheral and extracranial cerebrovascular work. The small-footprint sector or vector transducer, also called a phased array transducer, produces a pie slice-shaped image and is used for cardiac, transcranial, and some abdominal work (Fig. 1–3).

Although all modern PW transducers are arrays with multiple elements, technically a PW transducer only needs one piezoelectric element to send and receive sound. However, piezoelectric elements cannot send and receive simultaneously. Therefore, the PW transducer sends a pulse and then has to wait for it to return before sending the next pulse. The machine measures the travel time of the pulse and therefore knows the depth of the reflector, so it can be plotted on the display.

Image Storage

US images and data from other noninvasive testing devices must be archived in some fashion for future comparison and medicolegal purposes. US images may be stored either as a hard copy, meaning film or paper, or through digital storage, such as a hard drive or a picture archiving and communication system (PACS). The results from these studies must be made part of the patient's record for medicolegal purposes. Paper printouts may be part of the patient's hard copy file, or may be scanned into a digital reporting system.

Pulsed-wave   Continuous-wave

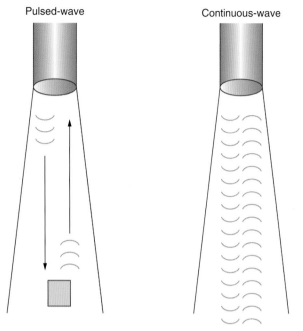

FIGURE 1–1. Pulsed-wave (PW) versus continuous-wave (CW) transducers. PW transducers need a minimum of one piezoelectric element to send and receive sound. Once the pulse is sent, the transducer must wait for that pulse to return before the next pulse is transmitted. CW transducers need a minimum of two elements: one to constantly send, and one to constantly receive. (Reproduced, with permission, from Fuster V, Harrington RA, Narula J, Eapen ZJ. *Hurst's The Heart,* 14th ed. New York, NY; 2017; Figure 15-27. Copyright © McGraw Hill.)

HEMODYNAMICS

Principles of Flow

The cardiac output of the heart is approximately 5–6 L/min, although that amount dramatically increases with exercise. Cardiac output, which helps to determine blood pressure, is equal

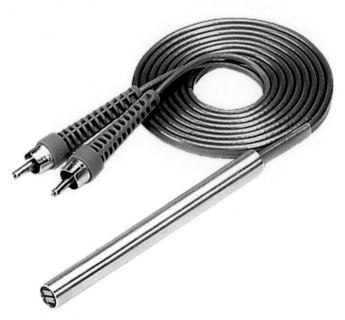

FIGURE 1–2. CW transducer. Dedicated CW pencil probe. Note the two piezoelectric elements for sending and receiving. (Reproduced, with permission, from Parks Medical Electronics, Inc., Las Vegas, NV.)

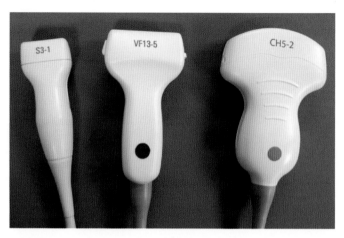

FIGURE 1–3. Ultrasound transducers. From left to right: Sector, or phased array transducer; linear transducer; curvilinear (or convex) transducer.

to the stroke volume times the heart rate (CO = SV × HR). The stroke volume is the amount of blood (in mL) pumped by the heart's every beat.

Blood flow (q) is defined as volume flow per unit time (e.g., L/min). Blood, like all liquids, moves from one point to another because of a difference in energy. In the body, that energy is pressure energy. Blood starts at the left side of the heart, where a substantial amount of potential energy exists. When the left ventricle contracts, that potential energy (in the form of blood pressure) is converted into kinetic energy (in the form of velocity) as the blood moves through the arterial system. The total, or net energy, never changes. If the potential energy goes up, the kinetic energy goes down, and vice versa. The blood pressure in the left heart is variable, but is typically around 120 mm Hg systolic. Blood flows when there is a pressure differential (ΔP, or P1 – P2) between two points along a blood vessel, where P1 is the first point and P2 is the second point. The greater the difference in pressures, the more flow through the vessel. Flow is offset by resistance, which will be explained in further detail later in the chapter.

It is important to differentiate between velocity and flow. Flow (Q) is the volume of flow per unit time, in mL/min or L/min. Velocity (V) is distance per unit time, in cm/s or m/s.

Bernoulli's Principle

The law of energy conservation states that energy cannot be created or destroyed. It may take a different form, such as the conversion of potential to kinetic energy, but the net energy never changes. Bernoulli wrote about the relationship between pressure and velocity. Pressure and velocity have an inverse relationship: if the velocity at a point increases, the pressure must decrease to preserve the net energy (Fig. 1–4).

Continuity Equation

The continuity equation states that flow (Q) is equal to the velocity (V) times the area (A) of the vessel, $Q = VA$. According to the equation, if the velocity increases, flow increases. If the

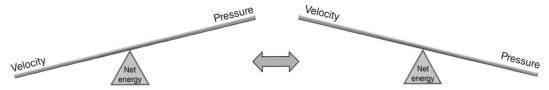

FIGURE 1–4. Bernoulli's see-saw. Pressure (potential energy) and velocity (kinetic energy) are inversely related. The net energy never changes, so if velocity increases, pressure decreases, and vice versa.

area of the vessel increases, flow increases. In reality, flow is a constant. The output of the heart does not change despite (non-hemodynamically significant) narrowing in a downstream vessel. Therefore, as the area of a vessel changes, it is the velocity that changes in order to preserve flow. In Figure 1–5, the area of the vessel narrows. Where the vessel is narrowed, the same volume of flow must go through the narrowed opening. In order to maintain volume flow through the vessel, the velocity must increase at this point.

Bernoulli's principle states that velocity and pressure have an inverse relationship. If the velocity goes up, the pressure must decrease. Therefore, at the point of a stenosis, there is a pressure drop, as evidenced by Figure 1–5. This is counterintuitive to what seems to be the case visually. It looks like the pressure should increase where the narrowed area is because it seems to be under pressure. However, remember that flow (Q) stays constant to allow the same volume of blood to get through the smaller space. Therefore, the velocity (kinetic energy) increases to maintain Q. Since energy cannot be created or destroyed, there is a pressure (potential energy) drop where the velocity increases. Notice the inverse relationship between velocity and pressure; the pressure does not increase in a stenosis, it decreases. Distal to the stenosis, the velocity decreases and the pressure goes back up, assuming a nonhemodynamically significant stenosis.

The short form of Bernoulli's principle is $\Delta P = 4(v_2)^2$, where ΔP is the pressure gradient and v is the velocity across a stenosis. This equation is often used when calculating the pressure drop across a stenotic heart valve.

Poiseuille's Law

Poiseuille's law was originally developed to describe a nonpulsatile, rigid, straight pipe containing a nonparticulate fluid. While the "pipes," or blood vessels, in the body do not meet this definition, the general principles still apply (Fig. 1–6).

As evidenced by the equation, the higher the pressure gradient, the more flow there is. The more viscous the fluid, the less flow there is. The longer the vessel, the less flow there is. It is tempting to think that a longer vessel would increase the amount of flow, but it is important to remember that the longer the vessel, the greater the frictional losses, and therefore, the greater the energy loss to heat. Anything that increases friction decreases flow. The more viscous a fluid is, the less flow there is. Viscosity, which is a fluid's resistance to flow, is generally considered to be a constant, but there are certain medical conditions that may increase the blood viscosity, such as polycythemia and sickle cell disease. The component of Poiseuille's law most subject to change is the radius, due to the innervation of the arterioles. Note that "radius" in the equation is to the fourth power. That is substantial, because if the radius is reduced to half, such as with thrombus or plaque, the amount of flow decreases 16 times.

Friction and Resistance

The blood vessels in the body are not frictionless. RBCs traveling along the blood vessel wall encounter friction from each other and from rubbing against the vessel walls. In a vessel with laminar flow, the RBCs immediately along the vessel wall are stationary as a result of the friction. The next level of RBCs

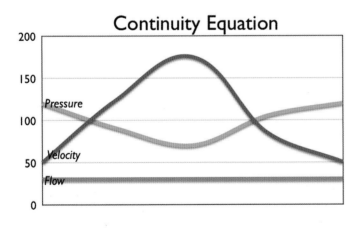

FIGURE 1–5. Continuity and Bernoulli. Flow (*blue line*) is a constant in a nonhemodynamically significant stenosis. Where the area decreases, the velocity (*red line*) increases. Where the velocity increases, the pressure (*yellow line*) decreases. Distal to the narrowing, the velocity goes back down and the pressure comes back up.

Poiseuille's Law	
Q = volume flow	
ΔP = pressure gradient, or P1-P2	$Q = \dfrac{\Delta P \pi r^4}{8 L \eta}$
L = length of vessel	
η = viscosity	

FIGURE 1–6. Poiseuille's law. Components and equation of Poiseuille's law.

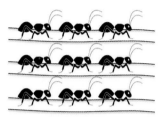

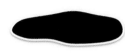

FIGURE 1–7. In-series resistance versus parallel.

move a little faster and the next level even faster, until the center of the vessel is reached. At the center of the blood vessel, the flow is fastest because this is the region with the least amount of friction.

Most resistance in the arterial system is as a result of the arterioles. These **innervated**, muscular-walled blood vessels are responsible for controlling downstream resistance through vasodilatation and vasoconstriction.

Poiseuille's law may be expressed as:

$$Q = \frac{\Delta P}{R}$$

This short form of Poiseuille's law is analogous to Ohm's law, used for discussing electronic circuitry. Ohm's law states that electron flow (current, or I) is equal to the pressure differences (voltage, or V) divided by resistance (R). Ohm's law is written as:

$$I = \frac{V}{R}$$

The resistance component in the short form of Poiseuille's law can further be broken down into the equation below:

$$R = \frac{8L\eta}{\pi r^4}$$

Resistance varies depending on whether vessels are in-series, or parallel. Vessels that are connected end to end are said to be in-series. In vessels that are in-series, the total resistance is equal to the sums of the resistance of each part of the system.

$$R_T = R_1 + R_2 + R_3 + \cdots$$

Vessels that are parallel have lower resistance because there are other pathways for blood to flow, not just one. An example of vessels in parallel occurs with collateral flow. The flow has another pathway through which to travel, so the resistance of the system is lower. The total resistance of vessels in parallel is equal to one divided by the resistance of each segment. The more vessels there are in parallel, the lower the total resistance. Think of it this way: the more collaterals there are, the more

pathways there are for blood to flow, and therefore the lower total resistance to flow.

$$R_T = \frac{1}{R_1} + \frac{1}{R_2} + \frac{1}{R_3} + \cdots$$

Figure 1–7 demonstrates the in-series versus parallel concepts. When the ants are in a line, one behind another, the ants do not get the whole group to the anthill as efficiently as the ants marching in parallel rows. In-series, one ant cannot move until the one before him moves. In parallel, the three rows of ants move simultaneously on multiple paths, which offer less resistance than the single path of the other ants.

Types of Flow

There are four types of flow patterns found in blood vessels: plug, laminar, disturbed, and turbulent (chaotic). Plug flow typically occurs at the entrance of large vessels and in the ascending aorta. With plug flow, the RBCs are all mostly traveling at the same velocity through the vessel. After some distance, friction causes an energy loss in the RBCs closest to the vessel wall, and they become motionless. This is called the boundary layer. The fastest flow is in the center of the vessel, which offers the least resistance to flow. This type of flow, in which the fastest flow is in the center and the slowest flow is toward the walls, is called laminar flow (Fig. 1–8). A laminar flow front has the appearance of a parabola, and is sometimes called parabolic flow, although, strictly speaking, with parabolic flow the average velocity is one-half the fastest flow. Laminar flow is considered

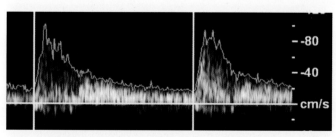

FIGURE 1–8. Spiky appearance of post-stenotic turbulence is seen in this spectral Doppler.

the most common type of flow found in the body, although the serpiginous nature of blood vessels does not allow for simple explanations.

The third type of flow, disturbed flow, occurs when flow is flowing down the vessel in the expected way, but the RBCs are not parallel to the vessel wall. An example of disturbed flow occurs at areas of soft plaque, where the RBCs are no longer parallel to the wall but still generally traveling down the vessel. Turbulence, also known as chaotic flow, occurs in both normal and abnormal vessels. Turbulent flow, in which the RBCs are no longer traveling in the expected direction, may be seen in areas of vessel widening, distal to a stenosis, and in tortuous vessels. Turbulence does not always signify pathology, and is normal in some vessels. It is up to the operator to know when turbulence is normal in a particular segment of a vessel. Poststenotic turbulence (PST) occurs distal to a stenosis and is a "shaggy" or "spiky" appearance to a waveform (Fig. 1–9).

Reynolds number (*Re*) is used to quantitate the presence of turbulence. A Reynolds number greater than 2,000 signifies the presence of turbulence.

$$Re = \frac{v2r\rho}{\eta}$$

Inertia

Inertial losses are caused any time blood flow changes direction, such as branching or at bifurcations. Newton's first law states that an object at rest stays at rest, and an object in motion stays in motion, unless acted on by an outside force. Inertia comes from an object's desire to resist change from its current state. As RBCs travel through the arterial system, arteries and arterioles branch as the blood travels toward the capillaries. This constant change in direction causes an energy loss, eventually resulting in decreased energy downstream. This reduced energy is important because, ultimately, the RBCs will reach the capillaries where the velocity needs to be slow enough for nutrient and waste exchange. Inertial losses also occur at the entrance and exit of a stenosis. Energy losses related to entrance and exit

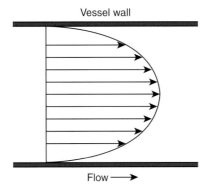

FIGURE 1–9. Laminar flow. Parabolic shape of laminar flow. Fastest flow is in the center of the vessel, with flow progressively slowing as it nears the walls. (Part B reproduced, with permission, from Barrett KE, Barman SM, Brooks HL, Yuan JJ. *Ganong's Review of Medical Physiology,* 26th ed. New York, NY; 2019; Figure 31-18. Copyright © McGraw Hill.)

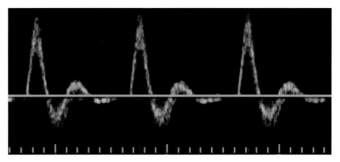

FIGURE 1–10. High-resistance flow. Multiphasic waveform indicative of a high-resistance distal bed.

effects are more significant than the length of the stenosis. For this reason, multiple stenoses in series have a more detrimental effect than one long stenosis.

Waveform Analysis

The shape, or morphology, of a waveform provides information about blood flow proximal and distal to the point of sampling. The heart has an effect on what the waveform looks like, in both venous and arterial flow. For example, elevated right heart pressures may alter venous waveforms, and changes in cardiac output or valvular problems can change the appearance of arterial waveforms. Downstream resistance can be evaluated by looking at the amount of diastolic flow present. Waveform classification is a topic certain to cause heated debate at any vascular conference. Numerous articles have been written about describing flow patterns and the appropriate terminology. In this text, the term "monophasic" implies forward flow throughout the cardiac cycle, and "biphasic" and "triphasic" will be replaced with "multiphasic" in order to eliminate the ambiguity between these two terms. High-resistance flow is represented by a multiphasic waveform and little to no diastolic flow (Fig. 1–10). There does not have to be return of flow above the baseline in diastole (formerly referred to as "triphasic"), although that may be seen. Low-resistance flow is represented by a monophasic waveform (Fig. 1–11), in which forward flow is present throughout all phases of the cardiac cycle. The resistive and pulsatility indices give quantitative information about the waveform that is more accurate than what the visual analysis alone provides.

The phasicity of the waveform (monophasic, multiphasic) provides information about the distal bed. If the distal bed is high-resistance, such as a resting lower extremity artery, then

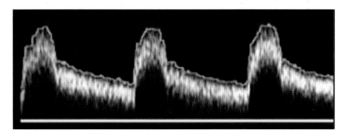

FIGURE 1–11. Low-resistance flow. Monophasic waveform indicative of a low-resistance distal bed.

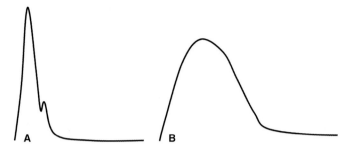

FIGURE 1–12. Upstroke shape. Healthy vessels have a sharp systolic upstroke **(A)**. With proximal disease, there is a delay in the upstroke called tardus parvus **(B)**.

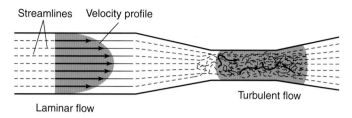

FIGURE 1–13. Laminar and turbulent flow. In a normal, straight vessel, laminar flow predominates. Distal to a stenosis, the flow will become turbulent. (Reproduced, with permission, from Mohrman D, Heller L. *Cardiovascular Physiology,* 9th ed. New York, NY; 2018; Figure 6-6. Copyright © McGraw Hill.)

a multiphasic waveform is expected. If a resting lower extremity artery is demonstrated to be monophasic, this implies distal arteriolar dilation, which is abnormal in a resting patient. If a normally low-resistance bed, such as the brain, is documented as high-resistance, that implies downstream obstruction, or, in the case of the brain, possibly cerebral edema or brain death.

The presence of proximal arterial disease can be diagnosed by examining the shape of the systolic upstroke. The systolic upstroke should be sharply vertical toward peak systole. When there is a delayed upstroke, called tardus parvus, it is indicative of a proximal obstruction (Fig. 1–12).

In July 2020, the Society for Vascular Medicine and Society for Vascular Ultrasound published a consensus statement to standardize nomenclature for arterial and venous waveforms. In this consensus document, the term *multiphasic* officially replaces "triphasic" and "biphasic." The baseline is now called the *zero-flow baseline,* although due to the timing of this publication, throughout this text you will still see the term "baseline." The definition of a multiphasic waveform is one that crosses the zero-flow baseline, while monophasic flow has forward flow in systole and diastole and does not cross the zero-flow baseline. The terms "high-resistance" and "low-resistance" were also further defined in this consensus statement, with high-resistance waveforms, whether monophasic or multiphasic, defined as having a "sharp upstroke and brisk downstroke." Waveforms described as low-resistance have a more drawn-out downstroke in late systole and forward flow throughout diastole. The reader of this text is encouraged to seek out this article (see Suggested Readings section at the end of the chapter) and review the new nomenclature.

Stenosis

In a nonhemodynamically significant stenosis, volume flow (Q) is preserved throughout the length of the vessel despite the area of narrowing. The continuity equation ($Q = VA$), previously discussed, describes how flow is preserved in a vessel with decreased area. The pressure drops in the region of the stenosis due to the velocity increase, as stated by Bernoulli's principle. Bernoulli's principle states that one energy increase has to be compensated by a corresponding energy decrease. When the velocity (kinetic energy) goes up, the pressure (potential energy) goes down. Distal to the stenosis, the pressure goes back up as the velocity decreases. Distal to the area of narrowing, there is PST as a result of widening of the vessel (Fig. 1–13). A stenosis that is hemodynamically significant may also be referred to as a "critical stenosis." Different vascular beds will have different criteria for what makes a critical stenosis. In the lower extremities, for example, a vessel may be non-hemodynamically significant at rest, but increased demands for flow during exercise make the stenosis critical. This will be discussed in more detail in the subsequent chapters. When evaluating a stenosis, know that a 50% diameter reduction corresponds to a 75% reduction in area. This is important because area reduction is used when discussing hemodynamic consequences of stenosis and diameter reduction is used when discussing clinical consequences. Unlike a nonhemodynamically significant stenosis, a critical stenosis will have decreased flow and pressure distal to the stenosis.

Flow Separation

When a blood vessel widens or makes a sharp turn, the blood flow along one wall of the vessel may no longer flow in a laminar flow pattern, but loop around in an eddy current consisting of forward and reverse flow. This is called flow separation (Figs. 1–14 and 1–15). Downstream from the flow separation, the flow resumes its laminar flow pattern. The wall of the vessel adjacent to the flow separation has low shear stress, and the wall opposite the flow separation has higher shear stress. This higher shear stress is a cause for endothelial damage and the formation of atherosclerosis.

Venous Hemodynamics

The venous system contains approximately two-thirds of all of the blood in the body. The venous system acts as a reservoir for blood, ready to be called into action when there is an increased demand for blood. In the venous system there is a pressure differential, albeit a much smaller one than found in the arterial system. The pressure gradient on the venous side is smaller than

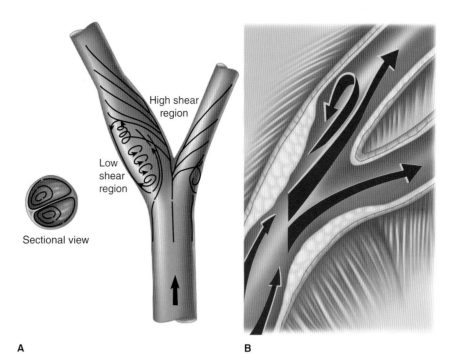

High shear region

Low shear region

Sectional view

FIGURE 1-14. Illustration demonstrating flow separation in a vessel. **(A)** Flow separation at an area of vessel dilatation with low-velocity vortices. **(B)** Flow separation at a bifurcation. (Reproduced, with permission, from Brunicardi F, Andersen DK, Billiar TR, et al. *Schwartz's Principles of Surgery,* 11th ed. New York, NY; 2019; Figure 23-14. Copyright © McGraw Hill.)

A

B

that of the arterial side, less than 15 mm Hg. In an erect patient, for blood to get back to the heart, it must overcome gravity. Hydrostatic pressure is the force that pulls blood downward. Dynamic pressure is much greater in the arterial system than in the venous system, whereas hydrostatic pressure is equal in both the arterial and venous systems because the only variable is distance from the heart. Hydrostatic pressure increases in the lower extremities with standing, thus making it a key contributor to a condition known as venous insufficiency, which will be discussed in detail in Chapter 5. The farther from the heart (i.e., the closer to the ground), the higher the hydrostatic pressure. Figure 1–16 is an illustration of hydrostatic pressure in the venous system with standing. The hydrostatic pressure in the raised hand is zero because the hand is above the level of the heart, and the vein walls collapse from the tissue pressure,

which is higher than the hydrostatic pressure. When a person is supine, the hydrostatic pressure in all segments is the same as the right heart, which is 0 mm Hg.

There are three ways that the venous system overcomes the hydrostatic pressure to return blood to the heart (Table 1–1).

The first tool the body has to aid venous return is the venous valves. The valves, when functioning properly, ensure that blood only travels in one direction: toward the heart. The second tool the body has is the soleal muscles, which act as pumps to force blood through the veins toward the heart. In a patient with normal venous valves, when the calf muscles contract, the blood

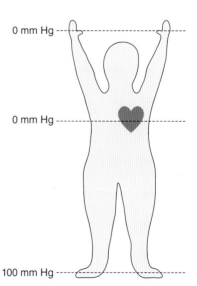

0 mm Hg

0 mm Hg

100 mm Hg

FIGURE 1-16. Illustration of hydrostatic pressure, which is highest closer to the ground and zero at the heart. Anything above the heart is also zero, because the veins are collapsed, although some books present this as a "negative pressure."

FIGURE 1-15. Color Doppler of flow separation in a vessel.

TABLE 1–1 • Table of How Venous Blood Returns to the Heart Despite Gravity
Venous Blood Return to the Heart
Venous valves
Calf muscle pump
Intrathoracic pressure changes

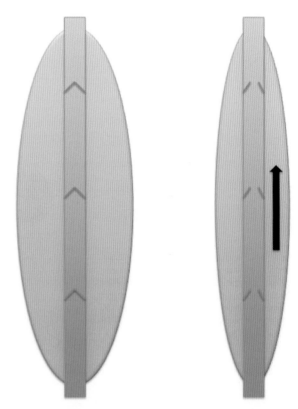

can flow toward the heart (Fig. 1–17). Lastly, blood gets into the heart through inspiration and expiration. During inspiration, the diaphragm drops, creating a negative pressure in the chest. This pulls in blood from the head and upper extremities into the thorax. During inspiration, there is a simultaneous increase in pressure below the diaphragm. During inspiration, venous flow below the diaphragm stops traveling toward the heart because of this increased pressure and compression on the inferior vena cava (IVC). During expiration, there is increased pressure in the thorax and decreased pressure below the diaphragm. Blood below the diaphragm moves toward the heart from the lower extremities and abdomen during expiration (Fig. 1–18).

FIGURE 1–17. Calf muscle pump. The calf muscle acts like a pump to send blood from the calves to the heart. Properly functioning venous valves ensure flow toward the heart.

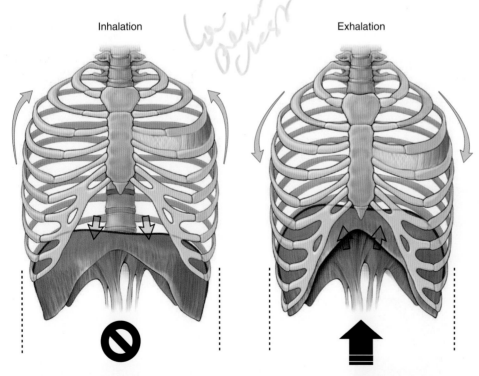

Inhalation

Increased intra-abdominal pressure
Blood returns to heart from
upper extremities and head

Exhalation

Lower intra-abdominal pressure
Blood returns to heart from
trunk and lower extremities

FIGURE 1–18. Movement of diaphragm and intrathoracic pressure. With inspiration, the diaphragm lowers, causing low pressure in the chest and increased intra-abdominal pressure. With expiration, the diaphragm rises and pressure in the abdomen decreases, causing flow from the legs and abdomen to flow toward the heart. (Reproduced, with permission, from Morton DA, Foreman K, Albertine KH. *The Big Picture: Gross Anatomy,* 2nd ed. New York, NY; 2019; Figure 3-4. Copyright © McGraw Hill.)

DOPPLER

Doppler Effect and the Doppler Equation

The Doppler effect is a change in the frequency of sound caused by a moving reflector (RBCs), when observed by a stationary source (the transducer). In the case of medical diagnostic US, the Doppler shift is caused by reflection from the RBCs. The Doppler shift is the difference between the frequency of sound being transmitted by the transducer and the frequency of the sound being received by the transducer.

If the RBCs are moving toward the transducer, there is an increase in the reflected frequency compared to the transmitted frequency. This is called a positive Doppler shift. If the RBCs are moving away from the transducer, the reflected frequency is less than the transmitted frequency. This is called a negative Doppler shift. Figure 1–19 shows the difference in received frequencies based on flow direction. Because the Doppler shift (F_D) is in the audible range of sound, what is heard over the speaker or headphones of a Doppler system is not the sound of the blood flow, but the Doppler shift itself.

The Doppler shift is measured by the machine using the Doppler equation:

$$F_D = \frac{2fv(\cos\theta)}{c}$$

In the Doppler equation, F_D is the Doppler shift, f is the frequency of the transducer, $\cos\theta$ represents the cosine of the Doppler angle, and c is propagation speed. In real-life application, the sonographer is not interested in the Doppler shift, but the velocity of the blood. The machine is able to measure the Doppler shift because it knows the transmitted frequency and it knows the received frequency. With this information, the machine calculates the velocity of the blood using the following equation:

$$v = \frac{(c)F_D}{2f(\cos\theta)}$$

In the Doppler equation, the propagation speed is a constant, assumed at 1,540 m/s. The frequency (f) of the transducer and the Doppler angle are the only two variables. Frequency and Doppler shift are directly related. That means if the frequency increases (i.e., you switch to a higher frequency transducer), the Doppler shift goes up. The Doppler equation does not use the Doppler angle itself, but the cosine of the angle. This is important, because the cosine of the angle is inversely related to the angle itself. In other words, as the Doppler angle increases, the cosine of the angle decreases. This will be important when aliasing is discussed.

The strongest Doppler shift is at 0 degrees, and there is no Doppler shift at 90 degrees. The lack of a Doppler shift perpendicular to flow is the reason Doppler cannot be used at 90-degree angles. The most accurate angle for spectral Doppler is 0 degrees because the higher the Doppler angle, the higher the degree of error. The Doppler angle should never exceed 60 degrees, or the degree of error will be too excessive. Many vascular studies are performed utilizing an angle between 30 and 60 degrees, although it varies study to study.

Pulsed-Wave Spectral Doppler

PW spectral Doppler operates on the same principles as 2D grayscale (B-mode) imaging: a pulse is sent out and the machine waits until that pulse has returned before sending out the next pulse. Pulses cannot be sent out too rapidly or depth ambiguity will occur, and the machine will not know where the return echoes originated. The pulse repetition frequency (PRF) is the number of pulses transmitted in 1 second and in grayscale imaging is controlled by the depth control.

PW spectral Doppler has a distinct advantage over its CW counterpart: range resolution, which is the ability to pick a sample depth. With PW Doppler, the operator selects a sample depth by placing a range gate in the area of interest. The area within the range gate, the sample volume, is adjustable in order to sample vessels of different sizes. The biggest disadvantage of PW Doppler is an artifact called aliasing (Fig. 1–20). Aliasing is a wraparound of the spectral waveform as a result of insufficient sampling speed. If the sampling speed is too low, an incorrect waveform is displayed, causing positive shift information to be displayed as a negative. Aliasing occurs when the Doppler shift exceeds one-half the PRF, a value termed the Nyquist limit. In order to eliminate the aliasing, either the PRF needs to increase or the Doppler frequency shift needs to decrease. Increasing the PRF can be accomplished by increasing the Doppler PRF (or scale) or decreasing the depth. There are several different ways to reduce the Doppler shift. One way is to lower the operating

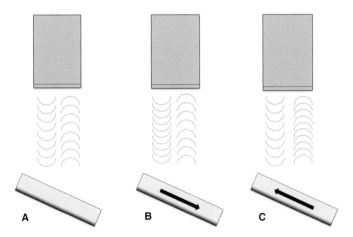

FIGURE 1–19. Doppler shift. With no motion of the reflectors, the received frequency equals the transmitted frequency **(A)**. With reflector motion away from the transducer, the received frequency will be less than the transmitted frequency **(B)**. With reflector motion toward the transducer, the received frequency will be greater than the transmitted frequency **(C)**.

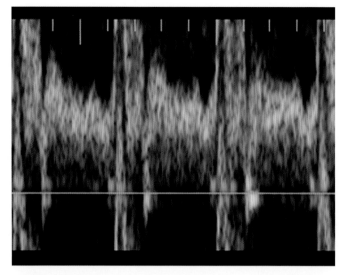

FIGURE 1–20. Aliasing of the spectral signal. When the Doppler shift exceeds the Nyquist limit, aliasing occurs.

frequency of the transducer. Another method for eliminating aliasing is to increase the Doppler angle. Note that increasing the angle reduces aliasing, which at first seems odd since it appears to be directly proportional to frequency shift. However, the Doppler equation does not use the Doppler angle, but the cosine of the Doppler angle. Therefore, increasing the Doppler angle will lower the Doppler shift (Table 1–2). If aliasing cannot be eliminated with these methods, the only alternative is CW spectral Doppler. CW Doppler has no velocity limit, although it may not be practical for all studies.

PW Doppler Controls

PRF/Scale—The PRF or scale setting adjusts the sensitivity of the Doppler and the size of the displayed spectral waveform. High PRF/scale should be used for higher velocity flow, and low PRF/scale settings should be used for slower flow.

Range Gate—The range gate is part of the PW spectral Doppler cursor that allows the operator to select the vessel to be

TABLE 1–2 • Methods to Reduce or Eliminate Aliasing. Aliasing Can be Reduced or Eliminated by Increasing the Nyquist Limit or Decreasing the Doppler Shift	
Reduce Aliasing by Increasing Nyquist Limit (1/2 PRF)	**Reduce Aliasing by Decreasing Doppler Shift**
Increase Doppler PRF (scale)	Decrease operating frequency
Decrease depth	Increase Doppler angle
Use continuous wave (CW)	

insonated. The size of the gate is user selectable. The area within the gate is the sample volume.

Spectral Gain—The brightness of the spectral waveform can be increased or decreased as needed. Increasing the spectral gain too much may result in over-measurement of the velocity.

Baseline—The baseline of the spectral waveform is user-adjustable. If there is the appearance of aliasing it may be because the baseline is too high, assuming the PRF is set correctly.

Angle Correction—With PW Doppler, it is possible to angle-correct so the angle to flow can be plugged into the Doppler equation in order to calculate the velocity.

Color Doppler

Color Doppler, a PW technique, uses Doppler shift information to display mean velocities as a color. The color, usually red or blue, provides information on magnitude and direction of flow. It is not possible to obtain accurate velocity information with color Doppler due to the slower processing technique it uses, called autocorrelation. Color Doppler places a color pixel where movement is detected. The color scale presents positive shifts as whatever color is above the baseline on the color scale, and negative shifts as the color below the baseline. The black in the middle of the color scale, the baseline, represents the absence of Doppler shift information.

Because color Doppler uses PW technology, it is susceptible to aliasing. Color aliasing, like spectral aliasing, is a wraparound of shift information in which positive shift information is displayed as a negative.

Color Doppler Controls

PRF/Scale—The PRF or scale setting adjusts the sensitivity of the Doppler. Decrease the scale for slower flow, increase for faster flow, or if aliasing is present.

Gate—The gate is the user-selectable area. For color Doppler, a smaller gate provides a better frame rate. With a linear transducer, the gate can be steered left, right, or center to avoid a 90-degree angle and obtain the best color flow image.

Color Gain—Color gain can be increased to fill a vessel with color, but if the gain is too high the color pixels will "bleed" out of the vessel. If the color gain is too low the vessel will not fill with color.

Packet Size—The packet size, also called the ensemble length, is the number of pulses sent per scan line, and can be increased to measure slow flow, at the cost of a decreased frame rate. Newer machines may not have a user-selectable packet size, but instead this setting is controlled in the background when the presets are changed.

Persistence—Also known as temporal compounding, a high persistence setting leaves color pixels on the screen as new color information is added. High persistence settings are used for slow flow or in the presence of excessive image noise in order to fill a vessel better.

Priority—The priority setting lets the operator add more weight to displaying the color pixels versus the grayscale pixels, and vice versa. A low priority setting will display grayscale pixels instead of color pixels, even if there is a Doppler shift present. High priority settings are used for slow flow situations, when color pixels are preferred over grayscale information.

Power Doppler

Power Doppler, sometimes known as color Doppler energy (CDE), color power angio (CPA) or amplitude Doppler, is a Doppler technique that has more sensitivity than color Doppler to slow flow. Instead of displaying the Doppler shift, power Doppler displays the strength, or amplitude of the Doppler shift. The amplitude of the Doppler shift is analogous to the number of RBCs in the blood. The more RBCs in the vessel, the stronger the amplitude of the shift. Unlike spectral Doppler and color Doppler, power Doppler does not provide either velocity information or information about direction of flow. The benefit of power Doppler is its sensitivity to flow in small vessels and its nondependence on angle.

Continuous-Wave Doppler

CW Doppler uses a minimum of two elements to obtain a Doppler signal. Piezoelectric elements cannot send and receive at the same time, so one element is constantly ("continuously") transmitting sound while another is always receiving. There is no time to stop and time how long it takes the pulses to return, so with CW Doppler there is depth (range) ambiguity. In other words, there is no image with a two-element CW Doppler, just a spectral waveform. The lack of range resolution means that the operator cannot tell what vessel is being insonated. In fact, CW probes have very large sample volumes and may be sampling multiple vessels at the same time. The displayed spectral waveform is a composite of all of the blood flow within that large sample volume. With CW Doppler there is also no angle correction, so a zero-degree angle is assumed. The advantage that CW Doppler has is the ability to measure very high velocities, as CW Doppler is immune to aliasing that occurs with PW Doppler.

The controls for CW Doppler are the same as for PW spectral Doppler except that the sample volume is not user-adjustable, and there is no angle correction.

Indices

The pulsatility index (PI) and resistive index (RI) are commonly used to evaluate the vascular bed being fed by a blood vessel. The RI quantifies the peripheral resistance to flow. The PI is indicative of how dampened a waveform is. For some studies, there are published charts with normal PI and/or RI values.

The RI is determined by subtracting the end-diastolic (ED) velocity from the peak-systolic (PS) velocity, and dividing the result by the PS velocity. The PI is determined by subtracting the ED velocity from the PS velocity, and dividing the result by the mean velocity. The mean velocity is obtained by tracing the waveform from the ED velocity of one waveform to the ED velocity of the next waveform (Fig. 1–21).

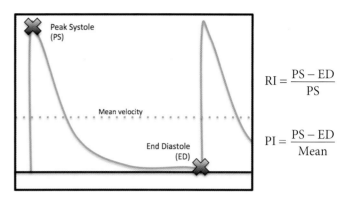

$$RI = \frac{PS - ED}{PS}$$

$$PI = \frac{PS - ED}{Mean}$$

FIGURE 1–21. Doppler indices. Resistive index (RI) and pulsatility index (PI) calculations.

> **Pro-Tip**
>
> Tracing the waveform will provide peak-systolic velocity (PSV), end-diastolic velocity (EDV), RI, PI, systolic/diastolic (S/D) ratio, heart rate, and other potentially useful values. If using auto-measure, always review the tracing to ensure it is adequate. High-wall filters, arrhythmias, and poor spectral gain settings can alter the values obtained.

ARTIFACTS

Artifacts are anomalies of the image that are not real. Artifacts occur in grayscale imaging as well as spectral and color Doppler. There are different causes for the different artifacts, and it is important to know why the artifact is present in order to try and correct for it.

Grayscale Artifacts

Reverberation is one of the most common grayscale artifacts. It is caused by sound bouncing repeatedly between two strong specular reflectors, such as the face of the transducer and wall of a blood vessel. On the image, it appears as equally spaced parallel echoes deep to the strong specular reflector (Fig. 1–22).

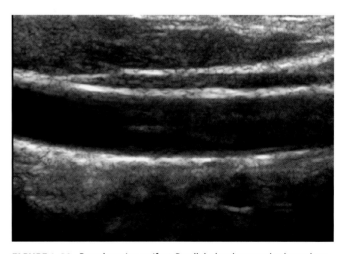

FIGURE 1–22. Reverberation artifact. Parallel, closely spaced echoes deep to a strong specular reflector.

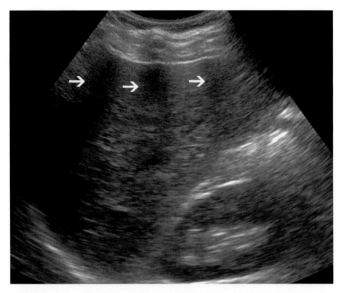

FIGURE 1–23. Shadowing artifact. Shadows occur deep to highly attenuative structures, such as bones or calcifications.

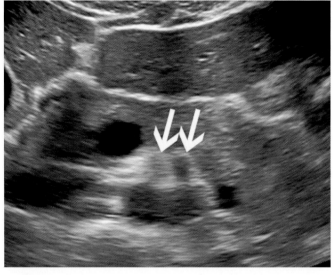

FIGURE 1–25. Ghost image. Ghost image is a refraction artifact commonly seen in the midline of the upper abdomen. It is a result of refraction off of the rectus muscles.

Reverberation artifact can be minimized through the use of tissue harmonic imaging.

Shadowing is caused by sound going through a strongly attenuating structure, such as calcified plaque or bone. Figure 1–23 is a shadow caused by ribs anterior to the liver.

Slice-thickness artifact (partial volume thickness artifact) is caused by an elevational plane that is too thick or is overlapping a blood vessel as well as its adjacent tissue. Tissue harmonic imaging can help eliminate this artifact. In Figure 1–24, image A is a sagittal view of the radial artery. It appears to be filled-in with echoes because the beam width in the elevational (slice-thickness) plane is greater than the size of the vessel at that depth. In transverse (image B), it is apparent that the vessel is patent. The newest transducers that are available utilize virtual beam forming, and have a razor thin beam, greatly reducing or eliminating this artifact.

Ghost image is a refraction type of artifact in which the sound refracts off of the rectus muscles and causes a duplication of anatomy. Figure 1–25 is an example of ghost image, with artificial duplication of the aorta and SMA vessels evident.

Spectral Doppler Artifacts

Aliasing, described previously, occurs when the frequency shift (F_D, or the difference between transmitted frequency and received frequency) exceeds one-half of the PRF, previously described as the Nyquist limit.

Mirror-image artifact occurs in spectral Doppler when either the spectral gain is too high or the beam is too close to a 90-degree angle. Reduce the spectral gain or change the Doppler steering in order to eliminate mirror-image artifact (Fig. 1–26).

Clutter is an artifact that occurs as a result of wall motion. With clutter, there is noise along the baseline of the spectral waveform. Using a wall filter will eliminate clutter but will also eliminate any useful Doppler information near the baseline.

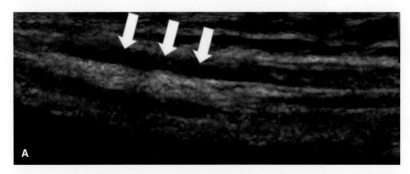

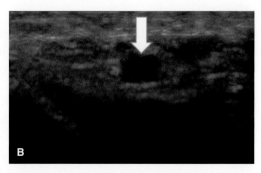

FIGURE 1–24. Partial volume thickness artifact, also known as slice-thickness artifact, occurs when the beam in the elevational (slice-thickness) plane is displaying tissue adjacent to the vessel, making it appear that the vessel contains echoes **(A)**. The solution to this artifact is to turn on the vessel and examine it from another plane **(B)**.

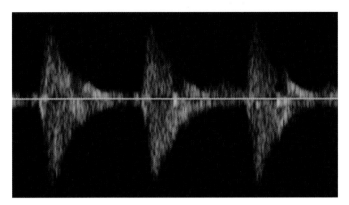

FIGURE 1–26. Mirror-image artifact. Mirror image occurs when the Doppler angle is too close to 90 degrees or the spectral gain is too high.

For this reason, the wall filter is commonly set to a low setting for slow-flow studies (Fig. 1–27).

Color Doppler Artifacts

Color Doppler is a PW technique, and as such it is susceptible to the same artifacts as PW spectral Doppler. Aliasing occurs with color Doppler and appears as a wraparound of the color signal to the opposite side of the scale. As with PW spectral aliasing, increasing the scale/PRF will reduce or eliminate color aliasing (Fig. 1–28).

Mirror-image artifact also occurs in color Doppler, commonly in the subclavian vessels although it may also occur with other vessels. Like spectral mirror-image artifact, color mirror-image artifact occurs when either the color gain is too high or the beam is too close to a 90-degree angle. Reduce the color gain or change the gate steering in order to eliminate mirror-image artifact (Fig. 1–29).

Bleeding of color pixels outside of the vessel wall occurs when the color gain is too high. Reduce the color gain to eliminate this artifact (Fig. 1–30).

Flash artifact may occur with color or power Doppler as a result of motion of the vessel or adjacent tissue (Fig. 1–31).

A color bruit, a nonvascular Doppler signal, is present when there are color pixels in the soft-tissue and the color gain is appropriately set. This useful artifact commonly occurs as a result of a stenosis in a nearby vessel causing a thrill in the adjacent tissue. The movement of the tissue causes a Doppler shift that appears as color pixels in the tissue (Fig. 1–32).

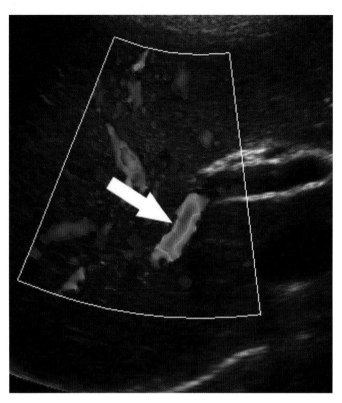

FIGURE 1–28. Color aliasing. Color Doppler is a PW technique, so aliasing will occur if the scale is set too low for the velocity being sampled.

ADVANCES IN TECHNOLOGY IN ULTRASOUND IMAGING

Ultrasound is a rapidly changing field from a technology perspective. This section will highlight some newer technologies available at the time of publication.

Superb Micro-vascular Imaging (SMI), by Canon Medical Systems, is a newer technique that uses advanced noise suppression and processing algorithms to visualize very small blood vessels (Fig. 1–32a).

Noted author Dr. Frederick Kremkau describes a "new paradigm" in ultrasound imaging that upends the physics sonographers have been studying for decades, and erases some of the tried and true mantras of image optimization like "depth, gain, focal zone." In this "new paradigm," the "one pulse is a scan line"

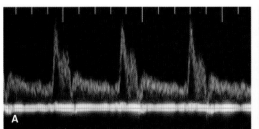
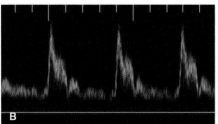
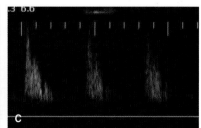

FIGURE 1–27. Clutter artifact. Clutter artifact **(A)** occurs near the baseline of a spectral Doppler waveform and can be eliminated with wall filters **(B,C)**. If the wall filter is set too high, useful information may be eliminated. Low-wall filters should be used whenever slow flow is being sampled.

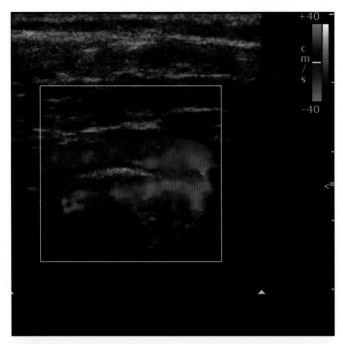

FIGURE 1–29. Mirror-image artifact with color Doppler. Mirror image occurs when the Doppler angle is too close to 90 degrees or the color gain is too high.

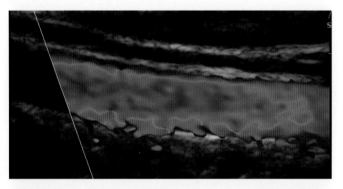

FIGURE 1–30. Color bleeding. Bleeding of color pixels outside the vessel occurs when the color gain is set too high.

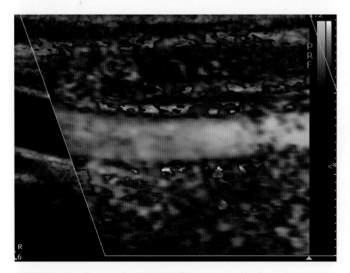

FIGURE 1–31. Flash artifact. Flash artifact occurs with color and power Doppler, but is more common with power Doppler, shown here, due to power Doppler's sensitivity to motion.

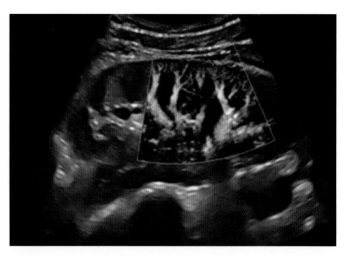

FIGURE 1–32A. SMI image of renal vasculature. Notice the detail of the smaller blood vessels of the cortex.

model is replaced by multiple pulses sent out simultaneously. Focal zones are gone as the entire image is in focus. Frame rates of 5-20 Hz seem novel when up to 6,000 Hz is now possible, and ultrafast Doppler allows for rapid acquisition of color and spectral Doppler at very high frame rates. This newer type of ultrasound imaging utilizes the virtual beam forming mentioned previously in the chapter.

Another newer technique for blood flow visualization is vector flow, which is a form of quantitative color Doppler. Whereas color Doppler only shows direction of flow and mean flow velocity information, vector flow shows flow as a series of arrows, or vectors, each of which can represents an actual velocity (not just a mean velocity) at that point in the blood flow (Fig. 1–32b).

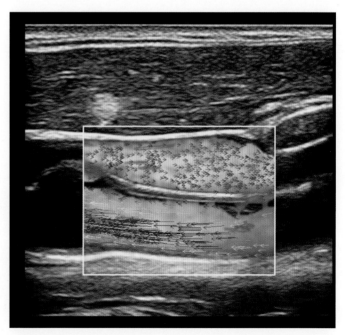

FIGURE 1–32B. V-flow image showing arrows as individual vectors representing direction and velocity of flow and multiple points within the vessel. (Reproduced, with permission, from Mindray North America, Mahwah, NJ.)

OTHER IMAGING TESTS

Conventional Angiography

Angiography and digital subtraction angiography (DSA) use ionizing radiation (x-ray) and x-ray contrast in a real-time fashion to image the lumen of the blood vessels (Fig. 1–33). Angiographic studies are considered the "gold standard" test for many vascular systems because of angiography's ability to visualize blood vessels without interference from the overlying anatomy. With arterial angiography, also called arteriography, a large bore needle is inserted into an artery, typically the common femoral artery, and

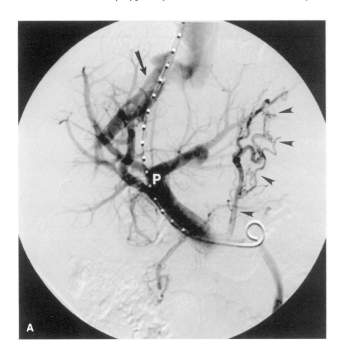

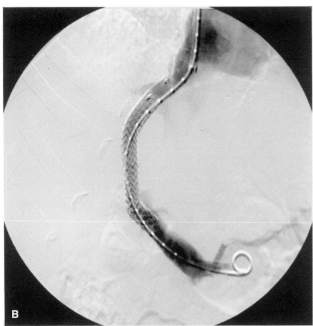

FIGURE 1–33. **(A,B)** Angiogram of the mesenteric vessels. (Reproduced, with permission, from Hall JB, Schmidt GA, Wood LDH. *Principles of Critical Care,* 3rd ed. New York, NY; 2005; Figure 101-5. Copyright © McGraw Hill.)

a guidewire is inserted through the needle to the vessels of interest. After a catheter is inserted over the guidewire and the guidewire removed, contrast is injected as a bolus and the vessels are imaged from different angles using x-ray. Multiple injections are frequently necessary until the entire area of interest is adequately documented. Angiography has an advantage in that bones and bowel gas are not barriers, unlike ultrasound. Another advantage is that if a stenosis is identified, an angioplasty or stent procedure can be performed at that point. In other words, diagnosis and intervention are possible in the same study. The disadvantages of angiography include substantial exposure to ionizing radiation; the invasiveness of the procedure, which includes a postprocedure recovery period; as well as exposure to x-ray contrast, which may cause complications. Another disadvantage of angiography is that it only provides information on the lumen of the blood vessels, and not on the vessel walls. Complications of angiography include pseudoaneurysm or arteriovenous fistula at the injection site, stroke from air or thrombus embolus, and anaphylactic reaction or renal dysfunction from the contrast media.

Magnetic Resonance Angiography

Magnetic resonance angiography (MRA) is a technique based on magnetic resonance imaging (MRI) in which the blood vessels are imaged using a strong magnetic field and radiofrequency waves (Fig. 1–34). A gadolinium-based contrast agent may be used, although renal function may be evaluated before administration of certain types of agents due to its potentially

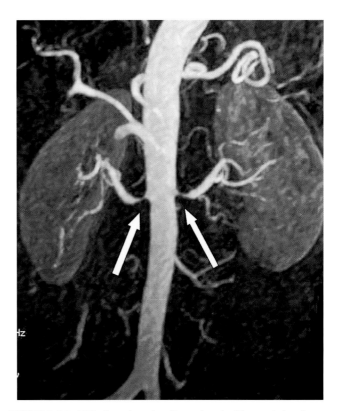

FIGURE 1–34. MRA of renal arteries. (Reproduced, with permission, from Brunicardi F, Andersen DK, Billiar TR, et al. *Schwartz's Principles of Surgery,* 11th ed. New York, NY; 2019; Figure 23-47. Copyright © McGraw Hill.)

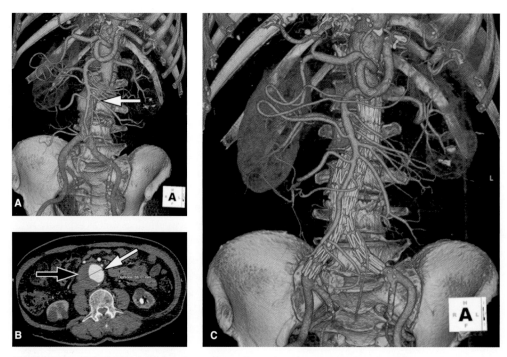

FIGURE 1–35. (A,B,C) CTA of abdominal vasculature. (Reproduced, with permission, from Doherty GM. *Current Diagnosis & Treatment: Surgery,* 15th ed. New York, NY; 2020; Figure 36-19. Copyright © McGraw Hill.)

toxic effects on the kidneys. In addition, several recent studies have demonstrated the presence of residual gadolinium concentrations in the brain following the administration of the contrast agent. The clinical significance of these findings is still unknown and being studied further. MRA is a very sensitive tool for evaluating blood vessels, and is able to image in all planes plus 3D reconstruction. Its limitations include a contraindication related to any metal in the body and claustrophobia related to the machine's small bore.

Computed Tomography Angiography

Computed tomography angiography (CTA) is a technique based on computed tomography (CT) in which x-rays and an x-ray contrast agent are used to image the patient's anatomy in multiple planes (Fig. 1–35). With CTA, 3D reconstruction of the images is used to provide very detailed images in three dimensions. Disadvantages of CTA include its use of ionizing radiation and x-ray contrast, the latter of which has issues related to renal dysfunction and anaphylaxis.

Both CTA and MRA provide detailed views of the blood vessels and permit 3D reconstruction, but, unlike angiography, also permit visualization of the vessel walls and surrounding organs. For this reason, CTA and MRA have replaced angiography as the preferred screening tool for vascular disease in many cases, although angiography still has the ability to offer therapeutic intervention in the presence of significant disease.

Questions

1. **Tardus parvus indicates which of the following?**

   (A) Severe outflow disease

   (B) Severe inflow disease

   (C) Downstream arteriolar dilatation

   (D) Showering emboli

2. **The venous system contains what percent of all of the blood in the body?**

   (A) 20% to 30%

   (B) 50%

   (C) 60% to 70%

   (D) 99%

3. **With inspiration, which of the following is true?**

   (A) Abdominal pressure increases and intrathoracic pressure decreases

   (B) Abdominal pressure decreases and intrathoracic pressure increases

   (C) Abdominal pressure increases and intrathoracic pressure increases

   (D) Abdominal pressure decreases and intrathoracic pressure decreases

4. **As the blood vessel decreases in size, which of the following is true?**

   (A) There is an increase in velocity and an increase in pressure

   (B) There is a decrease in velocity and a decrease in pressure

   (C) There is an increase in velocity and a decrease in pressure

   (D) There is a decrease in velocity and an increase in pressure

5. **Which of the following is true in the presence of a nonhemodynamically significant stenosis?**

   (A) There is a corresponding pressure increase at the point of stenosis

   (B) There is a corresponding pressure decrease distal to the point of stenosis

   (C) There is a corresponding pressure increase proximal to the point of stenosis

   (D) There is a corresponding pressure decrease at the point of stenosis

6. **Monophasic flow in a resting lower extremity artery**

   (A) Is indicative of normal flow

   (B) Is indicative of moderate to severe disease

   (C) Is normal if the patient is >60 years of age

   (D) Is normal with ABIs of 0.9 or greater

7. **Which of the following will increase the hemodynamic resistance?**

   (A) Decrease the viscosity of the blood

   (B) Increase volumetric flow rate

   (C) Decrease the vessel length

   (D) Increase vessel length

8. **With laminar flow in a straight vessel, what part of the flow is said to be the fastest?**

   (A) The center of the stream

   (B) At the boundary layer

   (C) Velocities are the same across the stream

   (D) Toward the edges

9. **In the venous circulation, which of the following is the only variable of hydrostatic pressure?**

   (A) Height

   (B) Gravity

   (C) Density

   (D) Viscosity

10. **Which of the following occurs with deep inspiration?**

    (A) There is an increase in blood flow from the lower extremities to the right heart

    (B) There is an increase in blood flow from the upper extremities and head to the right heart

    (C) There is a decrease in subdiaphragmatic pressures

    (D) There is an increase in pressure in the thorax

11. **A delay in the systolic upstroke is termed**

    (A) Monophasic flow

    (B) Laminar flow

    (C) Turbulence

    (D) Tardus parvus

12. **According to Poiseuille's law, an increase in the pressure difference causes**

    (A) A decrease in flow
    (B) An increase in viscosity
    (C) An increase in flow
    (D) An increase in resistance

13. **Which of the following will have the greatest impact on resistance in a vessel?**

    (A) Viscosity
    (B) Pressure difference
    (C) Vessel length
    (D) Vessel radius

14. **If the radius of a blood vessel is halved, what is the corresponding change in flow?**

    (A) The flow is one-fourth of what it was before the narrowing
    (B) The flow is one-half of what it was before the narrowing
    (C) Blood flow is decreased by a factor of 16
    (D) Blood flow is decreased by a factor of 20

15. **What effect does increasing vessel length have on flow?**

    (A) The longer the vessel, the more flow there is
    (B) The longer the vessel, the lower the flow
    (C) The longer the vessel, the fewer the frictional losses
    (D) The longer the vessel, the less resistance there is

16. **According to Bernoulli,**

    (A) There is no relationship between pressure and velocity
    (B) Velocity increases as pressure increases
    (C) Pressure and velocity are inversely related to each other
    (D) Velocity and pressure are directly related to each other

17. **What type of flow is commonly seen at the entrance of large vessels?**

    (A) Laminar
    (B) Parabolic
    (C) Chaotic
    (D) Plug

18. **Figure 1–36 waveform exhibits characteristics consistent with**

    (A) A distal low-resistance bed
    (B) A distal high-resistance bed
    (C) A multiphasic waveform
    (D) Turbulent flow

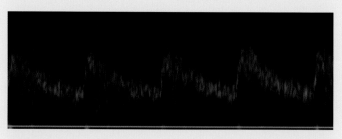

FIGURE 1–36.

19. **What is the type of flow most commonly seen in vessels in the body?**

    (A) Laminar
    (B) Turbulent
    (C) Plug
    (D) Stenotic

20. **When tardus parvus is present, it indicates**

    (A) Mild disease more distally
    (B) Normal flow
    (C) Disease proximal to the point of sampling
    (D) Severe disease distal to the point of sampling

21. **Which of the following increases as vessel area decreases?**

    (A) Pressure
    (B) Velocity
    (C) Flow
    (D) Cardiac output

22. **The stationary RBCs along the vessel walls are called the**

    (A) Viscosity layer
    (B) Boundary layer
    (C) Friction layer
    (D) Cellular layer

23. **Distal to a nonhemodynamically significant stenosis,**

    (A) The velocity decreases and the pressure increases
    (B) The velocity and pressure decrease
    (C) There is a pressure drop
    (D) The velocity increases and the pressure decreases

24. Ohm's law is analogous to Poiseuille's law, where current is represented by

    (A) Flow
    (B) Resistance
    (C) Pressure difference
    (D) Gravity

25. Increasing resistance has what effect on flow?

    (A) Flow is increased with an increase in resistance
    (B) Flow is decreased with an increase in resistance
    (C) Flow and resistance are unrelated
    (D) There are too many other variables to tell

26. In which blood vessels do nutrient and waste exchange occur?

    (A) Arterioles
    (B) Capillaries
    (C) Venules
    (D) Arteries

27. Which of the following is true about hydrostatic pressure?

    (A) In a supine patient, the hydrostatic pressure is greater at the ankles than at the heart
    (B) In a standing patient, with arm raised over head, the arm has a positive hydrostatic pressure
    (C) In a completely supine patient, the hydrostatic pressure is zero across all levels
    (D) In a standing patient, the hydrostatic pressure at the heart is 100 mm Hg

28. Which of the following can be predicted by Poiseuille's law?

    (A) Volume flow in a tube
    (B) Flow velocities in a tube
    (C) Pulsatility in arteries
    (D) Turbulence distal to a stenosis

29. Blood loses energy as it is forced to change direction in branching vessels. This is called

    (A) Bernoulli's principle
    (B) Inertia
    (C) Poiseuille's law
    (D) Continuity principle

30. A 50% reduction in diameter is equal to what percent reduction in area?

    (A) 10%
    (B) 25%
    (C) 50%
    (D) 75%

31. Why is blood slowest in the capillaries?

    (A) To permit maximum exchange of nutrients and wastes
    (B) To be slow enough to enter the venules
    (C) Due to increased right heart pressures
    (D) Due to decreased left heart pressures

32. Spectral broadening is

    (A) An abnormal flow pattern
    (B) Common in tortuous vessels
    (C) Unusual in the carotid bulb
    (D) Never seen with CW Doppler

33. Which of the following is representative of normal lower extremity peripheral venous flow?

    (A) Pulsatile flow
    (B) Respiratory phasicity
    (C) High transmural pressure
    (D) Nonspontaneous flow

34. RBCs increase scatter by 16 times if the frequency is doubled because they are

    (A) Weak reflectors
    (B) Raynaud's scatterers
    (C) Rayleigh scatterers
    (D) Specular reflectors

35. In order to eliminate mirror-image artifact, which of the following techniques can be employed?

    (A) Increase angle closer to 90 degrees
    (B) Increase color or spectral gain
    (C) Increase acoustic power
    (D) Reduce angle to flow

36. The spectral waveform is too dark. Which of the following would be the best method to improve the image?

    (A) Increase the output power
    (B) Increase the spectral gain
    (C) Decrease the spectral gain
    (D) Increase the PRF

37. A sonographer switches to a higher frequency transducer. What effect will that have on aliasing?

    (A) Increased risk of aliasing
    (B) Decreased risk of aliasing
    (C) Aliasing will definitely not occur
    (D) Transducer frequency does not affect aliasing

38. Which of the following will reduce the risk of aliasing?

    (A) Increase the depth
    (B) Decrease the PRF
    (C) Increase the Doppler angle
    (D) Lower the scale control

39. All of the following are components of the Doppler shift equation except for

    (A) Frequency
    (B) Spatial pulse length
    (C) Doppler angle
    (D) Propagation speed

40. Which of the following is a processing technique used to formulate the spectral waveform?

    (A) Fast Fourier transform (FFT)
    (B) Autocorrelation
    (C) Zero crossing detection
    (D) Phase waveform processing

41. Which of the following will occur with an increase in the ensemble length?

    (A) There will be more sensitivity to slow flow
    (B) The mean velocities will be less accurate
    (C) There will be less acoustic exposure to the patient
    (D) The temporal resolution will be improved

42. Aliasing occurs for which of the following reasons?

    (A) The velocities are too low
    (B) The PRF is too high
    (C) The sampling rate is too slow
    (D) The sampling rate is too high

43. Increasing the pulse repetition frequency

    (A) Decreases the number of cycles in a pulse
    (B) Decreases the number of pulses per second
    (C) Increases the imaging depth
    (D) Increases the measurable frequency shift

44. Power Doppler uses

    (A) Frequency shift information to generate directional information
    (B) Frequency shift information to generate velocity information
    (C) Amplitude information to generate a signal
    (D) Amplitude information to generate velocity and direction information

45. What effect does increasing the packet size have on color Doppler?

    (A) Ability to examine faster flow
    (B) More accurate mean velocities
    (C) More accurate maximum velocities
    (D) Improves frame rate

46. Which of the following does not provide direction of flow information?

    (A) Spectral Doppler
    (B) Color Doppler
    (C) Power Doppler
    (D) CW Doppler

47. With CW Doppler, how many transducer elements are needed at a minimum?

    (A) One
    (B) Two
    (C) Four
    (D) There is no minimum

48. What is the biggest advantage of PW Doppler?

    (A) Ability to select sample depth
    (B) There are no effective velocity limits
    (C) There are no depth limits
    (D) Lower acoustic output compared to B-mode

49. A sonographer is performing a renal arterial Doppler study. The sonographer wishes to more accurately measure acceleration time. Which control needs to be adjusted so the waveform can be stretched out to permit a more accurate measurement?

    (A) Doppler gate
    (B) Scale
    (C) Wall filter
    (D) Sweep speed

50. **Which of the following causes the most acoustic energy exposure to the patient?**

    (A) Spectral Doppler
    (B) Color Doppler
    (C) Grayscale imaging
    (D) M-mode

51. **Which of the following Doppler modes does not use the Doppler frequency shift information to generate the signal?**

    (A) Spectral Doppler
    (B) Color Doppler
    (C) CW Doppler
    (D) Power Doppler

52. **Why is it important for the spectral Doppler gain to be adjusted appropriately?**

    (A) If the gain is too low, the velocities will be over-measured
    (B) If the gain is too low, the risk of aliasing is increased
    (C) If the gain is not adjusted properly, the velocities may be measured inaccurately
    (D) If the gain is too high, the velocities will be under-measured

53. **Which of the following is true about color Doppler?**

    (A) It is a continuous-wave technique
    (B) It is subject to aliasing
    (C) It is commonly used because of the improvement in frame rate
    (D) It can accurately measure peak-systolic and end-diastolic velocities

54. **In order to decrease the Doppler shift, which of the following must be increased?**

    (A) Doppler angle
    (B) Transducer frequency
    (C) Velocity of blood
    (D) Packet size

55. **The transmitted frequency is 5.0 MHz. The received frequency is 5.0 MHz. Which of the following is true?**

    (A) The reflector is moving toward the transducer
    (B) The reflector is moving away from the transducer
    (C) The reflector is moving parallel to the beam
    (D) The reflector is not moving with respect to the transducer

56. **In the equation to calculate the Doppler shift, what does "c" in the equation represent?**

    (A) Frequency shift
    (B) Propagation speed
    (C) Velocity of blood
    (D) Transducer frequency

57. **If the frequency of the transducer is increased, what happens to the Doppler shift?**

    (A) The Doppler shift increases
    (B) The Doppler shift decreases
    (C) The Doppler shift stays the same
    (D) It depends on the direction of flow

58. **At which angle will the Doppler shift be at a maximum?**

    (A) 0 degrees
    (B) 90 degrees
    (C) 60 degrees
    (D) 15 degrees

59. **At which Doppler angle will the Doppler shift be at its lowest?**

    (A) 0 degrees
    (B) 90 degrees
    (C) 60 degrees
    (D) 15 degrees

60. **What angle to flow is the most accurate?**

    (A) 0 degrees
    (B) 90 degrees
    (C) 60 degrees
    (D) 15 degrees

61. **What is considered to be the largest angle permissible in order to avoid a large measurement error?**

    (A) 0 degrees
    (B) 90 degrees
    (C) 60 degrees
    (D) 45 degrees

62. **Which of the following describes the relationship between velocity and pressure?**

    (A) Doppler effect
    (B) Bernoulli principle
    (C) Poiseuille's law
    (D) Spectral effect

63. **What will occur if the sample volume is large relative to the size of the vessel?**

    (A) Aliasing

    (B) Loss of diastolic flow information

    (C) Inaccurate peak systolic measurement

    (D) Spectral broadening

64. **Color pixels are seen outside of the vessel walls. What control should be adjusted to eliminate this artifact?**

    (A) Decrease the gate size

    (B) Decrease the color gain

    (C) Decrease the PRF

    (D) Increase the PRF

65. **The PRF is 2,500 Hz. Above what Doppler shift will aliasing occur?**

    (A) 1,250 Hz

    (B) 1,500 Hz

    (C) 2,500 Hz

    (D) 5,000 Hz

66. **What is the most optimal angle for 2D, grayscale imaging?**

    (A) 0 degrees

    (B) 90 degrees

    (C) 60 degrees

    (D) 15 degrees

67. **An RBC is moving toward a stationary transducer. What can be said about the frequency of the reflected sound compared to the frequency of the incident sound?**

    (A) It is not possible for the machine to measure incident frequency

    (B) The frequencies will be identical

    (C) The incident frequency will be greater than the reflected frequency

    (D) The reflected frequency will be greater than the incident frequency

68. **What is the Doppler shift when a reflector is not moving compared to the stationary observer?**

    (A) The Doppler shift is zero

    (B) The Doppler shift is very high

    (C) The Doppler shift cannot be calculated

    (D) The Doppler shift is negative

69. **What is the Doppler shift when the transducer is 90 degrees to the direction of flow?**

    (A) It is zero

    (B) It is at a maximum

    (C) It is most accurate

    (D) It is very high

70. **A negative Doppler shift occurs when**

    (A) Both reflector and observer are stationary

    (B) The velocity of the reflector is negative

    (C) A reflector is moving away from a stationary observer

    (D) A reflector is moving toward a stationary observer

71. **Aliasing occurs because the sampling rate is too _____**

    (A) Fast

    (B) Slow

    (C) High

    (D) Expensive

72. **The higher the Doppler angle, the _____ the degree of measurement error.**

    (A) Greater

    (B) Lesser

    (C) Harder to calculate

    (D) Harder to reproduce

73. **For venous flow, a _____ setting should be used to look for slower flow.**

    (A) Lower gain

    (B) Lower scale

    (C) Higher scale

    (D) Lower persistence

74. **In one type of Doppler, mean velocity and direction of flow are displayed as a color. What type of Doppler technique is this?**

    (A) Power Doppler

    (B) Spectral Doppler

    (C) Amplitude Doppler

    (D) Color Doppler

75. **When must angle correction be used in spectral Doppler when performing vascular exams?**

    (A) At all times

    (B) Any time CW Doppler is used

    (C) Whenever arterial flow is measured

    (D) When velocity information is needed

76. Which of the following is representative of the PI?

(A) Peak-systolic velocity minus end-diastolic velocity divided by the end-diastolic velocity

(B) Peak-systolic velocity minus end-diastolic velocity divided by the peak-systolic velocity

(C) Peak-systolic velocity minus end-diastolic velocity divided by the mean velocity

(D) Peak-systolic velocity times end-diastolic velocity minus the peak-systolic velocity

77. You are imaging a carotid artery and aliasing is noted. Which of the following techniques would best eliminate the aliasing?

(A) Increasing the operating frequency

(B) Increasing the scale

(C) Increasing the gain

(D) Lowering the baseline

78. Which of the following has no influence on aliasing?

(A) Gain

(B) Pulse repetition frequency

(C) Operating frequency

(D) Angle of flow

79. Which of the following is directly related to the amplitude of the Doppler shift?

(A) The Doppler angle

(B) The operating frequency

(C) The velocity of flow

(D) The number of RBCs present

80. Which of the following has no effect on the Doppler shift?

(A) Operating frequency

(B) Pulse repetition frequency

(C) Propagation speed

(D) Velocity of the blood

81. The frequency of the transducer is increased while performing a carotid ultrasound. What will be the effect on the Doppler frequency shift?

(A) It increases

(B) It decreases

(C) It does not change

(D) It depends on the PRF

82. Aliasing is present while performing a PW lower extremity arterial examination. Which of the following is needed in order to eliminate the aliasing?

(A) Increase the Doppler shift

(B) Decrease the PRF

(C) Decrease the PRP

(D) Decrease the scale

83. Compared to a higher frequency transducer, a lower frequency transducer

(A) Increases the risk of aliasing

(B) Decreases the risk of aliasing

(C) Improves the spatial resolution of the image

(D) Increases the velocities

84. If the blood pressure represents the potential energy in the system, what represents the kinetic energy?

(A) Velocity of the blood

(B) Pressure in a stenosis

(C) Radius of the vessel

(D) Flow volume

85. PW Doppler is used for transcranial Doppler studies because

(A) CW is too sensitive

(B) CW does not permit selection of sample volume depth

(C) CW cannot accurately measure high velocities

(D) CW has too many artifacts associated with it

86. Bernoulli's principle describes

(A) Flow volume as it relates to resistance

(B) Frictional losses from vessel length and viscosity

(C) Inverse relationship between velocity and pressure

(D) Direct relationship between velocity and pressure

87. A vessel that is feeding a low-resistance bed will likely have which type of flow?

(A) Tardus parvus

(B) Monophasic

(C) Multiphasic

(D) Diastolic flow reversal

88. Flow that has low-velocity systolic "thumps" with no diastolic flow is indicative of which of the following?

(A) Normal arterial flow

(B) Proximal stenosis

(C) Distal obstruction or edema

(D) Distal arteriovenous fistula

89. Which setting can be adjusted to permit color Doppler twinkling artifact as an aide in identifying small calcifications?

    (A) Scale

    (B) Frequency

    (C) Priority

    (D) Persistence

90. Which artifact is seen in Figure 1–37?

    (A) Ghost image

    (B) Reverberation

    (C) Electronic noise

    (D) Mirror-image

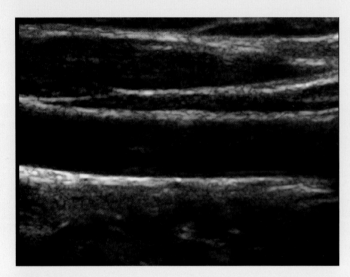

FIGURE 1–37.

91. In Figure 1–38 an artifact is present near the baseline. This artifact is called

    (A) Blooming

    (B) Aliasing

    (C) Mirror-image

    (D) Clutter

92. The y-axis of the spectral waveform may represent all of the following EXCEPT

    (A) Frequency shift

    (B) Velocity

    (C) Doppler shift

    (D) Time

93. In this image (Fig. 1–39), the gate is relatively large compared to the size of the vessel. Therefore, the spectral waveform is exhibiting

    (A) Mirror-image artifact

    (B) Spectral broadening

    (C) Clutter

    (D) Aliasing

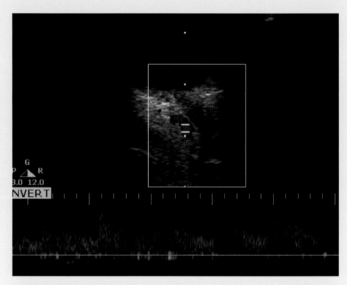

FIGURE 1–39.

94. If the Doppler shift is said to be negative, what does that mean regarding flow?

    (A) Flow is traveling away from the transducer

    (B) Flow is in the venous system

    (C) Flow is retrograde

    (D) Flow has a poor attitude

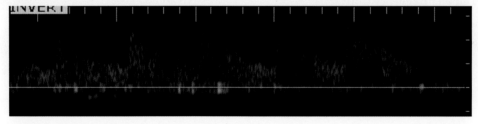

FIGURE 1–38.

95. If there is no Doppler shift, which of the following is true?

   (A) The vessel is stenosed
   (B) 90-degree angle of incidence
   (C) Spectral gain is too low
   (D) Flow is away from the transducer

96. Which of the following, if increased, will NOT increase the amount of flow?

   (A) Pressure gradient
   (B) Length of vessel
   (C) Radius of vessel
   (D) Area of vessel

97. Which of the following is a constant and does not change in a nonhemodynamically significant stenosis?

   (A) Area
   (B) Velocity
   (C) Flow
   (D) Pressure

98. The Doppler shift is in which range of sound?

   (A) Audible sound
   (B) Infrasound
   (C) Ultrasound
   (D) Medical diagnostic ultrasound

99. Figure 1–40 has spectral broadening. What might be one way to eliminate the spectral broadening in this image?

   (A) Open spectral gate wider
   (B) Decrease the spectral gain
   (C) Elevate the baseline
   (D) Increase the PRF

100. In Figure 1–41 there is a blue vessel. Based on the information given, this is

   (A) A vein
   (B) An artery
   (C) Flow toward the transducer
   (D) Flow away from the transducer

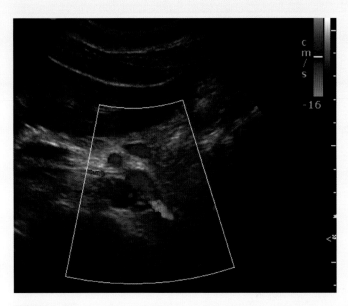

FIGURE 1–41.

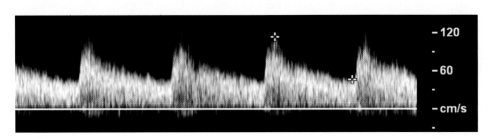

FIGURE 1–40.

Answers and Explanations

1. **(B)** Tardus parvus is the waveform appearance in which the systolic upstroke is delayed. This waveform shape is indicative of severe proximal, or inflow, disease.

2. **(C)** The venous system holds approximately 66% of the blood in reserve at any one time.

3. **(A)** With inspiration, the diaphragm moves inferior, compressing the IVC and causing increased abdominal pressure. At the same time, the intrathoracic pressure decreases, causing blood to be sucked into the thorax from the upper extremities and head.

4. **(C)** The continuity equation ($Q = VA$) indicates that where area decreases, velocity increases. According to Bernoulli, where velocity increases, pressure decreases.

5. **(D)** Pressure decreases at the point of a stenosis. In a nonhemodynamically significant stenosis, the pressure returns to normal distal to a stenosis because the velocity decreases to the prestenotic velocity.

6. **(B)** Phasicity of the arterial waveform indicates the resistiveness of the distal bed. In a resting lower extremity, the distal arterioles are high-resistance. Therefore, a high-resistance multiphasic waveform is expected. Monophasic flow indicates dilatation of the distal arterioles, indicative of moderate to severe disease.

7. **(D)** If resistance increases, flow decreases. Resistance is caused by a decrease in vessel radius, an increase in vessel length, or an increase in viscosity.

8. **(A)** In laminar flow, blood travels fastest in the center of the vessel, and becomes progressively slower as it nears the edges.

9. **(A)** In the venous system, height, or distance from the heart, is the only variable in the equation.

10. **(B)** With deep inspiration, there is increased flow from the upper extremities and head as a result of decreased pressure in the chest.

11. **(D)** Tardus parvus is a sloped, or delayed systolic upstroke as a result of proximal arterial disease. Healthy arteries should have a sharp systolic upstroke.

12. **(C)** Poiseuille's law relates flow to changes in pressure, the radius of the vessel, the length of the vessel, and viscosity of the blood. As the pressure difference (i.e., gradient) increases, flow increases.

13. **(D)** In Poiseuille's law, the radius component is to the fourth power (r^4). Therefore, changes in radius will have a dramatic impact in flow.

14. **(C)** In Poiseuille's law, the radius component is to the fourth power (r^4). A change in radius by one-half is equivalent to a 16-fold decrease in flow.

15. **(B)** Length is directly related to resistance. The longer a vessel, the more resistance there is due to frictional losses, and therefore, decreased flow.

16. **(C)** Bernoulli's principle states that pressure and velocity have an inverse relationship as part of the law of conservation of energy.

17. **(D)** Plug flow, which resembles a flat wave front before the flow assumes a more parabolic shape, is typically seen in the proximal aorta and at the entrance of large vessels.

18. **(A)** The displayed waveform is monophasic with a large amount of diastolic flow, indicative of a distal low-resistance bed.

19. **(A)** Laminar flow is considered to be the predominant type of flow present within the blood vessels of the body. In laminar flow, blood is fastest in the center, with flow slowing progressively toward the vessels' walls.

20. **(C)** Tardus parvus is a delayed systolic upstroke consistent with proximal arterial disease. The normal arterial waveform has a sharp upstroke.

21. **(B)** According to the continuity equation ($Q = VA$), velocity increases where area decreases.

22. **(B)** The boundary layer is a stationary layer of RBCs adjacent to the vessel wall. RBCs progressively increase in velocity until the fastest flow in the center of the vessel is reached.

23. **(A)** Distal to a nonhemodynamically significant (or "critical") stenosis, the velocity decreases (i.e., returns to normal), and there is a corresponding pressure increase consistent with Bernoulli's principle.

24. **(A)** Ohm's law ($I = V/R$) is analogous to Poiseuille's law ($Q = \Delta P/R$). Pressure is represented by voltage, flow is current, and resistance is the same for both.

25. **(B)** Poiseuille's law ($Q = \Delta P/R$) states that flow is inversely proportional to resistance. As resistance increases, flow decreases.

26. **(B)** Capillaries are the microscopic vessels connecting arterioles and venules, and are the location for nutrient/waste exchange.

27. **(C)** Hydrostatic pressure is based on vertical distance from the heart (the effect of height in the equation). When supine, everything is the same level as the heart, so the hydrostatic pressure is 0 mm Hg. When standing, anything below the heart is a positive hydrostatic pressure and anything at the level of the heart or above is 0 mm Hg.

28. **(A)** Poiseuille's law predicts volume flow (Q) when the radius and length of the vessel, viscosity of the blood, and pressure gradient are known.

29. **(B)** Inertia is the tendency of an object at rest to stay at rest and an object in motion to stay in motion, assuming to interaction from an outside source (like gravity). This is known as Newton's first law of motion.

30. **(D)** A 50% reduction in diameter results in a 75% reduction in area.

31. **(A)** Capillaries are about the same size as RBCs. The friction caused by the RBCs touching the vessel walls causes the cells to move very slowly, permitting maximum exchange of nutrients and wastes.

32. **(B)** Spectral broadening is seen whenever many flow velocities are present in a sample volume. Spectral broadening is common with the use of large spectral gates and CW Doppler, and also in the presence of turbulence, which may be a result of stenosis, areas of vessel dilatation, and tortuous vessels. Spectral broadening will also be seen if the spectral gain is too high.

33. **(B)** Lower extremity peripheral venous flow should be spontaneous, have respiratory phasicity, be noncontinuous, and be nonpulsatile. Veins typically have low transmural pressure, and will appear elliptical when supine due to the increased pressure outside the vessel compared to the pressure inside the vessel.

34. **(C)** Rayleigh scatterers are very small reflectors compared to the wavelength of the beam. RBCs, which are a type of Rayleigh scatterer, scatter to the fourth power of the frequency, so a doubling of frequency causes 16 times more scatter. Scatter is a type of attenuation because the sound energy is directed into all directions, leaving less energy to be transmitted through the tissue.

35. **(D)** Mirror-image artifact occurs when there is a close to 90-degree angle to flow, or when the color/spectral gain is too high.

36. **(B)** Spectral gain is the control that makes the spectral waveform brighter or darker. Increase the spectral gain if the spectral signal is too dark, but be careful not to increase the spectral gain too much.

37. **(A)** Frequency shift (F_D) is directly proportional to operating frequency (f). The higher the frequency shift, the greater the risk for aliasing. Aliasing occurs when the frequency shift exceeds the Nyquist limit, equal to one-half of the PRF.

38. **(C)** In the Doppler equation, frequency shift (F_D) is directly proportional to the cosine of the Doppler angle ($\cos \theta$). Increasing the angle causes the cosine of the angle to decrease, resulting in a lower frequency shift. Decreasing the frequency shift reduces the risk of aliasing.

39. **(B)** The Doppler equation includes everything listed except spatial pulse length. In addition to frequency, Doppler angle, and propagation speed, the Doppler equation also includes frequency shift and velocity of the blood.

40. **(A)** FFT is a processing technique used to convert complex frequency information into the spectral signal with which the sonographer is familiar. Autocorrelation is used for color Doppler processing.

41. **(A)** Ensemble length, also known as packet size, is the number of pulses per scan line used to make the color Doppler image. The higher the ensemble length, the better the ability to document slow flow, and the more accurate the measured mean velocities. The tradeoff of higher ensemble length is a slower frame rate (i.e., worse temporal resolution).

42. **(C)** Aliasing occurs due to an insufficient sampling rate. If the sampling rate is too slow, aliasing will occur. Increasing the PRF (scale) will increase the number of pulses sent per second, reducing the risk of aliasing.

43. **(D)** Increasing the PRF (scale) increases the Nyquist limit. The higher the Nyquist limit, the higher the measurable frequency shift without aliasing.

44. **(C)** Power Doppler uses the amplitude of the Doppler shift in order to generate a color signal, but is not able to measure velocities or determine direction of flow.

45. **(B)** A higher packet size, also known as ensemble length, enables more accurate mean velocities and better ability to measure slow flow, but at the expense of frame rate.

46. **(C)** Power Doppler does not permit measuring of velocity or direction of flow.

47. **(B)** With CW Doppler, two piezoelectric elements are needed: one to continuously transmit sound and one to continuously receive. PW transducers only need one element to send and receive because these actions are not happening simultaneously, as they are with CW.

48. **(A)** The ability to select an angle-corrected sample depth and selectively choose the vessel to sample is PW Doppler's greatest advantage. PW Doppler is limited by aliasing, which means it cannot sample high velocities in deep vessels. PW Doppler uses more cycles per pulse, and therefore puts more acoustic energy into the patient than grayscale (B-mode) imaging.

49. **(D)** The sweep speed adjusts how many waveforms are displayed on the screen at one time. Use a fast sweep speed to have fewer waveforms displayed, and a slower sweep speed to have more waveforms displayed.

50. **(A)** Spectral Doppler is an unscanned mode. In scanned modes (2D grayscale, color Doppler), the beam is swept across a path and the energy is spread out over a wider area. In unscanned modes (M-mode, spectral Doppler), the energy is concentrated to one scan line, and therefore concentrated to a smaller area. This permits less time for heat dissipation, potentially causing increased bioeffects.

51. **(D)** Power Doppler does not use the frequency shift itself to obtain color data, but the amplitude of the shift. This enables power Doppler to be very sensitive to slow flow and not angle dependent like spectral or color Doppler.

52. **(C)** Spectral gain makes the spectral waveform brighter or darker. Over-gaining the spectral waveform causes over-measurement of the velocities whereas under-gaining the spectral waveform causes under-measurement of the velocities.

53. **(B)** Color Doppler is a PW technique, and therefore is subject to aliasing.

54. **(A)** Increasing the Doppler angle decreases the cosine of the angle. Cosine of the Doppler angle is directly related to frequency shift. Therefore, if the angle is increased, the cosine of the angle is decreased, and therefore the frequency shift is decreased.

55. **(D)** Doppler shift is the difference between transmitted frequency and received frequency. If the difference between the two frequencies is zero, the Doppler shift is zero, indicating no movement with respect to the transducer.

56. **(B)** The letter "c" is always used to represent speed. In ultrasound, "c" is propagation speed, which is assumed to be 1,540 m/s.

57. **(A)** Frequency shift and operating frequency are directly related. If the operating frequency is increased, the Doppler shift is increased.

58. **(A)** The Doppler shift is highest at a 0-degree angle. The cosine of zero is one, so multiplying the Doppler equation by one does not change the result.

59. **(B)** The Doppler shift is lowest at a 90-degree angle. The cosine of 90 is zero, and multiplying an equation by zero causes the result to be zero.

60. **(A)** A 0-degree angle is most accurate. At angles higher than 0 degrees, the degree of error progressively increases.

61. **(C)** Angles should not be used greater than 60 degrees because above that point, the degree of error is considered to be too high.

62. **(B)** The Bernoulli principle describes the inverse relationship between velocity and pressure.

63. **(D)** Spectral Doppler gates that are large include a wide variety of velocities into the signal. Spectral broadening is seen when there are many velocities present.

64. **(B)** Color gain controls the "bleeding" of pixels outside the vessel wall. If the vessel is not filling to the walls, increase the color gain. If the color pixels are bleeding outside the walls, decrease the color gain.

65. **(A)** The Nyquist limit is half the PRF. Above the Nyquist limit is when aliasing occurs. The Nyquist limit in this example is 1,250 Hz.

66. **(B)** Grayscale imaging is best imaged at a 90-degree angle. Spectral and color Doppler cannot be performed at 90 degrees.

67. **(D)** A positive Doppler shift occurs when a reflector is moving toward a stationary source, which in the case of ultrasound is the transducer. With a positive shift, the reflected frequency is greater than the transmitted frequency.

68. **(A)** The Doppler shift is the difference between transmitted and received frequencies. A stationary reflector will have a Doppler shift of 0.

69. **(A)** There is no Doppler shift at a 90-degree angle.

70. **(C)** When the reflector moves away from the transducer, there is a negative Doppler shift; the reflected frequency is less than the transmitted frequency. The Doppler shift is the reflected frequency minus the transmitted frequency.

71. **(B)** Aliasing occurs when the sampling rate is too slow. There needs to be at least two to three samples per cycle to avoid aliasing.

72. **(A)** The higher the Doppler angle, the greater the degree of inaccuracy. Remember: the most accurate angle is 0 degrees, and the degree of error increases as angle increases.

73. **(B)** Slow venous flow requires sensitivity. Therefore, the scale should be decreased when looking for slow venous flow. Some veins may have faster flow, such as in the presence of an arteriovenous fistula. The scale should be adjusted according to the velocity to be measured.

74. **(D)** Color Doppler is a Doppler technique in which mean velocity and direction of flow are displayed as color pixels on top of grayscale information.

75. **(D)** Angle correction is possible with PW spectral Doppler. Angle correction permits peak-systolic and end-diastolic flow velocities to be measured. Angle correction is not limited to arterial flow, as there are some studies where venous velocities need to be measured. Angle correction is not possible with CW Doppler.

76. **(C)** The PI is PS-ED/Mean, or peak-systolic velocity minus end-diastolic velocity divided by the mean velocity.

77. **(B)** Increasing the scale increases the PRF, which reduces the risk of aliasing. Increasing the operating frequency will worsen aliasing. Lowering the baseline if it is too high should be the first step but if there is aliasing it is probably because the scale is too low.

78. **(A)** Gain does not influence aliasing, but operating frequency, PRF, and angle of flow may increase or decreases the risk of aliasing.

79. **(D)** The number of RBCs present represents the amplitude of the Doppler signal.

80. **(B)** Changing the PRF does not change the Doppler shift. PRF does affect whether there is aliasing in that the Nyquist limit (1/2 PRF) must be greater than the Doppler shift.

81. **(A)** The Doppler shift is directly proportional to operating frequency. If the frequency is increased, the Doppler shift is increased.

82. **(C)** Decreasing the PRP is the same as increasing the PRF because PRP and PRF are reciprocals. Therefore, decreasing the PRP will reduce the risk of aliasing.

83. **(B)** To eliminate aliasing, the Doppler shift needs to be reduced below the Nyquist limit. Operating frequency is directly related to Doppler shift, so if the frequency is decreased, the Doppler shift is decreased, reducing the risk of aliasing.

84. **(A)** Kinetic energy is the velocity of the blood.

85. **(B)** With CW Doppler, there is no user-selectable sample volume. Therefore, sampling depth cannot be selected. PW Doppler permits sample depth adjustment.

86. **(C)** Bernoulli's principle describes the inverse relationship between velocity and pressure. If velocity increases, pressure decreases because of energy conservation rules.

87. **(B)** Monophasic flow implies forward flow through all phases of the cardiac cycle. Low-resistance flow beds typically have monophasic flow when normal.

88. **(C)** Occlusive "thumping" may occur proximal to severe edema or occlusion. There is very low velocity systolic flow and absent diastolic flow. This flow pattern is called "thumping" because of the noise heard over the Doppler speaker.

89. **(C)** The priority setting allows color pixels to replace grayscale pixels or grayscale pixels to replace color pixels, as selected by the operator.

90. **(B)** Reverberation is a common artifact deep to a specular reflector, in this case, the common carotid artery. It can be mistaken for thrombus or plaque.

91. **(D)** Clutter is an artifact that occurs when there is noise near the baseline. It can be eliminated with wall filters.

92. **(D)** The y-axis of the spectral waveform usually represents frequency shift or velocity. Time is along the x-axis.

93. **(B)** Spectral broadening occurs with large gates relative to the vessel and causes loss of the spectral window.

94. **(A)** A negative Doppler shift means the reflectors are traveling in a relative direction that is away from the transducer.

95. **(B)** Absence of a Doppler shift may result from no movement of reflectors, or the inability to detect a Doppler shift related to a 90-degree angle of incidence.

96. **(B)** Length of vessel is a component of resistance, the enemy of flow. If the resistance is increased, flow is decreased.

97. **(C)** Flow is a constant and does not change in a nonhemodynamically significant stenosis.

98. **(A)** The actual Doppler shift (reflected frequency–transmitted frequency) is in the audible range of sound. The noise coming from the speaker of a Doppler instrument is the Doppler shift itself.

99. **(B)** In this image, the spectral gain is too high, causing spectral broadening. Decreasing the gain may decrease the spectral broadening unless the broadening is being caused by other reasons, such as turbulence.

100. **(C)** Color only indicates direction of flow, not artery or vein. In this example, the vessel is blue. According to the color scale given, "blue" is toward the transducer.

Suggested Readings

1. Barrett KE, Barman SM, Boitano S, et al. *Ganong's Review of Medical Physiology.* 24th ed. New York, NY: McGraw-Hill; 2012.

2. Brunicardi FC, Andersen DK, Billiar TR, et al. *Schwartz's Principles of Surgery.* 11th ed. New York, NY: McGraw-Hill; 2019.

3. Fuster V, Walsh RA, Harrington, RA. *Hurst's The Heart.* 13th ed. New York, NY: McGraw-Hill; 2011.

4. Ridgeway D. *Introduction to Vascular Scanning: A Guide for the Complete Beginner.* 4th ed. Pasadena, CA: Davies Publishing; 2014.

5. Knoop KJ, Stack LB, Storrow AB, et al. *The Atlas of Emergency Medicine.* 3rd ed. New York, NY: McGraw-Hill; 2010.

6. Kremkau F. *Sonography Principles and Instruments.* 10th ed. St. Louis, MO: Elsevier Saunders; 2020.

7. Mohrman DE, Heller JH. *Cardiovascular Physiology.* 8th ed. New York, NY: McGraw-Hill; 2014.

8. Pellerito JS, Polack JF. *Introduction to Vascular Sonography.* 7th ed. Philadelphia, PA: Elsevier; 2020.

9. Penny SM, Fox TB, Herring Godwin C. *Examination Review for Ultrasound: Sonographic Principles & Instrumentation (SPI).* 2nd ed. Philadelphia, PA: Lippincott Williams & Wilkins; 2017.

10. Scissons R. Characterizing triphasic, biphasic, and monophasic Doppler waveforms: should a simple task be so difficult? *J Diagn Med Sonography.* 2008;24(5):269–276.

11. Scissons R. Traditional peripheral arterial Doppler waveform descriptors are they still worth teaching? *J Diagn Med Sonography.* 2012;28(2):51–57.

12. Szabo TL. *Diagnostic Ultrasound Imaging: Inside Out.* 2nd ed. San Diego, CA: Elsevier; 2014.

13. Thrush A, Hartshorne T. *Vascular Ultrasound: How, Why, When.* 3rd ed. London, UK: Churchill Livingstone; 2010.

14. Wood MM, Romine LE, Lee YK, et al. Spectral Doppler signature waveforms in ultrasonography: a review of normal and abnormal waveforms. *Ultrasound Q.* 2010;26(2):83–99.

15. Kim ES, Sharma AM, Scissons R, et al. Interpretation of peripheral arterial and venous Doppler waveforms: A Consensus Statement from the Society for Vascular Medicine and Society for Vascular Ultrasound. *Vascular Medicine.* 2020;1–26.

2

Extracranial Cerebrovascular

CEREBROVASCULAR ANATOMY

Vessel Anatomy and Basic Hemodynamics

Arteries are tubular structures that carry blood away from the heart to the surrounding tissues. They start as large arteries (the aorta being the largest) and progressively get smaller, becoming arterioles and eventually capillaries. The capillaries communicate with the venules which are the smallest component of the venous system that eventually allows blood to flow back to the heart. This is what makes up the closed loop of the circulatory system. Arteries provide a mechanism to deliver gases and nutrients to the body's surrounding tissues. This transfer of gases and nutrients occurs at the level of the capillaries. The arterial system is a high-pressure system with a typical intraluminal pressure of 80 to 100 mm Hg. This higher pressure is due to the pumping action of the heart and the higher volume of blood flowing through the arterial system.

Arteries have three distinct layers. Each layer is composed of slightly different materials and varies in thickness. The three layers are:

- Tunica intima—Thin innermost layer of the arteries composed of endothelial cells and connective tissue
- Tunica media—Thicker middle layer of the arteries composed of smooth muscle and connective tissue
- Tunica adventitia—Outermost layer of the arteries composed of fibrous connective tissue; generally thinner than the media layer but thicker than the intima layer; usually contains the vasa vasorum that is responsible for providing a blood supply to the walls of the larger arteries.

The pattern of flow through the arterial system is determined by the location and size of the vessels containing the flow. The majority of the cerebral vessels have laminar blood flow in their normal state. Turbulent flow can occur when disease is present as the flow travels through a stenosis; however, it also exists in normal vessels due to tortuosity. The primary extracranial cerebral blood vessels are the common carotid arteries (CCAs), which bifurcate into the internal carotid arteries (ICAs) and external carotid arteries (ECAs) on each side of the neck. The ICAs receive the majority of the blood flow (70% to 80%) provided by the CCAs. The ICAs are responsible for providing blood flow to the anterior and middle portions of the brain. The other two primary extracranial cerebral vessels are the vertebral arteries (VAs) located on either side at the back of the neck. They join intracranially to form the basilar artery and provide blood flow to the posterior portion of the brain. The ECA has eight branches that provide blood flow to portions of the face and neck.

The brain receives approximately 15% of the body's blood supply produced by the heart through the cerebral vessels. It has very little circulatory reserve due to its high metabolic rate, which makes it completely dependent on the vascular system for maintenance, meaning that even the slightest interruption to flow can cause symptoms.

Extracranial Anatomy

Aorta

The aorta originates from the left ventricle and is the longest artery in the body. The aorta is divided into four main segments. The first portion is the ascending aorta that arises from the left ventricle. As the aorta curves in a downward fashion, it becomes the second segment known as the aortic arch. The aorta continues down the thoracic cavity as the third segment known as the descending aorta, also known as the thoracic aorta. Once the aorta transverses the diaphragm, it then becomes the fourth segment known as the abdominal aorta.

There are three main branches that arise from the aortic arch which supply blood flow to the brain and both arms.

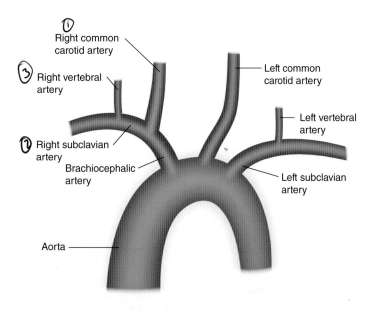

FIGURE 2–1. Illustration of the thoracic aortic arch.

The main branches in ascending to descending order include the following:

- Innominate or brachiocephalic artery
- Left CCA
- Left subclavian artery

The first branch that arises from the arch is the innominate artery, also referred to as the brachiocephalic artery. This branch then typically bifurcates into the right CCA and the right subclavian artery. The next branch of the arch is typically the left CCA, followed by the left subclavian artery (Fig. 2–1). This is the most typical anatomical configuration; however, there can be anatomical variants to this configuration with the most common being a common origin of the innominate and the left CCA (Fig. 2–2).

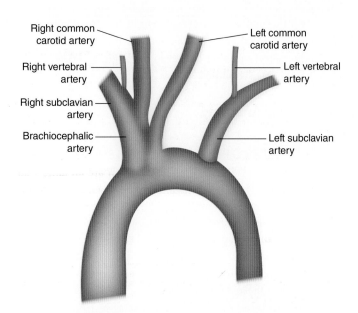

FIGURE 2–2. Illustration of thoracic aortic arch with anatomical variant of common origin or brachiocephalic and left common carotid arteries.

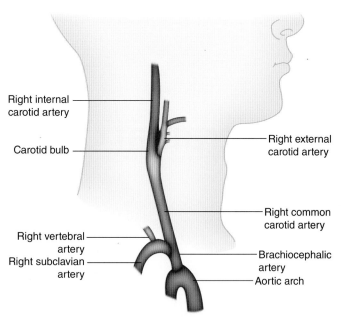

FIGURE 2–3. Illustration of extracranial cerebrovascular arteries.

Vascular Anatomy of the Neck

The CCAs originate from the aortic arch with the right CCA as a branch of the innominate, and the left CCA the second main branch of the arch. Both CCAs continue cephalad from the base of either side of the neck to about the angle of the mandible where they bifurcate into the ICA and the ECA. Somewhere along the course of these vessels, the carotid bulb area can be identified as a slightly dilated area most commonly at the bifurcation; however, its location can vary among patients (Fig. 2–3). The "flow divider" is another name for the spot where the bifurcation occurs. The ICA most commonly courses lateral to the ECA and continues through the base of the skull intracranially to provide blood flow to the anterior and middle portions of the brain. The ICA typically does not have any extracranial branches. The ECA most commonly courses medial to the ICA and does not provide blood flow to the brain in a normal patient; however, can serve as an important collateral pathway when disease is present which will be discussed later in this chapter. The ECA supplies blood to portions of the face, neck, and scalp through eight extracranial branches (Fig. 2–4). The eight branches arising from the ECA are the following:

- Superior thyroid artery
- Ascending pharyngeal artery
- Lingual artery
- Facial artery
- Occipital artery
- Posterior auricular artery
- Superficial temporal artery
- Maxillary artery

The first branch arising from the ECA is the superior thyroid artery which is readily identified on ultrasound. Identification of

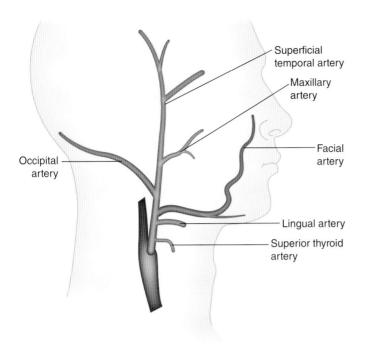

FIGURE 2–4. Illustration of external carotid artery branches.

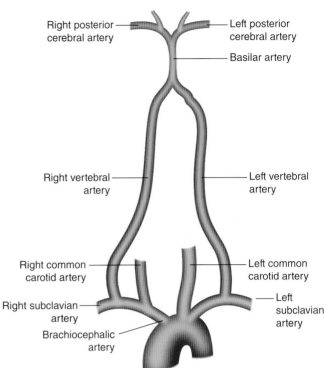

FIGURE 2–5. Illustration of vertebral and basilar arteries.

this branch is one of the methods used to distinguish between the ECA and ICA since the ICA typically does not have extracranial branches.

> **Pro-tip**
>
> The ICA is usually, but not always, more LATERAL, more POSTERIOR, LARGER in diameter and more likely to have DISEASE compared to the ECA. Naturally, this is not always the case so each vessel must be interrogated carefully. With color Doppler, look at the bifurcation – the ICA should have flow in all phases of the cardiac cycle; whereas, the ECA has a more staccato nature because it usually has a multiphasic pattern. Also, with color Doppler, look for ECA branches.

The VAs originate from the proximal portions of the right and left subclavian arteries and course along the posterior aspect of both sides of the neck through the foramen of the transverse processes of the cervical spine and eventually join together intracranially to form the basilar artery (Fig. 2–5). The VAs provide blood flow to the posterior portion of the brain.

PATHOLOGY OF THE EXTRACRANIAL CEREBROVASCULAR SYSTEM

Cerebrovascular Events

Transient Ischemic Attack

A transient ischemic attack (TIA) is a neurological event in which the symptoms resolve in less than 24 hours. The duration of a TIA can vary from minutes to hours and can be considered a precursor to a stroke in a large percentage of patients especially for those who have TIAs lasting a few hours. TIAs are most often caused by an embolic event where a clot or other debris such as plaque originate in another part of the body, travel through the blood stream, and get lodged in the cerebral arteries causing a temporary interruption of blood flow that results in neurological symptoms. Common origins for these emboli are the heart and carotid arteries.

Cerebrovascular Accident

A cerebrovascular accident (CVA), otherwise known as a stroke, is a neurological deficit that is permanent. The symptoms associated with a stroke are the same as those of a TIA. The difference is that the symptoms do not resolve. Similar to a TIA, the main source of a stroke is an embolic event. Strokes can also be hemorrhagic in nature caused by bleeding in the brain; however, this is far less common. There are various causes of hemorrhagic strokes. Some of the most common are an abnormal connection between the arteries and veins known as an arteriovenous malformation (AVM) or a ruptured cerebral aneurysm.

Atherosclerosis (Stenosis)

Atherosclerosis is a chronic disease process that affects the walls of the arteries and is commonly seen at areas where vessels bifurcate. For this reason, the most common area for atherosclerosis to occur in the cerebrovascular system is at the bifurcation of the ICA and ECA. Atherosclerosis starts with the

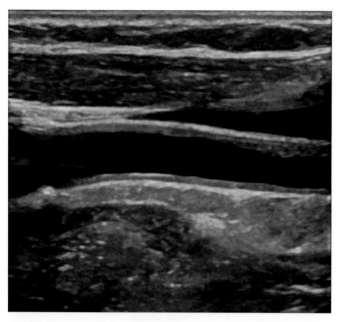

FIGURE 2–6. Longitudinal image of the common carotid artery showing evidence of intima media thickening.

accumulation of plaque causing a thickening of the arterial wall beneath the intima layer. Plaque is composed of lipids known as fatty streaks (Fig. 2–6). Over time the disease might progress to include more lipids as well as fibrous material and collagen. This is commonly referred to as fibrous plaque. This type of plaque typically contains a fibrous cap that separates the contents of the plaque from the lumen of the vessel (Fig. 2–7). As plaque continues to accumulate, it will start to invade more of the vessel lumen leading to what is known as a stenosis, which is the narrowing of the blood vessels that leads to diminished flow. Some plaques may also contain more complex materials such as calcium and cellular components. The characteristics of the plaque are oftentimes identified on ultrasound by their echogenicity which will be discussed in further detail later in this chapter. In addition to different composition, plaques may

also contain ulcerations as well as intraplaque hemorrhage. Ulceration within a plaque is defined as a complete loss of the vascular endothelium, whereas an intraplaque hemorrhage is exactly as the name describes, bleeding within the plaque. Both can be identified on ultrasound as a sonolucent area within the plaque; however, this finding has not proven to be a very reliable method of identifying either. Plaques with ulcerations and intraplaque hemorrhage are considered unstable and increase the chances of an embolic event and neurological symptoms.

Thromboembolic Disease

Embolic strokes are caused by debris that forms somewhere else in the body, travels through the blood stream, and gets lodged in the smaller cerebral arteries causing them to become completely thrombosed, thus restricting blood flow to that area of the brain. Emboli can be solid, liquid, or a gas and may originate from different areas of the body with the heart being the most common. Emboli originating from the heart can be caused by atrial fibrillation, left ventricular dysfunction, and paradoxical emboli through a patent foramen ovale. A paradoxical embolism is a rare event; it occurs when a deep vein thrombosis embolizes and passes through a septal defect in the heart into the arterial system and ends up in the brain causing a stroke. Patients with atrial fibrillation are at a much higher risk for an embolic stroke and are often placed on oral anticoagulants to help reduce that risk. Another source of emboli is anywhere an atherosclerotic lesion is located. Common areas of atherosclerotic plaque are the carotid arteries as well as the aortic arch making them common areas for emboli to originate.

Other Cerebrovascular Pathology

Carotid Body Tumor

A carotid body tumor is a paraganglioma tumor that arises from the paraganglionic cells of the carotid arteries at the area of the carotid bifurcation (Fig. 2–8). These solid masses are highly vascular and are generally benign, receiving the majority of their blood supply from the branches of the ECA. Carotid body tumors can become rather large before becoming symptomatic, and are treated by surgical excision, ECA branch embolization, and occasionally radiation therapy.

Symptoms of large carotid body tumors can include difficulty swallowing and a large pulsating mass at the area of the carotid bifurcation.

Fibromuscular Dysplasia

Fibromuscular dysplasia (FMD) is a nonatherosclerotic disease process affecting the median layer of arteries that is caused by the abnormal development of cells. Unlike atherosclerosis, which occurs predominantly in the origin and proximal segments of arteries, FMD affects the middle and distal portions of the arteries, causing multiple focal areas of stenosis with slight dilatation in between the stenotic areas. FMD can best be visualized with angiography due to its characteristic appearance as

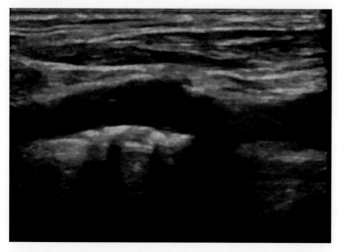

FIGURE 2–7. Longitudinal image of the internal carotid artery showing evidence of smooth fibrous plaque.

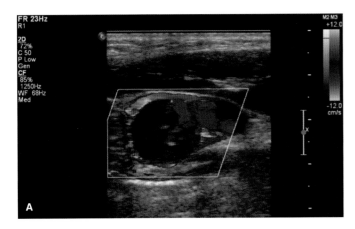

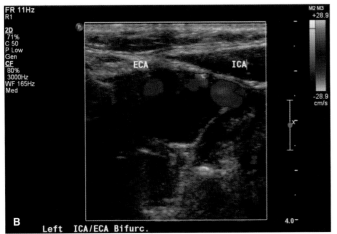

FIGURE 2–8. Sagittal **(A)** and transverse **(B)** images at the level of the carotid bifurcation demonstrating a highly vascular mass which is consistent with a carotid body tumor.

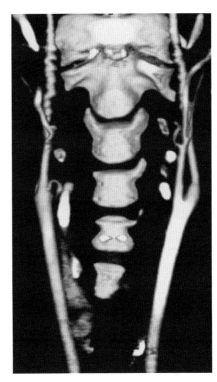

FIGURE 2–9. CT angiography image demonstrating a string of beads appearance within both internal carotid arteries which is a classic sign of fibromuscular dysplasia (FMD).

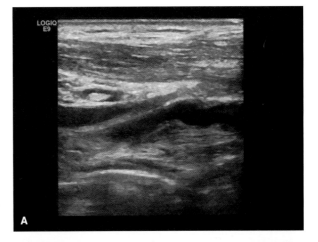

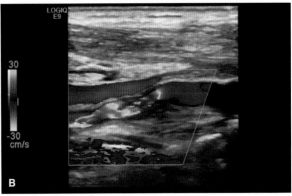

FIGURE 2–10. Longitudinal 2D **(A)** and color Doppler **(B)** images of an internal carotid artery status post carotid endarterectomy demonstrating thickening of the intimal layer consistent with neointimal hyperplasia.

a "string of beads." FMD is more common in younger women and primarily affects the renal and carotid arteries (Fig. 2–9), although it can also be found in many other arteries. The two subtypes of FMD are focal, which is more common in pediatrics, and multifocal, which is the more common subtype. Multifocal FMD means it is seen in more than one location. Some cases of ICA stenosis, especially in the distal ICA, are actually FMD and not from plaque. The distinction is important because the management is different, although a patient may have plaque and FMD in the same vessel.

Neointimal Hyperplasia

Neointimal hyperplasia is an intimal layer thickening caused by the accumulation of smooth muscle cells, typically occurring following a surgical intervention such as a carotid endarterectomy (CEA). Neointimal hyperplasia can result in a hemodynamically significant stenosis or even occlusion and is the most common reason for restenosis or failure within the first 2 years after a CEA (Fig. 2–10).

Dissection

A dissection is a tear in the intimal layer of an artery resulting in an intimal flap within the vessel lumen. The intimal flap within

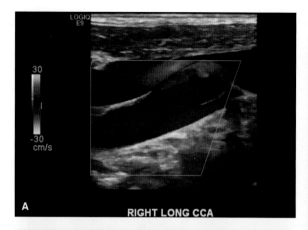

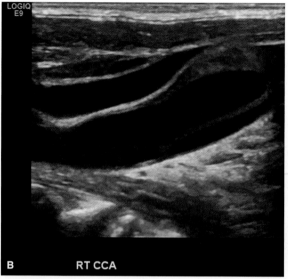

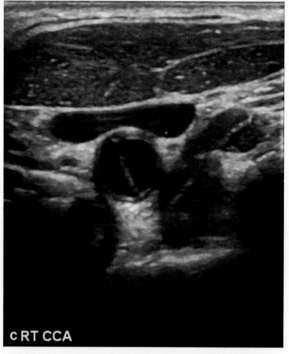

FIGURE 2–11. Color Doppler **(A)**, sagittal **(B)**, and transverse **(C)** images showing evidence of an intimal flap with the lumen of the common carotid artery. The color Doppler images demonstrate flow in both the true and false lumens.

the vessel oftentimes causes a false lumen where flow may be present (Fig. 2–11). Dissections are often caused by trauma to the artery. Dissections can be asymptomatic unless they begin to restrict flow or develop thrombus and become a source of emboli resulting in neurological symptoms. Dissections can occur from connective tissue disorders and from trauma, such as injury to the neck from a seatbelt during a motor vehicle accident.

Carotid Aneurysm

An aneurysm is defined as a focal dilation of an artery that is 50% greater than the diameter of its normal segment. Aneurysms are rarely found in the carotid arteries but when seen on ultrasound will have a sonographic appearance in the area representing the focal dilation (Fig. 2–12). The classic clinical presentation of a carotid aneurysm is a pulsatile mass in the neck.

One important note to make is that oftentimes a large carotid bulb or a tortuous proximal carotid artery is mistakenly suspected to be an aneurysm clinically.

Subclavian Steal Syndrome

Subclavian steal syndrome occurs when there is reversal of flow in the ipsilateral VA providing blood flow to the affected arm in the presence of a proximal subclavian artery or innominate artery obstruction. In order for subclavian steal syndrome to occur, the subclavian artery stenosis must be proximal to the origin of the ipsilateral VA (Fig. 2–13). It occurs more commonly on the left side due to the left subclavian artery origination directly from the aortic arch. The findings associated with subclavian steal syndrome are reversed or alternating flow in the ipsilateral VA and a drop in systolic blood pressure greater than 15-20 mm Hg in the ipsilateral arm when compared to the

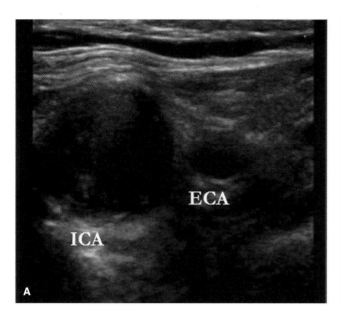
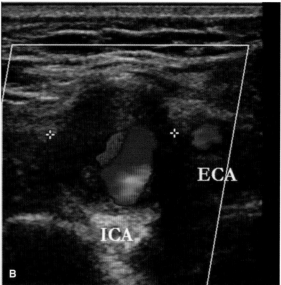

FIGURE 2–12. Transverse 2D **(A)** and color Doppler **(B)** images of the carotid bifurcation showing focal dilatation of the internal carotid artery consistent with an internal carotid artery (ICA) aneurysm.

contralateral side. Patients with subclavian steal syndrome are oftentimes asymptomatic; however, symptoms associated with vertebrobasilar insufficiency can result and may worsen with arm exercise.

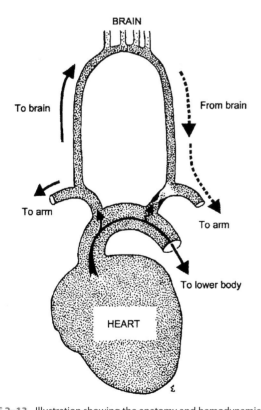

FIGURE 2–13. Illustration showing the anatomy and hemodynamics as a result of subclavian steal syndrome. With a hemodynamically significant stenosis proximal to the origin of the vertebral artery, there is antegrade flow in the contralateral flow and retrograde flow in the ipsilateral vertebral artery. (Reproduced, with permission, from Odwin CS, Fleischer AC. *Lange Review: Ultrasonography Examination,* 4th ed. New York, NY; 2012; Figure 12-5. Copyright © McGraw Hill.)

PATIENT ASSESSMENT AND INTEGRATION OF DATA

Risk Factors

Anyone at any age regardless of gender or race may have a stroke; however, there are certain conditions that contribute to a higher risk, some of which are controllable through lifestyle and/or medical therapy and some that are uncontrollable. The risk factors associated with stroke include:

- Hypertension—Also known as high blood pressure, hypertension causes increased strain on the arteries and has been known to contribute to the atherosclerosis process. According to the American Stroke Association (ASA), hypertension is the most important risk factor because it is the number one cause of stroke. Hypertension is a controllable risk factor when patients are appropriately medicated. The current normal values for blood pressure are: normal = less than 120/90 mm Hg, elevated blood pressure = 120-129 mm Hg systolic, stage 1 hypertension = 129-139 mm Hg systolic, and stage 2 hypertension = greater than 140 mm Hg systolic.

- Tobacco use—Damages the endothelial lining of blood vessels and contributes to atherosclerosis.

- Diabetes mellitus—A chronic metabolic disease that produces high blood sugar levels for prolonged periods of time and increased atherosclerosis of the arteries, including the cerebral arteries, leading to a high risk of stroke.

- Hyperlipidemia—High lipid levels in the blood contribute to an increase in atherosclerosis.

- Obesity—Patients who are inactive and/or obese have a higher rate of cardiovascular disease making them much more likely to have a stroke.

- Atrial fibrillation—Atrial fibrillation causes the chambers of the heart to beat ineffectively leading to an increased risk of thrombus formation and embolism. As mentioned earlier, placing patients on anticoagulation therapy can significantly reduce this risk factor.

- Uncontrollable risk factors—Risk factors such as age, gender, race, and heredity can increase the risk of stroke but are beyond control. Even though more women die each year from stroke, in general, men have a higher risk of stroke than women. The older you are the higher your risk. The risk of stroke increases with each year as you age. African Americans have a higher incidence of stroke and disability from a stroke than any other race. A history of stroke in the family indicates a higher risk for stroke as well.

Signs and Symptoms

ICA
ACA
MCA

Anterior Circulation Symptoms

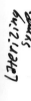

The anterior circulation is primarily composed of the ICA, anterior cerebral artery, and middle cerebral artery (MCA). These arteries are responsible for perfusion to the brain's cerebral hemispheres. Any disturbance to blood flow to one of the hemispheres can cause neurological symptoms on the contralateral side of the face or body. This is due to the fact that the right hemisphere controls the left side of the body and the left hemisphere controls the right side of the body. Therefore, with a left hemispheric stroke the symptoms would occur on the right side, except in the case of amaurosis fugax. These types of symptoms are what are known as lateralizing symptoms. Some of the most common lateralizing symptoms associated with the anterior circulation include:

- Hemiparesis/hemiparalysis—Unilateral weakness or partial or complete paralysis affecting the contralateral side.

- Hemiparesthesia—Unilateral numbness, tingling, or loss of feeling affecting the contralateral side.

- Dysphasia/aphasia—Dysphasia is slurred or impaired speech while aphasia is the inability to speak. These are considered hemispheric lateralizing symptoms because the left hemisphere is dominant for speech in right-handed people and vice versa for left-handed people. As a note of caution, do not mistake "dysphasia" for "dysphagia," which is difficulty swallowing.

- Amaurosis fugax—Temporary partial or complete blindness, typically in one eye. This symptom is often described as "a shade lowering down over the eye." The source of this symptom is often emboli through the ophthalmic artery from the ipsilateral ICA.

- Hemianopia—Blindness in one-half of the field of vision in one or both eyes commonly caused by occlusion of the MCA.

Posterior Circulation Symptoms

VA
Basilar
PCA

Non-lateralizing

The posterior circulation is primarily composed of the vertebral, basilar, and posterior cerebral arteries. These arteries are responsible for providing blood flow to the posterior portions of the brain including the cerebellum, occipital lobes, and the brainstem. Disturbance of blood flow to these areas of the brain causes symptoms that are nonlateralizing and affect the body as a whole. It is important to note that while 20% to 30% of ischemic event are the result of posterior circulation, symptoms involving these vessels can often times be vague and nonspecific.

Some of the most common symptoms associated with posterior circulation include:

- Ataxia—Unsteady gait.
- Diplopia—Double vision.
- Blurred vision.
- Hemianopia—Blindness in half your field of vision.
- Nystagmus or "Dancing eyes"—Uncontrollable eye movements.
- Dizziness or vertigo (in conjunction with other symptoms)—The inability to maintain equilibrium; often described as the room spinning around a person.
- Bilateral paresthesia—Numbness, tingling, or loss of feeling on both sides of the body. When paresthesia is not localized to one side of the body, it can oftentimes be the result of a disturbance to the posterior circulation.
- Difficulty ambulating.
- Loss of balance.

Nonlocalizing Symptoms

There are some symptoms of stroke that are considered rather vague in their presentation and cannot be linked to any specific area of the brain. Some of these symptoms are often the result of other disease processes as well. Nonlocalizing symptoms include:

- Syncope—Complete loss of consciousness. Presyncope is when the patient felt like they were going to pass out but did not. The patient may have dizziness, lightheadedness, heart palpitations, diaphoresis, etc.
- Confusion or change in mental status.
- Headaches.

Clinical Assessment

The clinical assessment of patients for cerebrovascular disease starts with evaluation of risk factors and is followed by the assessment of stroke-type symptoms, both of which were described in full detail previously in this chapter. The most common location for cerebrovascular disease to occur is in the carotid arteries. The challenge is that not all carotid artery lesions cause symptoms. A hemodynamically significant carotid stenosis can be symptomatic or asymptomatic. The only somewhat reliable screening tool other than carotid duplex is listening for a carotid bruit. A bruit is a noise that is produced by the vibrations of the surrounding tissues as the result of turbulent flow in the artery that is commonly heard with a hemodynamically significant stenosis. To check for a carotid bruit, a stethoscope is held to the patient's neck in the area of the carotid artery and the patient is instructed to take in a deep breath and hold it while the examiner listens for the bruit. A bruit cannot always be heard in patients with a hemodynamically significant stenosis and the presence of a bruit does not always solidify that one is present. Because of the low specificity of this examination it cannot serve as a reliable means for diagnosing carotid artery disease, but rather should be used as a tool to generate additional evaluation and testing.

PROTOCOLS

Carotid Duplex

Carotid duplex is a noninvasive method that uses 2D ultrasound combined with Doppler [typically both pulsed-wave (PW) spectral and color] to evaluate the extracranial cerebrovascular vessels including the common carotid, internal carotid, external carotid, and VAs. Carotid duplex can be used to identify and evaluate the extent of a carotid stenosis with a fair amount of accuracy, and because of its noninvasive nature it can be used as the primary modality to follow patients for the progression of disease.

Patient Positioning

The patient should be placed in a supine position with the neck area exposed by having the patient elevate their chin and turn their head slightly away from the side being examined. This

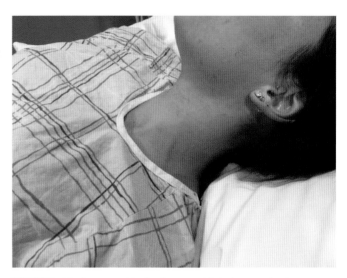

FIGURE 2–14. Proper positioning for a carotid duplex examination.

will allow the sonographer access to the vessels being imaged (Fig. 2–14).

Scanning Technique

The highest frequency transducer for better resolution without compromising penetration should always be selected for each examination. Typically, a 5-7 MHz linear transducer is used for a carotid duplex examination. The arteries are imaged in both longitudinal and transverse planes throughout their course. The image orientation for a sonographic image is always the same. In the longitudinal plane, with the transducer notch toward the head, the right side of the screen is always toward the patient's feet while the left is toward the patient's head. In the transverse plane, with the notch toward the patient's right, the right side of the screen is always the left side of the patient and the left side of the screen is always the right side of the patient (Fig. 2–15). Although there is often

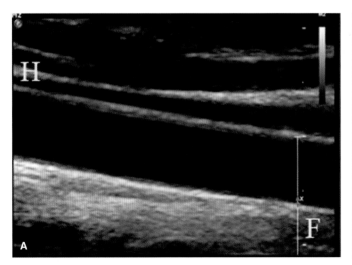

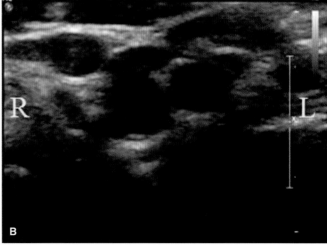

FIGURE 2–15. (A) Longitudinal ultrasound image showing the normal orientation with the notch of the transducer toward the head. **(B)** Transverse ultrasound image showing the normal orientation with the notch of the transducer toward the right of the patient.

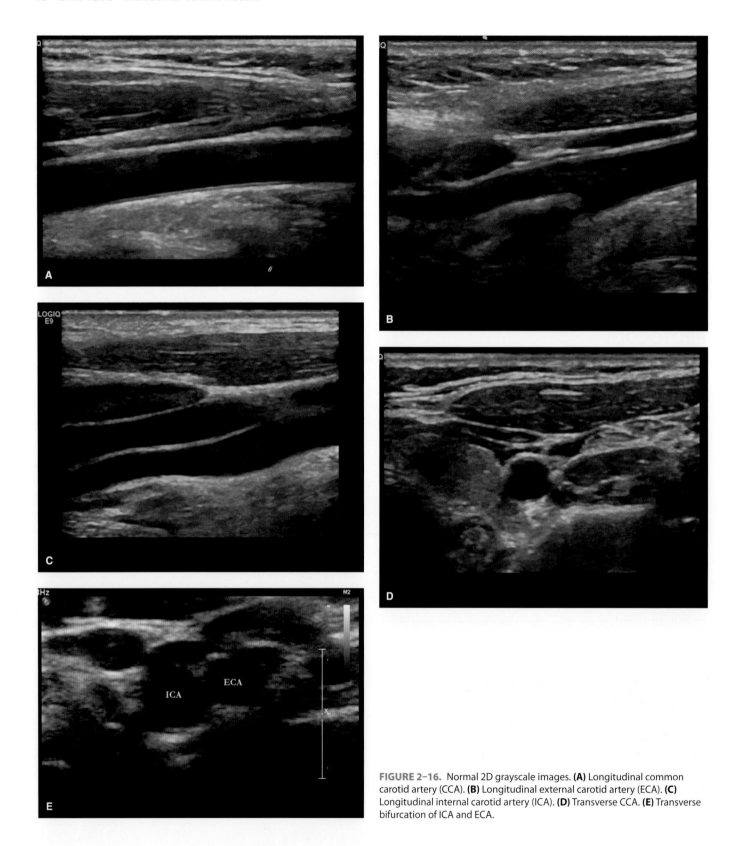

FIGURE 2–16. Normal 2D grayscale images. **(A)** Longitudinal common carotid artery (CCA). **(B)** Longitudinal external carotid artery (ECA). **(C)** Longitudinal internal carotid artery (ICA). **(D)** Transverse CCA. **(E)** Transverse bifurcation of ICA and ECA.

debate about whether to scan with the patient head up/feet down or feet up/head down, it is important to do whatever is comfortable for the sonographer.

The examination begins with 2D grayscale evaluation of the arteries at the base of the neck just above the clavicle where the most proximal portion of the CCA can be identified. The CCA is followed cephalad to the carotid bifurcation. At the area of the bifurcation, the origins of the ECA and ICA are identified. The ICA is then followed cephalad past the angle of the mandible as far as the extracranial ICA can be seen.

TABLE 2–1 • Common Characteristics Used to Determine ECA From ICA

Characteristics	ICA	ECA	Examples
Size	Usually larger than the ECA	Usually smaller than the ICA	
Location	Usually located more laterally	Usually located more medially	
Branches	No extracranial branches	Has eight extracranial braches *Sup. Thyroid AA modify scan*	
Waveform	Low-resistant waveform with broad peak systolic and high diastolic flow	Higher-resistant waveform with sharp peak systolic and low diastolic flow	

These 2D grayscale images are obtained in both longitudinal and transverse views (Fig. 2–16). It is important to differentiate the ICA from the ECA, and there are several characteristics that can help distinguish between the two. See Table 2–1 for a list of these characteristics. The arteries should be evaluated for any evidence of plaque or intimal thickening. Plaque is defined as a 50% focal increase in intima-media thickness (IMT) compared to a surrounding normal segment. The VA can be identified in the longitudinal plane by locating the CCA and angling posterior and lateral. The artery will be seen passing through the foramina of the transverse processes of the cervical spine, which are seen as shadows on ultrasound (Fig. 2–17). Color Doppler is typically used to locate the VA as well as to evaluate the direction of flow. Flow should always be cephalad (toward the head).

Color Doppler is used most commonly in the longitudinal plane to assist placement of the PW spectral Doppler gate. It can be very useful when significant disease is present in finding the highest velocity within a stenosis. PW spectral Doppler waveforms should be obtained throughout the carotid system and always obtained in the longitudinal plane in order to provide the best Doppler angle. In order to provide the most accurate results, the Doppler angle is extremely important and should never exceed 60 degrees. More importantly, the angle correction should always be parallel to the vessel walls in order to avoid over- or underestimation of disease. Sample volume size is typically 1-3 mm and placed in the center of each vessel (assuming a normal vessel). If a small sample volume size is used (assuming it is placed in the center of a normal vessel), the spectral waveform will be most optimized and a thin spectral envelope with an open window will be obtained. However, higher velocities may be missed if the sample volume is too small. Opening the gate wider will cause even normal waveforms to have spectral broadening,

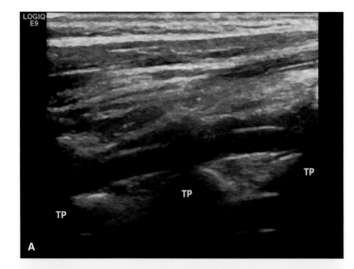

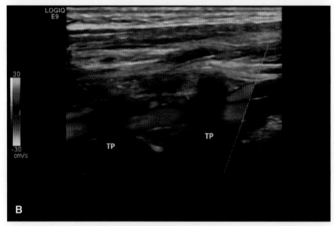

FIGURE 2–17. Longitudinal 2D **(A)** and color Doppler **(B)** images of the vertebral artery coursing through the transverse processes of the cervical spine (identified by the shadows of the images).

but you will be assured of obtaining the highest velocities present in the flow (Fig. 2–18).

Protocols may vary among institutions, particularly when disease is present. Although protocols vary by lab, labs accredited by the Intersocietal Accreditation Commission (IAC) requires, at a minimum: spectral Doppler waveforms from the proximal and mid/distal CCA, proximal and distal ICA (as cephalad as possible), the origin of the ECA, and one from the VA. If a carotid stent is present, waveforms must be obtained proximal, mid, and distal stent in addition to the native vessels.

Controversies in Ultrasound – The 60 degree Angle

There is often a misunderstanding regarding the needs for a 60 degree angle in ultrasound. True, when performing carotid ultrasounds, the angle should be around 60 degree, or at least between 45 degree and 60 degree. But it is not because the higher angle is more accurate. In fact, as you learned in physics, a 0 degree angle is the most accurate angle when performing Doppler. In the carotids, however, an angle approaching 60 degree is easier to obtain than a 0 degree angle. So, what happens when the distal ICA dives down and you need to use a 0 degree angle? Do you try and force a 60 degree angle because you were taught to "only use a 60 degree angle"? No. It is okay to use 0 degrees. The most important thing is that the angle correction is parallel to the wall and consistent from study to study. Some labs prefer to use an angle parallel to flow, but the key thing is reproducibility.

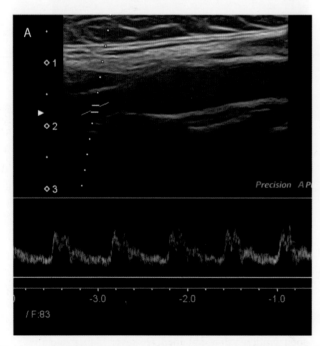

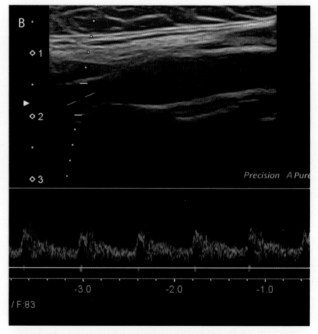

FIGURE 2–18. Open window versus spectral broadening. **(A)** Spectral Doppler image in center of vessel with small gate revealing "laminar" type waveform. **(B)** Same image with wider gate shows filling-in of the spectral window, called spectral broadening. There are many causes of spectral broadening.

Limitations

The limitations of carotid duplex are like those seen in other types of duplex examination and include:

- Patient body habitus—May limit ultrasound penetration.
- Calcified plaque—May hide underlying disease due to distal shadowing. Consider coming in from a different window, like the posterior neck approach.
- Access to anatomy—Dressings, braces, and IV lines are just some of the examples of items that can obstruct the anatomy being imaged.
- Patient cooperation—Any type of uncontrollable patient movement and erratic breathing patterns can limit the ability to complete the examination accurately.
- Patient anatomy—Tortuous vessels can cause increased velocities which may cause overestimation of disease.
- Disease process—Collateralized flow caused by different disease processes can cause increased velocities, which may cause overestimation of disease.
- Technologist technique—Ultrasound is a modality that is very operator-dependent, and results are only as accurate as the skill level of the sonographer performing the examination. Improper Doppler angle can cause over- or underestimation of disease, the inability to properly identify the highest velocity within a stenosis can cause underestimation of disease, and inability to recognize changes in waveform characteristics can cause missed diagnosis.
- Intraaortic balloon pumps (IABP)—Cause a distortion of the waveform as the balloon inflates and deflates through the cardiac cycle causing a second peak during systole and a decrease and reversal during diastole. The distortion of the waveforms limits the accuracy of the examination because of the inability to analyze the waveforms and their velocities.
- Left ventricular assist device (LVAD)—This is a mechanical pump implanted into the left ventricle in patients waiting for a heart transplant. The nature of the pump causes a waveform with minimal pulsatility and no flow reversal below the baseline (Fig. 2–19).

INTERPRETATION OF RESULTS

Normal 2D Grayscale Findings

In a normal 2D grayscale image of a carotid artery, all three distinct layers should be visualized intact and free of any intraluminal material such as plaque or thrombus (Fig. 2–20). The intima-media layer should be smooth with uniform thickness throughout the artery. Any signs of thickening should be identified. Increased IMT has been reported to increase the likelihood of developing coronary artery disease. There is a measurement that can be performed with specific calculation packages on some equipment known as IMT that has been used to rate risk of cardiovascular disease.

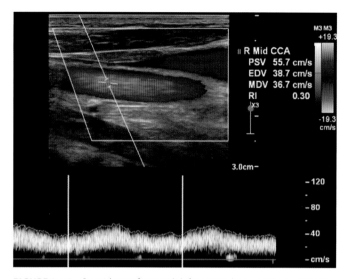

FIGURE 2–19. Carotid waveform with left ventricular assist device (LVAD). Flow within an LVAD may have low or absent pulsatility depending on the device used. As with the intraaortic balloon pump (IABP), the degree of stenosis present within the vessel may be underestimated.

Abnormal 2D Grayscale Findings

As the disease process first begins in the carotid arteries, it often appears as a thickening on the intimal-media layer. As the amount of plaque starts to increase, it will occupy more of the vessel lumen. As the amount of plaque in the artery increases, the diameter of the artery decreases, causing a stenosis. Stenosis is more accurately quantified using PW spectral Doppler and will be discussed in further detail later in this section. Plaque or thrombus may completely fill the lumen of an artery leading to a complete occlusion. The most common area for an occlusion to occur in the cerebrovascular system is the ICA. A complete occlusion can be identified using 2D imaging by echogenic material filling the lumen. It is also possible for an occlusion to appear anechoic depending on the composition of the plaque. It is important to note that both color and PW Doppler

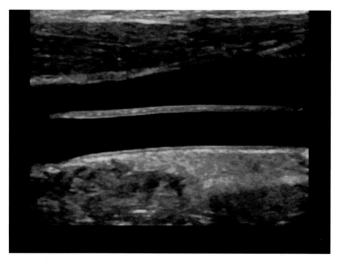

FIGURE 2–20. Normal longitudinal 2D grayscale image of the common carotid artery.

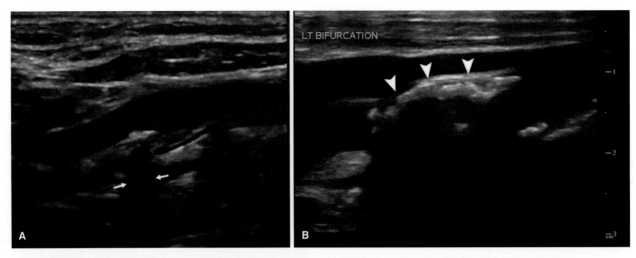

FIGURE 2–21. Shadowing plaque. **(A)** Calcific plaque in the proximal internal carotid artery (ICA). Arrows point to shadowing. **(B)** Anterior plaque with marked shadowing makes visualization of the vessel difficult. Try a more posterior approach to avoid the shadowing plaque.

should also be used to evaluate whether an artery is completely occluded or not.

Plaque can form in any portion of the common, ICA, or ECA; however, it is at the level of the bifurcation where the CCA leads into the ICA that disease is most common. As plaque is identified in the carotid arteries, it is important to attempt to characterize it in terms of content and surface. This characterization will assist the clinician to better evaluate the patient's risk of stroke. The internal contents of the plaque are determined on ultrasound by their echogenicity and are defined using subjective visual criteria. The intensity (or brightness) of the echoes should be evaluated when attempting to characterize plaque. Very low level or dark echoes are described as echolucent or hypoechoic and can suggest the presence of lipid materials. Echolucent areas within plaque can also suggest the presence of hemorrhage or thrombus in high-risk plaques. Increased echoes in the absence of calcifications

are described as isoechoic or hyperechoic and are most commonly associated with an increase in fibrous tissue. Hyperechoic plaque with areas of distal acoustic shadowing suggests the presence of calcifications. This acoustic shadowing makes it difficult to characterize the underlying plaque in many cases (Fig. 2–21). Plaque with echolucent/hypoechoic areas has a higher rate of ischemic event and therefore should be described as part of the characterization. Another aspect of characterizing plaque is homogeneity. Homogeneity refers to the overall distribution of the echo within the plaque. Homogeneous plaque refers to plaque that is uniform and is commonly associated with low-medium level echoes. This type of appearance indicates a high fibrous content and usually also demonstrates a fibrous cap between the plaque and the vessel lumen making it fairly stable (Fig. 2–22). Heterogeneous plaque refers to plaque with mixed echogenicities. Heterogeneous plaque will have a mixture of medium-high level echoes mixed with focal

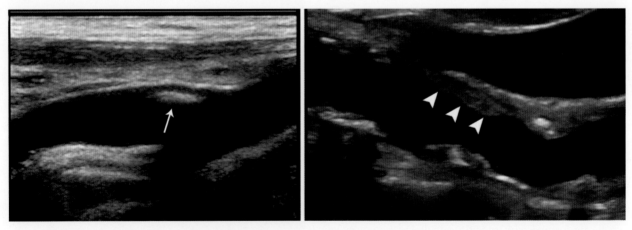

FIGURE 2–22. Homogeneous plaque. **(A)** Plaque (arrow) on the near-field wall of the internal carotid artery (ICA). **(B)** Common carotid artery (CCA) with mixed homogenous (arrowheads) and heterogeneous plaque.

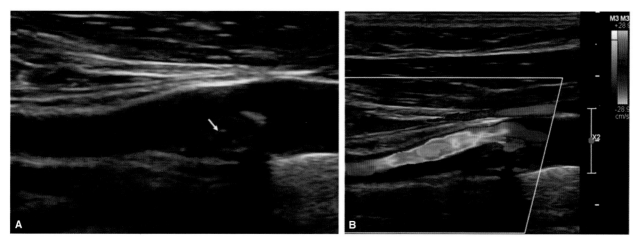

FIGURE 2-23. Heterogeneous plaque. **(A)** Grayscale image of the proximal ICA. Arrow points to anechoic area within mostly homogeneous plaque. **(B)** Color Doppler of same image showing irregular surface of plaque proximally.

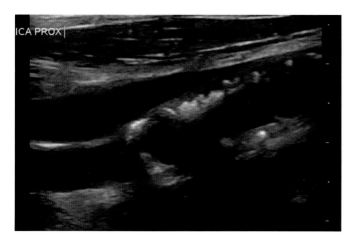

FIGURE 2-24. Extensive heterogeneous plaque in proximal internal carotid artery (ICA).

anechoic areas (Figs. 2–23 and 2–24). The anechoic areas seen within the contents of heterogeneous plaque often represent an intraplaque hemorrhage, rupture, or repair. The majority of plaques seen in symptomatic patients are heterogeneous in nature; however, homogenous plaques that are hypoechoic can also be vulnerable to patients. When an anechoic area is identified, it is important to identify if the endothelial lining or "surface" of the plaque is intact. The surface of plaque can be identified with ultrasound as either smooth or irregular. Plaque identified as having a smooth surface refers to plaque that has a fibrous cap and is more stable. Plaque with an irregular surface refers to plaque that has a possible rupture or ulceration and is considered unstable (Fig. 2–25). Both ruptured and ulcerated plaques increase the risk of an embolic event leading to a possible stroke. Larger ulcerations are more likely to be accurately detected by ultrasound than the smaller ones found in complex calcified plaques. Superb microvascular (or microflow) imaging (SMI) can be an aid in identifying potential areas of ulceration within a plaque (Fig. 2–26).

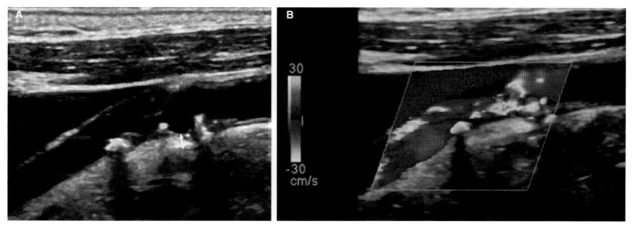

FIGURE 2-25. Heterogeneous plaque with potential ulceration. **(A)** Heterogeneous plaque in lumen of proximal internal carotid artery (ICA) with anechoic area within plaque suspicious for ulceration (arrow). **(B)** Color Doppler of same area.

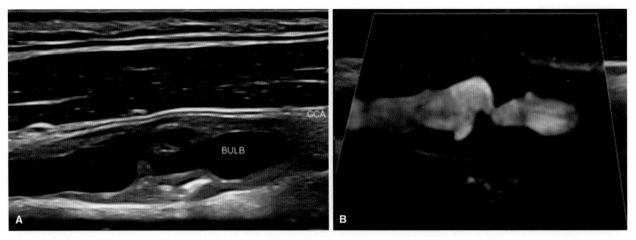

FIGURE 2–26. Ulcerated plaque. **(A)** Grayscale image of heterogeneous plaque with ulceration confirmed by angiography. **(B)** Superb microvascular imaging (SMI), also called microflow, of same vessel.

In addition to plaque, the carotid arteries should be evaluated for any other wall defects such as dissection, aneurysms, or pseudoaneurysms.

Normal Doppler Findings

Color Doppler

Color Doppler for the majority of the carotid vessels should show a laminar-type flow pattern with velocities increasing toward the center of the vessel and decreasing toward the vessel walls (Fig. 2–27). One exception is the carotid bulb. The carotid bulb has a helical-type flow pattern with flow in both directions separated by a flow separator (Fig. 2–28). At times, turbulent flow patterns can be seen in the carotid arteries. This is common when the vessels are tortuous (Fig. 2–29). Color Doppler is also used to assess the direction of blood flow in the extracranial cerebrovascular arteries. With the color box angled in one direction or the other, flow will be displayed as either going toward or away from the transducer. It is important to confirm that all the extracranial arteries have flow in the cephalic direction (toward the head). This is particularly important in the VAs to rule out the presence of subclavian steal syndrome (Fig. 2–30).

PW Spectral Doppler

The ICA is the main artery that provides blood flow to the majority of the brain. The brain is a very low-resistance vascular bed causing the ICA waveform to appear as a much more low-resistance waveform than the ECA and CCA. The ICA also shows broader peak systolic velocity (PSV) and higher diastolic velocity. The flow in a normal ICA should be laminar and therefore a normal ICA waveform should have a clear spectral window.

The ECA does not provide blood flow to the brain under normal circumstances. It is, however, responsible for providing blood flow to areas of the face and head. These areas have a higher resistance to flow than the brain, so the ECA waveform is going to appear as a high-resistance waveform. The waveform has a sharp peak with very little diastolic flow. It too should have normal laminar flow with a clear spectral window.

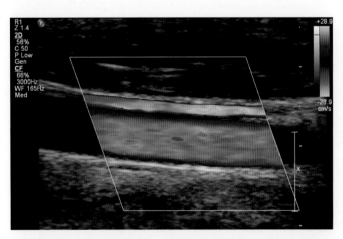

FIGURE 2–27. Normal color Doppler image of the common carotid artery demonstrating laminar flow with the higher velocities toward the center of the vessel and slower velocities along the vessel walls.

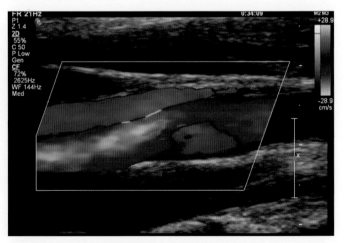

FIGURE 2–28. Normal color Doppler image of the carotid bulb area demonstrating helical flow.

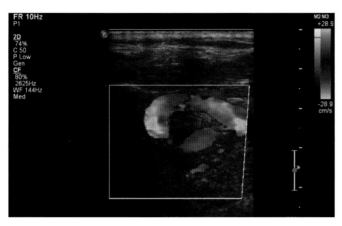

FIGURE 2-29. Normal color Doppler image of the internal carotid artery demonstrating aliasing caused by tortuous vessel course.

The CCA provides blood flow to both the ICA and the ECA, therefore should have a waveform with flow characteristics similar to each. The CCA should demonstrate a moderate amount of diastolic flow that is lower than that seen in the ICA but slightly higher than that seen in the ECA.

The VA is the main artery supplying blood to the posterior portions of the brain and should demonstrate a flow pattern similar to that of the ICA with slightly lower velocities. Normal vertebral artery velocities range from 40 to 64 cm/s on average. More than half of all patients have a dominate VA which can have a slightly larger diameter and higher velocities. This is most often the left VA.

Figure 2-31 demonstrates the normal spectral waveforms for each cerebrovascular artery.

Abnormal Doppler Findings

Color Doppler

The most common abnormal color Doppler finding associated with a stenosis is aliasing. With appropriate scale settings, aliasing will occur typically at areas of stenosis due to the frequency shift related to the increased velocities and turbulent flow at the exit point of the stenosis (Fig. 2-32). The absence of color can suggest the possibility of a total occlusion; however, standard color Doppler should be used in conjunction with 2D, power Doppler, and PW spectral Doppler to confirm. If blood flow is reversed, for example, when subclavian steal syndrome is present, flow will be displayed as retrograde or caudal (toward the feet) (Fig. 2-33). In situations where the steal has not yet manifested itself fully, there may be alternating flow directions in systole and diastole. This is known as a latent steal.

PW Doppler

As an arterial lumen narrows due to plaque accumulation, the velocity of blood flow through that vessel increases. This is one of the key elements of a stenosis that is identified by the Bernoulli's principle, described in Chapter 1. The spectral waveform that corresponds with a stenotic vessel will show elevated PSV and end-diastolic velocity (EDV). In addition to the elevated velocities, there will also be changes to the waveform distally in the form of spectral broadening. Spectral broadening refers to loss of the clear spectral window due to turbulent flow (Fig. 2-34). Spectral broadening can exist in normal vessels due to tortuosity as well as distal to a stenosis. In general, the narrower the stenosis, the higher the velocity and greater the spectral broadening.

With any stenosis, there are three areas of interest. They are (1) prestenotic area, (2) stenotic area, and (3) poststenotic area. The stenotic area was already addressed in this section; however, the pre- and poststenotic waveforms frequently offer just as much diagnostic information as the stenosis itself. Since most carotid artery disease occurs within the first 2 cm of the ICA, the prestenotic region is usually the CCA. Changes in waveform of the CCA help us predict more distal disease. Loss of the diastolic component in the CCA usually suggests the presence of a

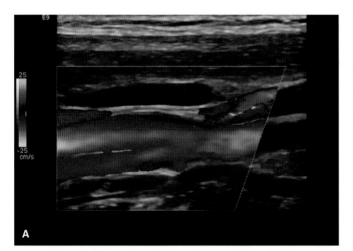

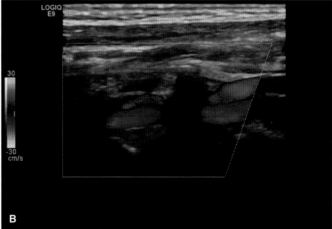

FIGURE 2-30. (A) Normal color Doppler images of the carotid bifurcation of the internal carotid artery and the external carotid artery demonstrating flow traveling away from the transducer toward the head. **(B)** Normal color Doppler images of the vertebral artery also demonstrating flow traveling away from the transducer toward the head.

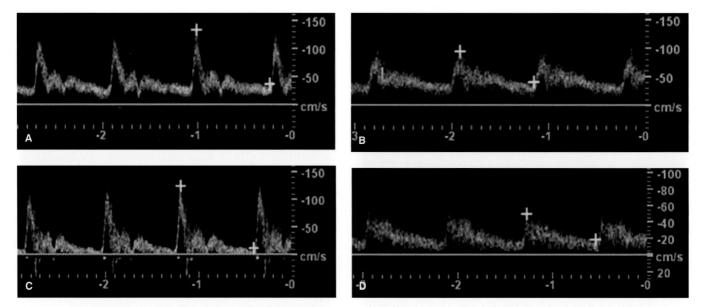

FIGURE 2–31. Normal pulse-wave spectral Doppler waveforms. **(A)** Common carotid artery (CCA). **(B)** Internal carotid artery (ICA). **(C)** External carotid artery (ECA). **(D)** Vertebral artery.

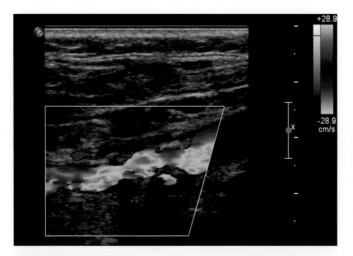

FIGURE 2–32. Color Doppler image of a stenosis within the internal carotid artery demonstrating aliasing consistent with high velocities and turbulent flow.

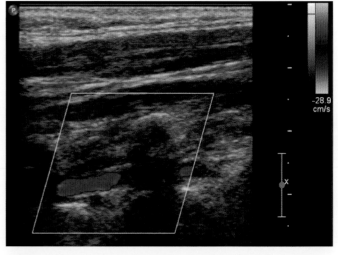

FIGURE 2–33. Color Doppler image of a vertebral artery with retrograde flow toward the transducer in a caudal direction.

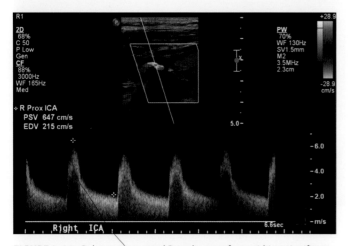

FIGURE 2–34. Pulse-wave spectral Doppler waveform within a significant stenosis demonstrating high velocities and spectral broadening.

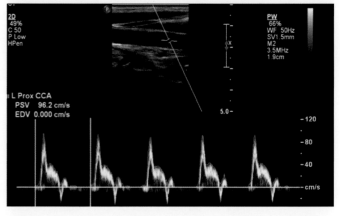

FIGURE 2–35. An abnormal pulse-wave spectral Doppler waveform of a common carotid artery demonstrating increased resistance due to the absence of diastolic flow suggesting a distal obstruction.

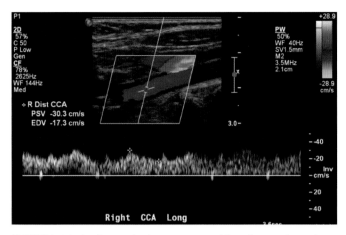

FIGURE 2–36. An abnormal pulse-wave spectral Doppler waveform of a common carotid artery demonstrating dampened flow with delayed acceleration to peak systolic suggesting a proximal obstruction.

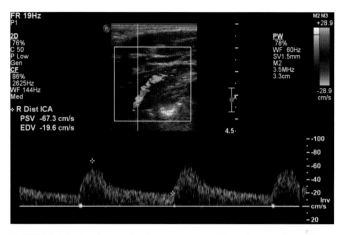

FIGURE 2–38. An abnormal pulse-wave spectral Doppler waveform of a distal internal carotid artery demonstrating dampened flow with delayed acceleration to peak systolic, a common finding with a critical stenosis at the origin of the internal carotid artery. This waveform is classically known as a tardus-parvus waveform.

distal ICA occlusion (Fig. 2–35). If the loss of diastolic flow is also present in the ipsilateral ICA, this may suggest the presence of occlusive disease even more distal such as the intracranial ICA or MCA. There are times when the CCA becomes the post-stenotic region where you will see diminished or turbulent flow as the result of an innominate or proximal CCA stenosis (Fig. 2–36). These presentations are typically unilateral in nature so the right and left CCA waveforms should always be compared to each other. If changes in waveforms occur bilaterally, then the cause is most likely cardiac. The typical poststenotic region in cerebrovascular disease occurs in the middle to distal ICA. The changes in waveform will depend on the severity of the disease as well as the proximity to the stenosis. The more severe the stenosis the more obvious the changes in the distal waveforms will appear. The waveform seen just distal to a significant stenosis will have a poststenotic turbulent waveform that is characterized by an elevated peak systolic with a characteristic "spiky" appearance (Fig. 2–37). Further downstream from a significant stenosis, the waveform will appear more dampened

with a rounded peak displayed and an increased acceleration time. This is a classic-type waveform known as "tardus parvus," meaning a slow-rising pulse (Fig. 2–38). In the event of a possible total occlusion of the ICA, it is important to still access the vessel with PW spectral Doppler for the presence of flow since a critical stenosis cannot be ruled out by just the absence of color Doppler. If a total occlusion is present, there will be absence of flow with PW spectral Doppler (Fig. 2–39). Loss of diastolic flow in the ipsilateral CCA as mentioned earlier can assist in confirming the presence of an ICA occlusion. Another finding that may be present with ICA occlusion is reversal of flow in the ipsilateral ECA. The ECA shares collateral branches with the ophthalmic artery in the eye, and reversed flow in the ECA may be seen with CCA occlusion or near occlusion, so called "internalizing" of the ECA. The ultrasound findings of CCA occlusion with ECA reversal of flow are that the ECA waveform will lose its dicrotic notch, demonstrate more diastolic flow, and flow in a direction that is away from the brain (Fig. 2–40).

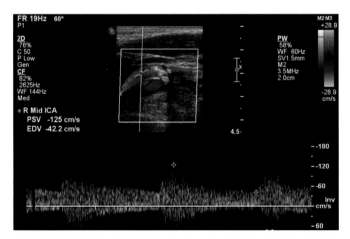

FIGURE 2–37. An abnormal pulse-wave spectral Doppler waveform of an internal carotid artery demonstrating turbulent flow distal to a hemodynamically significant stenosis.

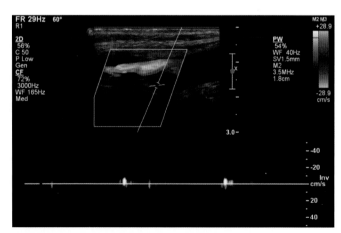

FIGURE 2–39. An abnormal pulse-wave spectral Doppler waveform of an internal carotid artery demonstrating lack of flow in the presence of a total occlusion.

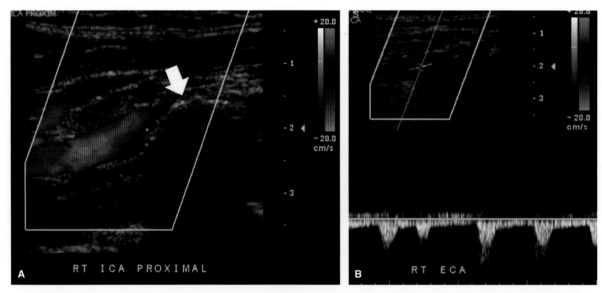

FIGURE 2–40. Reversal of ECA waveform. **(A)** Arrow points to large calcific plaque occluding the distal common carotid artery (CCA). **(B)** Spectral Doppler of the ipsilateral external carotid artery (ECA) shows reversal of flow, retrograde filling the internal carotid artery (ICA).

When a vertebral steal phenomenon exists, there will be changes to the spectral waveforms in the arteries supplying the compensating flow. When a proximal subclavian artery stenosis is present, the patient might experience subclavian steal syndrome. In this case, the ipsilateral VA flow may be paused, alternating, or fully reversed. The change is determined by the significance of the proximal stenosis and the distal resistance downstream (Fig. 2–41). With a significant lesion in the proximal subclavian artery, the spectral waveform may be paused which is a sign of early onset of subclavian steal. This waveform is often referred to as the "Bunny Sign" (Fig. 2–41A).

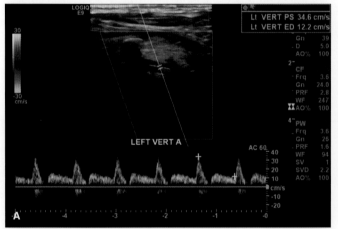

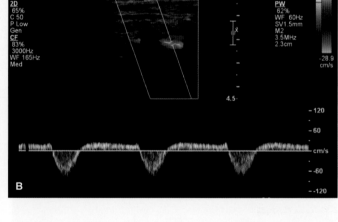

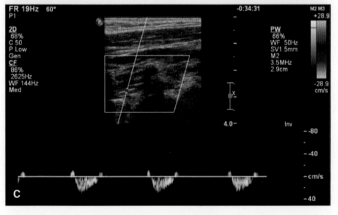

FIGURE 2–41. Abnormal pulse-wave spectral waveform within the vertebral artery during the different manifestations of subclavian steal syndrome. **(A)** Paused flow. **(B)** Alternating flow. **(C)** Complete reversal.

TABLE 2–2 • D.E. Strandness, M.D. From the University of Washington Criteria for Grading ICA Stenosis. It Is Important to Note that More Current Studies Have Shown that There Is No Reliable Way to Distinguish Between Different Percent Stenosis Below 50%			
Diameter Reduction	**Peak Systolic Velocity (PSV)**	**End-Diastolic Velocity (EDV)**	**Spectral Waveform Characteristics**
Normal	<125 cm/s	N/A	Minimal or no spectral broadening
1–15%	<125 cm/s	N/A	Spectral broadening present during deceleration phase of systole
16–49%	<125 cm/s	N/A	Spectral broadening throughout systole
50–79%	>125 cm/s	<140 cm/s	Marked spectral broadening
80–99%	>125 cm/s	>140 cm/s	Marked spectral broadening
Occluded	Absent	Absent	No flow signal in the internal carotid artery

Diagnostic Criteria

A variety of diagnostic criteria for characterizing carotid lesions into a percent stenosis have been developed over the years by comparing the results of the duplex examination to a different modality that is considered the "gold standard." Such examinations include conventional angiography, computed tomography angiography (CTA), and magnetic resonance angiography (MRA). It is important to note that there is no one criterion that is universally accepted and used in all laboratories. What is more important is that whichever criterion is chosen, it should be used consistently and validated through each laboratory's quality assurance program. It is also important to point out that the majority of the diagnostic criteria has only been validated for use in the first portion of the ICA and therefore cannot accurately be applied to other areas of the carotid system such as the CCA, ECA, or vertebral. The CCA, ECA, and vertebral use criteria similar to that of the peripheral arteries in which a doubling of the velocity is greater than a 50% stenosis. For measurement purposes, the carotid bulb is considered to be the distal CCA. For the VAs, most significant stenosis occurs at the origin where the artery originates from the subclavian artery. Other causes of elevated velocities within these arteries include compensatory flow, extrinsic compression, and vasculitis to name a few.

CCA and ECA stenosis can be inferred by the identification of plaque accompanied by a focal increase in PSV and poststenotic turbulence. One of the most widely adopted methods of its time for characterizing ICA stenosis was developed by D. E. Strandness, MD from the University of Washington (Table 2–2). These criteria are based on a standard 60-degree angle of insonation so it is important when adopting this protocol that close to a 60-degree angle be maintained throughout the examination.

In the 1990s, there were two pivotal trials that took place related to the care of patients with cerebrovascular disease and the efficacy of CEA. These two trials known as the Asymptomatic Carotid Atherosclerosis Study (ACAS) and the North America Symptomatic Carotid Endarterectomy Trial (NASCET) aided in the development of new interpretive criteria (Table 2–3). These trials looked at the benefits of endarterectomy treatment in patients who were asymptomatic (ACAS) as well as symptomatic (NASCET). The ACAS trial utilized PSV and EDV as their parameters for percent stenosis similar to Strandness criteria. The NASCET criteria implemented another parameter known as the ICA/CCA ratio. The ICA/CCA ratio is calculated by dividing the highest PSV in the ICA stenosis by the PSV in the ipsilateral mid to distal CCA. There are different standards for where the CCA velocity should be obtained for the ICA/CCA ratio calculation. It is important to note that whichever standard you use, it should be consistent, and in an area of the vessel where you can obtain a good laminar flow profile. It is also important to point out that in the presence of significant CCA disease the ICA/CCA ratio is not valid.

In 2002, a consensus panel of several different disciplines addressed the large variability with the performance and interpretation of carotid duplex examinations. The panel's goal was to develop a consensus on the criteria for the classification of ICA stenosis. Table 2–4 shows the recommended criteria from that panel. The consensus panel's recommendations are just the views and opinions of that panel and have not been validated in

TABLE 2–3 • NASCET and ACS Criteria for Grading ICA Stenosis		
Trial	**Trial Criteria**	**Diameter Reduction**
NASCET	ICA PSV/CCA PSV ratio ≥4	≥70%
ACAS	PSV ≥290 cm/s and EDV ≥80 cm/s	≥60%

TABLE 2–4 • Consensus Panel Recommended Criteria for Grading ICA Stenosis			
Diameter Reduction	Peak Systolic Velocity (PSV)	End-Diastolic Velocity (EDV)	ICA/CCA Ratio
Normal	<125 cm/s	<40 cm/s	<2.0
<50%	<125 cm/s	<40 cm/s	<2.0
50–69%	125–230 cm/s	40–100 cm/s	2.0–4.0
70–99%	>230 cm/s	>100 cm/s	>4.0
Near occlusion	High, low, or undetectable	Variable	Variable
Occluded	Absent	Absent	N/A

any one laboratory. They can however be used as a starting point and through each laboratory's quality assurance program be validated and adjusted as needed. Because of the variability from one laboratory to another, the recommendation of the panel was consistent use of broad ranges of percent stenosis for the ICA. They also suggested that PW Doppler cannot subcategorize a less than 50% stenosis and recommended that all less than 50% be reported under one category. In addition, it was recommended that the Doppler angle be maintained as close to 60 degrees as possible without exceeding that angle to reduce the variability in PSV measurements. EDV and ICA/CCA ratio was viewed as secondary parameters in the interpretation of ICA stenosis.

OTHER CEREBROVASCULAR TESTING

Cerebral Angiography

Angiography is a diagnostic procedure where a catheter is used to cannulate an artery (most commonly the common femoral or external iliac artery). The catheter is then threaded through the arterial system with the use of a guidewire to the point of interest. In the case of cerebral angiography that point of interest is typically the aortic arch. Contrast is injected at the site and fluoroscopy or cine film x-rays are used to obtain images of the vascular anatomy. Once all the images are obtained, the catheter is removed from the artery and pressure is held to the vascular access site to prevent bleeding out into the surrounding tissue. The patient is typically instructed to lie supine for 3-6 hours following the procedure to further avoid any bleeding complications. Because of its invasive nature as well as advances in other technologies such as CTA and MRA, cerebral angiography is not performed as routinely for diagnosis purposes as it once was. Instead it is usually utilized when an intervention is taking place such as a carotid artery stent or cerebral aneurysm coiling.

Normal vessels should appear to fill with contrast entirely (Fig. 2–42). If disease is present in any arteries, a "filling defect"

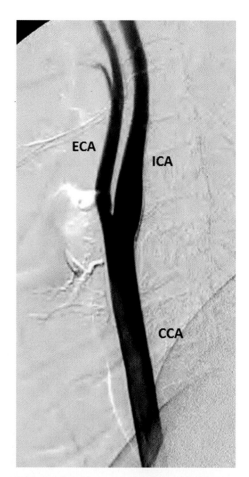

FIGURE 2–42. Normal cerebral angiogram demonstrating the common carotid, internal carotid, and external carotid arteries.

will appear where plaque has replaced the lumen (Fig. 2–43). A stenosis identified using angiography can be calculated as either percent diameter reduction or a percent area reduction. The formulas for these calculations are:

- Percent diameter reduction = $[1 - (d/D)] \times 100$
- Percent area reduction = $[1 - (d^2/D^2)] \times 100$

In these formulas, (d) is the residual lumen and (D) is the true lumen. The percent diameter reduction is obtained in the longitudinal plane, while the percent area reduction is obtained in the cross-sectional plane (Fig. 2–44). For a lesion to be considered hemodynamically significant, it must have at least a 50% diameter reduction which is equal to a 75% area reduction.

Computed Tomography and Computed Tomography Angiography

Computed tomography (CT), also known as a CT scan, uses ionizing radiation to produce cross-sectional images of structures in the body. These studies can be performed with or without the use of contrast. Neurological uses include cerebral infarct, tumors, and anatomical variants to name a few. Due to the speed of the examination, CT is the primary initial assessment for patients with a suspected stroke. CTA is virtually the same examination as a CT scan except it is always performed with IV contrast and

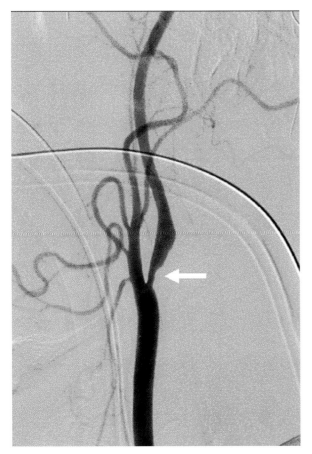

FIGURE 2–43. An abnormal cerebral angiogram demonstrating a hemodynamically significant stenosis at the origin of the internal carotid artery identified by the *white arrow*.

its focus is on the vascular structures and abnormalities. Neurological uses for CTA include extracranial and intracranial stenosis or occlusion, cerebral aneurysms, and AVMs.

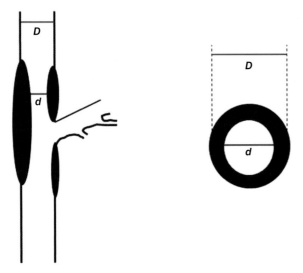

Percent diameter stenosis   **Percent area stenosis**

FIGURE 2–44. Illustration showing how the diameter measurements are obtained in order to calculate both the percent diameter and the percent areas stenosis.

Magnetic Resonance Imaging and Magnetic Resonance Angiography

Magnetic resonance imaging (MRI) uses high-frequency radio waves and a powerful magnetic field to produce images of structures in the body. Most MRI examinations can be done with and without IV contrast. Neurological uses are the same as CT, but MRI has been shown to detect evidence of a stroke earlier than CT. There have been some more recent neurological applications for MRI, such as functional MRI (fMRI) and spectroscopy. fMRI uses MRI imaging to measure brain activity by measuring changes in blood flow to different areas of the brain while the patient is asked to perform different tasks. Spectroscopy is the use of analytical software to measure the metabolic changes that occur in different disease processes in the brain. MRA is the same as MRI and like CTA focuses on the blood vessels. The neurological uses are the same as for CTA; however, CTA has proven to be more accurate in predicting the percent stenosis whereas MRA tends to overestimate disease.

TREATMENT OF CEREBROVASCULAR DISEASE

Treatment of Acute Ischemic Stroke

As mentioned earlier in this chapter, the majority (85%) of acute strokes are caused by ischemia. Acute stroke management has been and will continue to be rapidly evolving. It has been shown that for patients to have the best outcome early intervention is key. Patients presenting with acute stroke who do not have any contraindications should be treated immediately with drugs known as recombinant tissue plasminogen activators (rtPA). This treatment has been shown to be most effective within 4.5 hours of symptom onset. In additional, patients with large vessel occlusion should be considered for endovascular intervention up to 6 hours of symptom onset. One of the most notable breakthroughs in stroke management came in 2018 as a result of the DAWN trial which showed a significant benefit of endovascular thrombectomy in patient with large vessel occlusions in the anterior circulation up to 24 hours from the onset of symptoms.

Medical Therapy

Medical therapy can be in the form of controlling risk factors and/or pharmacological treatments. Oftentimes, it will include both. The following is a list of common medical therapies for cerebrovascular disease:

- Controlling hypertension—Hypertension is the number one cause of stroke. Patients who suffer with hypertension should be placed on antihypertensive medications to control their blood pressure. Classes of antihypertensives include beta blockers, angiotensin converting enzyme (ACE) inhibitors, angiotensin receptor blockers (ARBs), calcium channel blockers, diuretics, and others.

- Lifestyle modifications—Patients who use tobacco are at a higher risk for developing atherosclerosis and should be instructed to quit smoking. There are many smoking cessation classes and aides available to patients who wish to quit. Patients who are overweight should be instructed to modify their diets and follow a low-calorie, low-cholesterol diet.

- Anticoagulation therapy—Patients who suffer from atrial fibrillation are at great risk of stroke and these patients are placed on anticoagulation therapy to reduce that risk.

- Antiplatelet therapy—Patients can be placed on aspirin or another form of antiplatelet drug therapy to slow disease progression.

Carotid Endarterectomy

A CEA is the surgical removal of atherosclerotic plaque from the carotid artery, most commonly the ICA. Patients are typically evaluated and followed with duplex postoperatively to watch for restenosis. Restenosis may occur at any time following the procedure due to the progression of atherosclerosis or neointimal hyperplasia. Restenosis occurring within the first 2 years is usually a sign of neointimal hyperplasia rather than atherosclerosis. Figure 2–45 shows the surgical procedure to remove the intimal plaque.

Carotid Stenting

Carotid stenting is a less-invasive procedure than endarterectomy, in which a catheter is placed in the artery through an arterial puncture site typically located in the groin. A catheter is fed through the arterial system with a guidewire past the stenotic

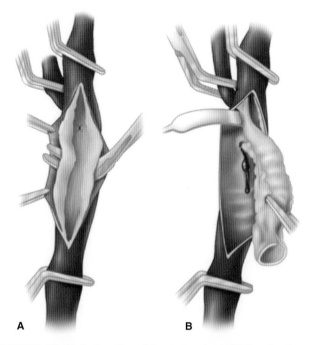

FIGURE 2–45. Illustration of carotid endarterectomy. **(A)** Opening the vessel and isolating the plaque from the carotid lumen. **(B)** Removal of the plaque. (Reproduced, with permission, from Brunicardi F, Andersen DK, Billiar TR, et al. *Schwartz's Principles of Surgery,* 11th ed. New York, NY; 2019; Figure 23-18. Copyright © McGraw Hill.)

lesion using contrast and fluoroscopy to find the area of interest. Next, a balloon is inflated to dilate the vessel and open the vessel with a technique known as angioplasty. Finally, a stent is deployed in the area to keep the narrowing open and the vessel patent (Fig. 2–46). Duplex is also used to evaluate and follow

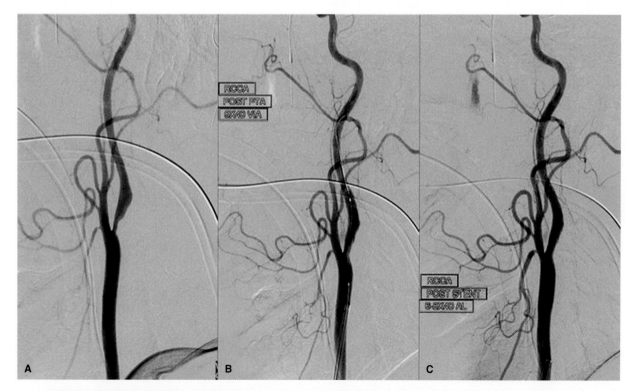

FIGURE 2–46. Cerebral angiogram demonstrating a hemodynamically significant stenosis of the internal carotid artery before and after angioplasty and stenting. **(A)** Preprocedure. **(B)** Postangioplasty. **(C)** Poststenting.

these patients postprocedure for the possibility of restenosis within or adjacent to the stent. Issues with the stent such as kinking, fracture, or deformation can be evaluated using duplex as well.

Evaluation of a carotid stent begins with grayscale imaging. Unlike a CEA, with a stent the plaque remains in situ. This results in decreased compliance of the vessel and higher velocities. Therefore, standard velocity criteria cannot be applied accurately to the poststented ICA (Fig. 2–47). There are several studies that have been completed and others are currently taking place to develop a standardized recommendation related to the proper velocity criteria to use for these patients; however, there are no concrete findings, so it is very important that the findings be validated in each laboratory. Patients with carotid artery stents usually will have a postprocedure evaluation after 1 month. At least 50% of patients will have restenosis after 18 months, so patients are usually scanned at 6-month intervals for the first 2 years followed by annual ultrasounds.

CEA Versus Stenting

For years, medical professionals were debating on which invasive procedure provided the most benefits to patients. In 2010, the CREST trial results were published which showed both procedures were associated with very similar outcomes which was carotid revascularization performed either way by highly

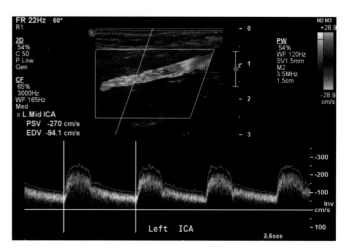

FIGURE 2–47. Pulse-wave spectral Doppler waveform demonstrating a normal elevation in peak systolic velocity within an internal carotid artery status poststent placement.

qualified physicians is effective and safe. A second trial, the CREST 2 trial, is currently underway and reaching its end. The purpose of this trial is different in that it is not comparing CEA to stenting. CREST 2 is a parallel multicentered trial to determine the best methods for preventing stroke in asymptomatic patients. This trial is comparing advanced medical treatments to stenting as well as advanced medical treatments to CEA. This trial is currently set to be completed by the end of 2020.

Questions

1. The term hemiparesis means

   (A) Paralysis on one side

   (B) Weakness on one side

   (C) Numbness on one side

   (D) Spasm of voluntary muscle on one side

2. All of the following may represent vertebrobasilar symptoms EXCEPT

   (A) Bilateral paresthesia

   (B) Vertigo

   (C) Ataxia

   (D) Amaurosis fugax

3. A stroke can be defined as

   (A) A neurological event with symptoms lasting less than 24 hours

   (B) A neurological event with symptoms lasting longer than 24 hours

   (C) A neurological event caused by increased blood flow to the brain

   (D) A neurological event occurring with no symptoms

4. Which of the following would NOT produce increased velocities within a vessel?

   (A) Narrowing of a normal stented ICA

   (B) Enlarged segment of the vessel at the level of the carotid bulb

   (C) Intraluminal 50% to 69% diameter stenosis within the ICA

   (D) Intraluminal 70% to 99% diameter stenosis within the ICA

5. All of the following may represent ICA symptoms EXCEPT

   (A) Contralateral hemiparesis

   (B) Aphasia

   (C) Amaurosis fugax

   (D) Ataxia

6. Which of the following is considered the number one controllable cause of stroke?

   (A) Hypertension

   (B) Smoking

   (C) Diabetes mellitus

   (D) Hyperlipidemia

7. The first branch of the ICA is the

   (A) Ophthalmic artery

   (B) Superior thyroidal

   (C) Supraorbital artery

   (D) ICA does not have branches

8. A TIA

   (A) Resolves within 24 hours

   (B) Does not resolve within 24 hours

   (C) Typically lasts longer than 1 hour

   (D) Resolves within 72 hours

9. The optimal Doppler angle for the extracranial cerebrovascular arteries is which of the following?

   (A) 0-degree angle to the artery walls

   (B) 60- to 80-degree angle to the artery walls

   (C) 25- to 45-degree angle to the artery walls

   (D) 45- to 60-degree angle to the artery walls

10. The first branch of the thoracic aortic arch is the

    (A) Right CCA

    (B) Left CCA

    (C) Brachiocephalic artery

    (D) Left subclavian artery

11. A normal ICA

    (A) Has a high-resistant spectral waveform

    (B) Has a low-resistant spectral waveform

    (C) Is the main source of blood supply to the posterior portions of the brain

    (D) Has a tardus parvus systolic upstroke

12. There is a significant amount of shadowing plaque overlying the proximal ICA. What is the best approach to overcome this?

    (A) Use a more posterior approach

    (B) Turn the acoustic power up

    (C) Use power Doppler instead of color Doppler

    (D) Nothing—plaque is like bone and attenuates sound

13. **A normal ECA**

    (A) Has less diastolic flow compared to the ICA

    (B) Has more diastolic flow compared to the ICA

    (C) Is the main source of blood supply to the posterior aspect of the brain

    (D) Both A and C

14. **What type of waveform would you most likely expect to see in the distal ICA with a focal 80% to 99% stenosis at the proximal ICA?**

    (A) Monophasic waveform

    (B) Tardus-parvus waveform

    (C) Normal waveform

    (D) Poststenotic turbulent waveform

15. **Which of the following describes plaque that is uniform and mostly composed of lipids?**

    (A) Homogeneous plaque

    (B) Heterogeneous plaque

    (C) Ulcerated plaque

    (D) Hemorrhagic plaque

16. **The innominate artery gives rise to which two arteries?**

    (A) Left common carotid and left subclavian arteries

    (B) Right common carotid and right subclavian arteries

    (C) Left and right CCAs

    (D) Left and right subclavian arteries

17. **Which of the following lesions is most likely to cause a subclavian steal syndrome?**

    (A) Left proximal ICA stenosis

    (B) VA occlusion

    (C) Left proximal subclavian artery stenosis

    (D) Left distal subclavian artery stenosis

18. **In the cerebrovascular system, atherosclerosis occurs most commonly in the**

    (A) Proximal area of a bifurcation

    (B) MCA

    (C) Proximal CCA

    (D) Brachiocephalic artery

19. **The most common cause of ischemic stroke is**

    (A) Occlusion of a carotid artery

    (B) Emboli

    (C) Hemorrhage

    (D) Dissection of the carotid artery

20. **A 75-year-old man is scheduled for a carotid duplex and presents with symptoms of complete loss of mobility in the left arm. In which vessel would you most likely find disease?**

    (A) Left ICA

    (B) Left CCA

    (C) Right ICA

    (D) Right VA

21. **The term paresthesia refers to**

    (A) Vertigo

    (B) Inability to speak

    (C) Loss of muscular control

    (D) Tingling sensation

22. **A patient arrives in your laboratory for a carotid duplex examination. Your findings are that the patient has a markedly dampened waveform in the right CCA with a PSV of 24 cm/s with an EDV of 14 cm/s. The left CCA had a normal waveform with a PSV of 126 cm/s with an EDV of 30 cm/s. The right VA had retrograde flow and the left VA had antegrade flow. Based on all the information, what is the most likely diagnosis?**

    (A) There is a stenosis of the left CCA

    (B) There is a stenosis of the right brachiocephalic artery

    (C) There is a stenosis of the right proximal CCA

    (D) There is a stenosis of the right proximal subclavian artery

23. **If a patient is experiencing vertigo, which vessel is most likely the cause of the symptoms?**

    (A) CCA

    (B) ICA

    (C) ECA

    (D) VA

Questions 24 through 35: Match the structures in Figure 2–48 with the names of the arteries in Column B.

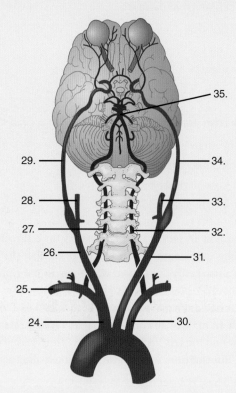

FIGURE 2–48. (Reproduced, with permission, from Doherty GM. *Current Diagnosis & Treatment: Surgery,* 15th ed. New York, NY; 2020; Figure 36-10. Copyright © McGraw Hill.)

COLUMN A	COLUMN B
24. _____	(A) Right CCA
25. _____	(B) Innominate artery
26. _____	(C) Left VA
27. _____	(D) Left subclavian artery
28. _____	(E) Right ECA
29. _____	(F) Left CCA
30. _____	(G) Left ICA
31. _____	(H) Right VA
32. _____	(I) Right subclavian artery
33. _____	(J) Left ECA
34. _____	(K) Basilar artery
35. _____	(L) Right ICA

36. A typical waveform in a CCA with an ipsilateral ICA occlusion may have

(A) Increased PSV

(B) Decreased or no diastolic flow

(C) Increased diastolic velocity

(D) A low-resistance waveform

Questions 37 through 39: Match the waveforms in Figure 2–49 with the names of the correct extracranial arteries.

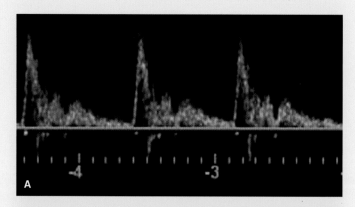

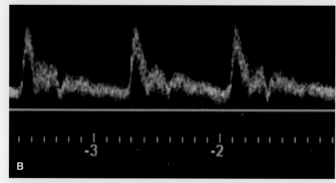

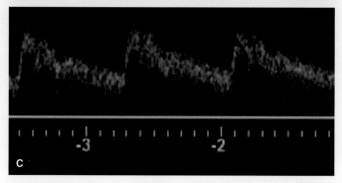

FIGURE 2–49.

37. ICA _____

38. CCA _____

39. ECA _____

40. A patient undergoes CEA. Within the first year following the surgery a carotid duplex is performed because of symptoms on the contralateral side. The follow-up carotid duplex shows that the operated ICA is significantly narrowed. The most likely cause is

    (A) Atherosclerotic plaque recurrence
    (B) Carotid dissection
    (C) Embolism
    (D) Neointimal hyperplasia

41. A normal VA should have what type of flow?

    (A) Caudal
    (B) Tardus parvus
    (C) Low resistant
    (D) Pulsus bisferiens

42. The VA in Figure 2–50 has what type of flow?

    (A) Retrograde
    (B) Antegrade
    (C) Alternating
    (D) Hesitating

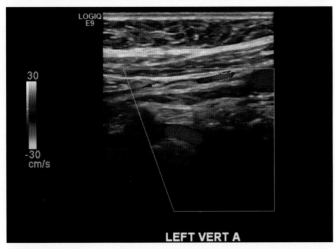

FIGURE 2–50.

43. The plaque seen in Figure 2–51 can be characterized as which of the following?

    (A) Heterogeneous
    (B) Homogeneous
    (C) Smooth
    (D) Lipid

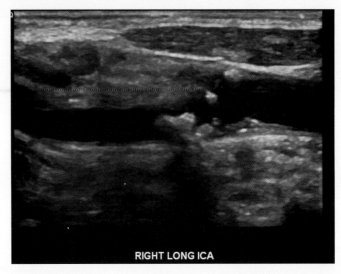

FIGURE 2–51.

44. The waveform in Figure 2–52 was obtained from the right CCA. Based just on this waveform, what might it suggest?

    (A) There is a possibility of a proximal CCA obstruction
    (B) There is a possibility of a distal ACA obstruction
    (C) There is a possibility of a brachial artery obstruction
    (D) There is an ICA occlusion

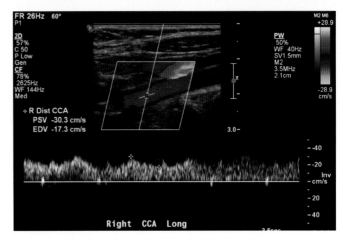

FIGURE 2–52.

45. The waveform in Figure 2–53 was obtained from a patient's right VA. Based just on this finding, what might this suggest?

    (A) Distal subclavian artery stenosis

    (B) Proximal subclavian artery stenosis

    (C) Proximal CCA stenosis

    (D) Basilar artery occlusion

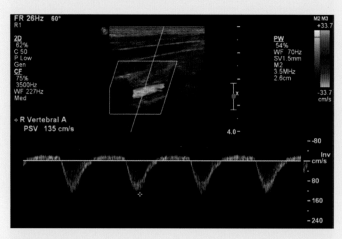

FIGURE 2–53.

46. With laminar flow, the velocity of blood is _____ in the center of the vessel and _____ at the vessel wall.

    (A) highest; lowest

    (B) lowest; highest

    (C) highest; reversed

    (D) lowest; indeterminate

47. The first branch of the ECA is which of the following?

    (A) Facial artery

    (B) Superior thyroid artery

    (C) Ascending pharyngeal artery

    (D) Superficial temporal artery

48. Which artery originated directly from the thoracic aortic arch?

    (A) Right CCA

    (B) Right subclavian artery

    (C) Left CCA

    (D) Left VA

49. Causes of turbulent flow, other than stenosis, in the carotid arteries include all of the following EXCEPT

    (A) Tortuous ICA

    (B) Laminar flow

    (C) Kinking of the ICA

    (D) Dilatation at region of bifurcation

50. A patient having a carotid duplex examination has the following velocities obtained. What is your diagnosis?

CCA PSV = 60 cm/s
EDV = 24 cm/s
ICA PSV = 300 cm/s
EDV = 100 cm/s

    (A) Normal

    (B) Less than 50% stenosis

    (C) 50% to 69% stenosis

    (D) Greater than 70% stenosis

51. A nonlocalized symptom resulting in complete loss of consciousness is known as

    (A) Syncope

    (B) Dizziness

    (C) Vertigo

    (D) Ataxia

52. The waveform in Figure 2–54 was obtained from the right CCA. This type of waveform suggests

    (A) Occlusion of the right ICA

    (B) Normal flow through the CCA

    (C) Occlusion of the proximal CCA

    (D) Occlusion of the ECA

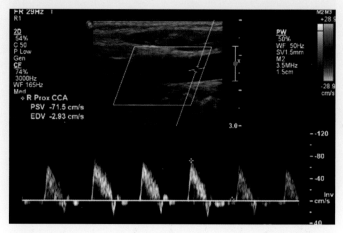

FIGURE 2–54.

Questions 53 through 55: Match the following color Doppler image with the names of the correct extracranial arteries in Figure 2–55.

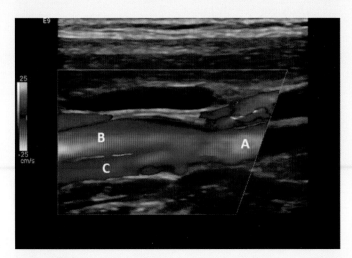

FIGURE 2–55.

53. ICA _____

54. CCA _____

55. ECA _____

56. The waveform in Figure 2–56

(A) Has poststenotic waveform characteristics

(B) Has a laminar flow pattern

(C) Was obtained just proximal to a stenosis

(D) Has no spectral broadening

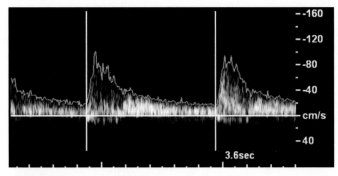

FIGURE 2–56.

57. An 80-year-old man arrives in the emergency department with a sudden onset of left hemiparalysis. Based on the pulse-wave sampling of the right ICA in Figure 2–57, what are your findings?

(A) More than 50% diameter stenosis of the right ICA

(B) 50% to 69% diameter stenosis of the right ICA

(C) More than 70% diameter stenosis of the right ICA

(D) Normal right ICA

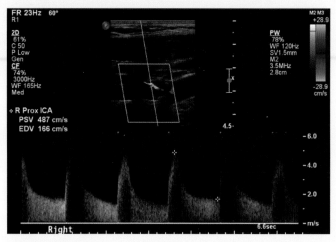

FIGURE 2–57.

58. What was the pivotal trial that took place related to the care of patients with symptomatic cerebrovascular disease and looked at the benefits of CEA treatment?

(A) ACAS

(B) NASCET

(C) Strandness Symptomatic Endarterectomy Trial

(D) North America Asymptomatic Carotid Endarterectomy Trial

59. Which of the following is a classic finding associated with subclavian steal syndrome?

(A) Retrograde flow in the contralateral VA

(B) Decreased flow in the contralateral VA

(C) Increased bilateral brachial arterial pressures

(D) 15 to 20 mm Hg decrease in pressure of the ipsilateral arm

60. A carotid stenosis identified by angiography can be calculated as either percent diameter reduction or a percent area reduction. A percent area reduction of 75% is symmetrical to what percent diameter reduction?

    (A) 25%

    (B) 75%

    (C) 50%

    (D) 90%

61. What is the most reliable method to differentiate between the ICA and the ECA with carotid duplex?

    (A) ICA is typically larger than the ECA

    (B) ICA is typically more lateral to the ECA

    (C) ECA has extracranial branches

    (D) ICA will not have oscillations with temporal tap maneuver

62. What is the pathology identified in the cervical angiographic image in Figure 2–58?

    (A) AVM

    (B) Hemodynamically significant stenosis of the ICA

    (C) FMD

    (D) Carotid aneurysm

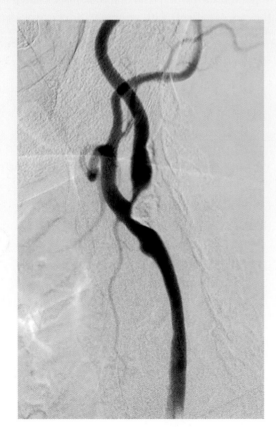

FIGURE 2–58.

63. What is the pathology identified in the carotid duplex image in Figure 2–59?

    (A) Hemodynamically significant stenosis of the ICA

    (B) Carotid body tumor

    (C) Total occlusion of the ICA

    (D) Carotid dissection

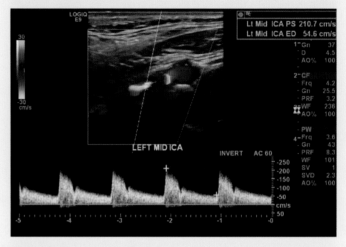

FIGURE 2–59.

64. The following color Doppler image was obtained on a 60-year-old man who underwent a right CEA 1 year ago. What would be your impression based just on the information obtained from the image in Figure 2–60?

    (A) Restenosis due to the progression of atherosclerosis

    (B) Restenosis due to neointimal hyperplasia

    (C) Normal ICA status post endarterectomy

    (D) Dissection of the ICA status post endarterectomy

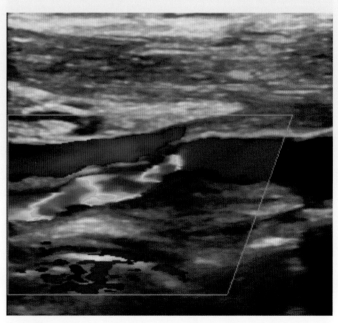

FIGURE 2–60.

65. What pathology is inferred by the carotid duplex image in Figure 2–61?

(A) Hemodynamically significant stenosis of the ICA

(B) AVM

(C) Findings consistent with a normal ICA

(D) Total occlusion of the ICA

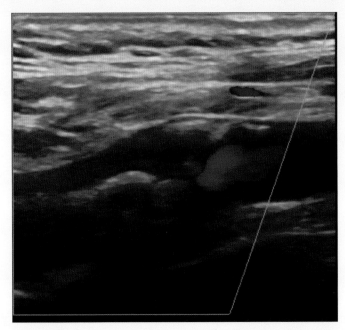

FIGURE 2–61.

66. The pressure gradient across a stenotic segment as it increases from a 50% narrowing to a 90% narrowing

(A) Decreases

(B) Does not change

(C) Is unaffected

(D) Increases

67. A rare event where a venous clot passes through a patent septal defect in heart and embolizes to the brain causing a stroke is known as

(A) Arteriovenous fistula

(B) Subarachnoid hemorrhage

(C) Paradoxical embolism

(D) FMD

68. A neurological symptom that is described as "a shade lowering down over the eye" often caused by emboli through the ophthalmic artery from the ipsilateral ICA is known as

(A) Hemiparalysis

(B) Hemianopia

(C) Diplopia

(D) Amaurosis fugax

Questions 69 through 71: Match the layer of the vessel wall with the correct description.

69. Tunica media _____

70. Tunica intima _____

71. Tunica adventitia _____

(A) Thin innermost layer

(B) Outermost layer containing the vasa vasorum

(C) Thicker middle muscular layer

72. What percentage of blood flow from the CCA is received by the ICA?

(A) 20% to 30%

(B) 50% to 60%

(C) 70% to 80%

(D) 10% to 15%

73. The arteries that originate from the proximal portions of the subclavian arteries and course along the posterior aspect of both sides of the neck through the foramen of the transverse processes of the cervical spine are known as the

(A) VAs

(B) Cervical arteries

(C) ECAs

(D) Posterior cerebral arteries

74. This waveform is from a right CCA in a patient with severe CHF. What does the waveform indicate (Fig. 2–62)?

(A) The patient has a severe proximal stenosis

(B) The patient has a severe distal stenosis

(C) The patient has aortic regurgitation

(D) The patient is on an intraaortic balloon pump

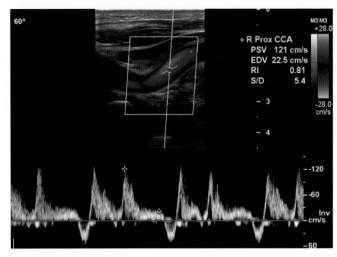

FIGURE 2–62.

75. **A normal spectral Doppler waveform of a CCA should include all of the following characteristics EXCEPT**

    (A) Clear spectral window
    (B) Laminar flow pattern
    (C) Little to no diastolic flow
    (D) Rapid rise to peak systolic

76. **A 57-year-old man was sent to your laboratory with symptoms of difficulty swallowing. What would be your findings based on the information obtained from the transverse image in Figure 2–63?**

    (A) FMD
    (B) Carotid artery aneurysm
    (C) Carotid body tumor
    (D) Carotid artery pseudoaneurysm

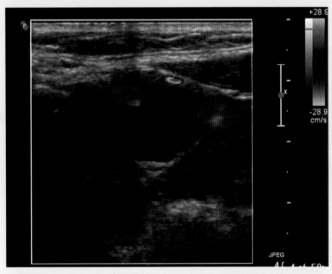

FIGURE 2–63.

77. **A 28-year-old woman was in a motor vehicle accident and taken to the emergency department by ambulance. She presents to your laboratory for a carotid duplex with symptoms of aphasia. What would be your findings based on the information obtained from the image in Figure 2–64?**

    (A) FMD
    (B) Intraplaque hemorrhage
    (C) Carotid dissection
    (D) Intimal hyperplasia

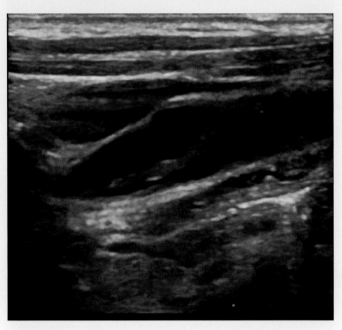

FIGURE 2–64.

78. **The color Doppler image in Figure 2–65 represents**

    (A) Abnormally turbulent blood flow within the carotid bulb
    (B) Normal flow pattern for the carotid bulb
    (C) Abnormal flow reversal in carotid bulb
    (D) Stenosis in carotid bulb

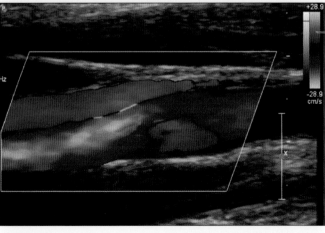

FIGURE 2–65.

79. The easiest way to determine ECA from ICA in the color Doppler image in Figure 2–66 is

    (A) Size
    (B) Location
    (C) Pulsatility
    (D) Branches

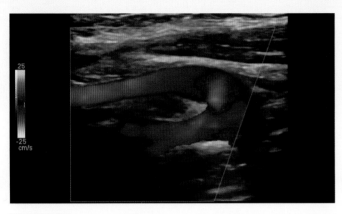

FIGURE 2–66.

80. A noise that is produced by the vibrations of the surrounding tissues as the result of turbulence in the artery that is commonly heard with a hemodynamically significant stenosis is known as

    (A) An oscillation
    (B) A bruit
    (C) Aliasing
    (D) A thrill

81. All of the following are considered lateralizing symptoms EXCEPT

    (A) Dysphasia
    (B) Hemiparalysis
    (C) Vertigo
    (D) Amaurosis fugax

82. According to SRU consensus criteria, which of the following corresponds to a 50% to 69% stenosis?

    (A) PSV < 125 cm/s, EDV < 40 cm/s
    (B) PSV 125-230 cm/s, EDV 40-100 cm/s
    (C) PSV > 230 cm/s, EDV > 100 cm/s
    (D) PSV absent, EDV absent

83. The type of flow pattern that exists in most of the normal carotid arteries is

    (A) Turbulent
    (B) Laminar
    (C) Plug
    (D) Helical

84. Aliasing with color Doppler in a normal vessel is least likely to occur in the carotid arteries with which of the following attributes?

    (A) Tortuous vessels
    (B) A hemodynamically significant stenosis
    (C) Low PRF settings
    (D) High PRF settings

85. The VAs join to form which vessel intracranially?

    (A) Posterior cerebral artery
    (B) Carotid siphon
    (C) Basilar artery
    (D) Posterior communicating artery

86. A patient underwent a CT angiogram of the carotid arteries that showed a greater than 70% right ICA stenosis. A comparative duplex was performed which agreed with the CTA findings. Which of the following diagnostic parameter measurements were most likely obtained from the duplex study?

    (A) PSV 125 cm/s, EDV 40 cm/s, ICA/CCA ratio 2.0
    (B) PSV 229 cm/s, EDV 82 cm/s, ICA/CCA ratio 3.0
    (C) PSV 317 cm/s, EDV 142 cm/s, ICA/CCA ratio 4.2
    (D) PSV 193 cm/s, EDV 74 cm/s, ICA/CCA ratio 3.5

87. During a routine carotid duplex examination with an indication of carotid bruit, there is an incidental finding of subclavian steal syndrome on the left side. What symptoms will this patient most likely be experiencing?

    (A) Dizziness
    (B) Left hemiparalysis
    (C) Vertigo
    (D) The patient will most likely be asymptomatic

88. **The flow within a normal ICA will have which of the following characteristics?**

    (A) Flow consistent with a low-resistant vascular bed

    (B) Multiphasic flow pattern

    (C) Low to no diastolic flow

    (D) Turbulent flow

89. **A 50-year-old woman with a history of atrial fibrillation and hypertension was experiencing symptoms consistent with a TIA. Based on the duplex findings in Figure 2–67, what is most likely the cause of her symptoms?**

    (A) The duplex demonstrates a hemodynamically significant stenosis

    (B) The duplex demonstrates normal flow suggesting another cause such as a thromboembolic event

    (C) The duplex scan demonstrates reduced diastolic flow suggesting distal disease

    (D) The duplex demonstrates a delayed acceleration time suggesting proximal disease

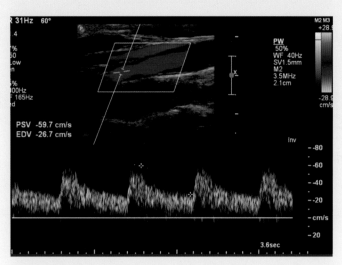

FIGURE 2–67.

90. **A patient with impaired speech has**

    (A) Dysphagia

    (B) Hemiplegia

    (C) Dysphasia

    (D) Hemianopia

91. **All of the following are branches of the ECA EXCEPT**

    (A) Basilar artery

    (B) Superior thyroid artery

    (C) Ascending pharyngeal artery

    (D) Occipital artery

92. **What is the nonatherosclerotic disease process affecting the median layer of arteries that is caused by the abnormal cellular development and is often diagnosed with angiography due to its classic appearance as a string of beads?**

    (A) Neointimal hyperplasia

    (B) Myointimal hyperplasia

    (C) Vasospasm

    (D) FMD

93. **All of the following conditions increase your risk of stroke EXCEPT**

    (A) Hypotension

    (B) Hyperlipidemia

    (C) Obesity

    (D) Diabetes

94. **A patient comes to your lab after having a severe lateralizing CVA. The right proximal ICA has a sharp systolic upstroke and no diastolic flow. Which of the following is most likely?**

    (A) Patient has a severe brachiocephalic artery stenosis

    (B) Patient has subclavian steal syndrome

    (C) Patient has low blood pressure

    (D) Patient has a distal occlusion

95. **Which of the following is generally not a part of a carotid protocol?**

    (A) Transverse 2D grayscale images

    (B) Longitudinal 2D grayscale images

    (C) Diameter measurements of stenotic areas

    (D) Spectral and color Doppler of CCA, ICA, ECA, and vertebrals

Questions 96 through 99: Match the following plaque characteristics with the correct images in Figure 2–68.

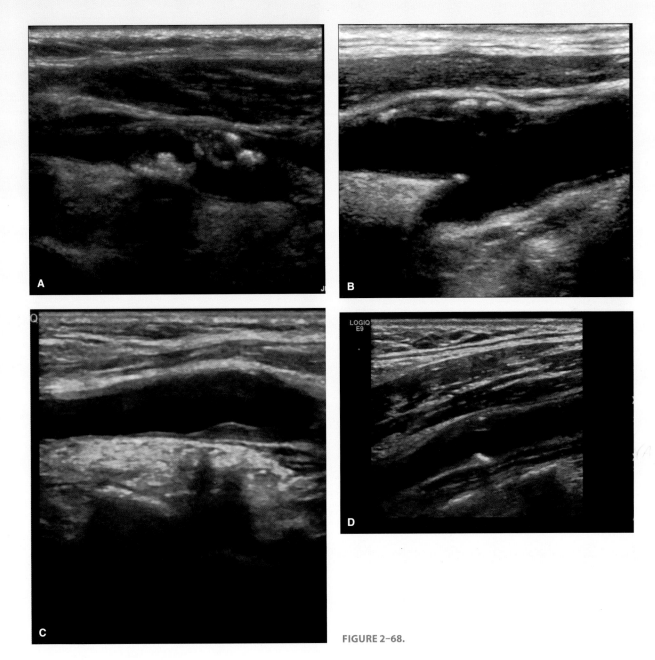

FIGURE 2–68.

96. Heterogeneous and smooth surface _____

97. High suspicion of ulceration _____

98. Homogeneous and smooth surface _____

99. Heterogeneous and irregular surface _____

100. **All of the following are true regarding the color Doppler image in Figure 2–69 EXCEPT**

    (A) Aliasing is present

    (B) It represents turbulent blood flow

    (C) This aliasing is most likely due to a narrowing of the blood vessel

    (D) This aliasing is most likely due to tortuosity

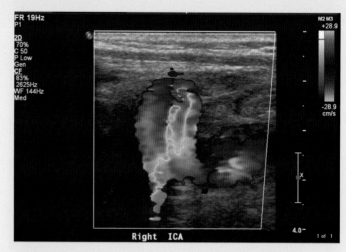

FIGURE 2–69.

Answers and Explanations

1. **(B)** Hemiparesis is a neurological symptom that refers to unilateral weakness that occurs on the contralateral side of the body to the affected side of the brain.

2. **(D)** Bilateral paresthesia, vertigo, and ataxia are all symptoms that affect the body as a whole and therefore are related to the posterior circulation. Amaurosis fugax is a lateralizing symptom that is most commonly caused by emboli to the ophthalmic artery through the ipsilateral ICA.

3. **(B)** A CVA, or stroke, is defined as a neurological event lasting longer than 24 hours. By comparison, a TIA is a resolving deficit that lasts less than 24 hours.

4. **(B)** Any stenosis within a vessel will cause an increase in velocity. The normal narrowing that occurs when a stent is placed in a vessel will also cause an increase in velocity. The natural enlargement of a vessel at the area of the carotid bulb will create a helical-type flow pattern that does not have increased velocities.

5. **(D)** Ataxia is a neurological symptom that is defined as an unsteady gait and is associated with the posterior circulation.

6. **(A)** According to the ASA, hypertension is the number one controllable risk factor for stroke.

7. **(A)** The first branch of the ICA occurs intracranially and is the ophthalmic artery.

8. **(A)** The symptoms of a TIA resolve within 24 hours. Typically, they resolve within 30 minutes to an hour.

9. **(D)** The optimal Doppler angle for the extracranial carotid arteries is between 45 and 60 degrees allowing the angle to be parallel to the vessel walls.

10. **(C)** The first branch arising from the aortic arch is the brachiocephalic artery. The brachiocephalic artery then bifurcates into the right subclavian and right CCAs.

11. **(B)** The ICA should have a low-resistant monophasic spectral waveform with flow throughout the cardiac cycle. It is also the main source of blood supply to the middle and anterior portions of the brain.

12. **(A)** A more posterior approach may help if the plaque is mostly located on the anterior surface of the vessel. Turning up the power and using power (amplitude) Doppler will not help because plaque is very attenuating. Changing windows is the best approach.

13. **(A)** The ECA should have less diastolic flow when compared to the ICA and does not provide blood flow to the brain under normal circumstances.

14. **(B)** The type of waveform commonly seen distal to a critical (80% to 99%) stenosis will have delayed rise to peak systolic and low velocities. This type of waveform is referred to as a tardus-parvus waveform.

15. **(A)** Homogeneous plaque refers to plaque with uniform low-level echogenicity and is mostly composed of lipids.

16. **(B)** The innominate artery originates from the thoracic aortic arch and then bifurcates into the right subclavian and CCAs.

17. **(C)** Both an innominate artery and proximal left subclavian artery stenosis are likely to cause a subclavian steal syndrome because they would be proximal to the origin of the VAs. A stenosis in the distal left subclavian artery would be past the origin of the VA, thus not resulting in a steal.

18. **(A)** Atherosclerosis in the cerebrovascular system occurs most commonly at the area of the bifurcation and the first few centimeters of the ICA.

19. **(B)** Most ischemic strokes are caused by emboli that travel from another location in the body through the blood stream to one of the cerebral arteries resulting in occlusion.

20. **(C)** Complete loss of mobility on one side of the body is a lateralizing symptom that is associated with ICA disease and since the left side of the body is controlled by the right cerebral hemisphere the vessel that would most likely have disease would be the right ICA.

21. **(D)** Paresthesia is described as numbness, tingling, or loss of feeling.

22. **(B)** The brachiocephalic artery gives rise to the right subclavian and right CCAs. A stenosis of the brachiocephalic artery would affect the flow of both the right subclavian artery as well as the right CCA. The reduced flow through to the right subclavian is what would cause the reversal of flow in the ipsilateral vertebral.

23. **(D)** Vertigo is a nonlateralizing symptom and is usually associated with vertebrobasilar disease.

24. **(B)** Innominate artery

25. **(I)** Right subclavian artery

26. **(A)** Right CCA

27. **(H)** Right vertebral

28. **(E)** Right ECA

29. **(L)** Right ICA

30. **(D)** Left subclavian artery

31. **(F)** Left CCA

32. **(C)** Left VA

33. **(J)** Left ECA

34. **(G)** Left ICA

35. **(K)** Basilar artery

36. **(B)** Normally the CCA has a moderate amount of diastolic flow because it is providing blood flow to both the ICA and the ECA. When a distal occlusion occurs, the resistance to flow may increase resulting in a decrease of diastolic flow on the same side as the occlusion. It is common to see little to no diastolic flow in a CCA with an ipsilateral ICA occlusion.

37. **(C)** ICA

38. **(B)** CCA

39. **(A)** ECA

40. **(D)** When restenosis occurs within the first 2 years following a CEA, it is most commonly the result of neointimal hyperplasia not atherosclerosis.

41. **(D)** The VAs should normally have low-resistant flow toward the head (cephalic) since they provide the posterior portion of the brain with blood.

42. **(B)** The VA in Figure 2–50 has antegrade flow going toward the transducer toward the head.

43. **(E)** The plaque in Figure 2–51 is heterogeneous because it has mixed echogenicity and its surface is irregular.

44. **(A)** The waveform in Figure 2–52 shows a delayed rise to peak systolic suggesting more proximal disease. In this case, proximal disease could be either proximal CCA or distal innominate artery.

45. **(B)** The waveform in Figure 2–53 represents alternating flow in the right VA, which suggests the presence of a latent subclavian steal syndrome caused by a proximal right subclavian artery stenosis.

46. **(A)** Laminar flow has a parabolic velocity profile with the highest velocities in the center of the vessel and the lowest velocities at the vessel walls.

47. **(B)** The ECA has eight extracranial branches, the first being the superior thyroid artery.

48. **(C)** The three main branches of the thoracic aortic arch are the brachiocephalic, left common carotid, and left subclavian arteries.

49. **(B)** Areas of dilatation, kinking, or tortuosity can all cause turbulent blood flow in a normal vessel. Laminar flow is smooth flow with a parabolic velocity profile.

50. **(D)** A PSV of 300 cm/s with an end-diastolic velocity of 100 cm/s is consistent with a greater than 70% stenosis by most criteria.

51. **(A)** Syncope is a nonlocalized symptom that results in complete loss of consciousness.

52. **(A)** The spectral waveform in Figure 2–54 of the right CCA represents a high-resistant signal with no diastolic flow. This type of waveform suggests distal disease. It is most likely an ipsilateral ICA occlusion because of the loss of diastolic flow normally present in the CCA.

53. **(B)** ICA

54. **(A)** CCA

55. **(C)** ECA

56. **(A)** The waveform demonstrated in Figure 2–56 is a classic poststenotic turbulent waveform that is commonly found just distal to a stenosis. It is characterized by a spiky waveform and spectral broadening.

57. **(C)** A PSV of 487 cm/s and an end-diastolic velocity of 166 cm/s are consistent with a greater than 70% stenosis.

58. **(B)** The North American Symptomatic Carotid Endarterectomy Trial (NASET) was the pivotal trial that took place related to the care of patients with symptomatic cerebrovascular disease and looked at the benefits of CEA treatment.

59. **(D)** Retrograde flow in the ipsilateral VA, increased flow in the contralateral vertebral, and a decrease in pressure in the ipsilateral arm are all findings consistent with a subclavian steal syndrome.

60. **(C)** A 75% area reduction is equivalent to a 50% diameter reduction. The formula used to calculate percent diameter reduction is $[1 - (d/D)] \times 100$ whereas the formula for percent area reduction is $[1 - (d^2/D^2)] \times 100$.

61. **(C)** Although size, location, and waveform are tools in determining the ICA versus ECA, the presence of extracranial branches is the strongest indicator of the ECA. It is very uncommon for the ICA to have extracranial branches.

62. **(B)** The cerebral angiogram image in Figure 2–58 shows a significant filling defect at the origin of the ICA consistent with a hemodynamically significant stenosis.

63. **(A)** A PSV of 210 cm/s is consistent with a hemodynamically significant ICA stenosis.

64. **(B)** The image in Figure 2–60 is consistent with a hemodynamically significant stenosis. Restenosis that occurs within the first 2 years following a CEA is usually the result of neointimal hyperplasia not atherosclerosis.

65. **(D)** The image in Figure 2–61 shows the absence of color Doppler within the ICA which suggests the presence of a total occlusion. It is important to note that the absence of color Doppler can only suggest the presence of a total occlusion. Pulse wave spectral Doppler set to maximum sensitivity is more conclusive, although the patient would still need a CTA or conventional angiogram to prove occlusion versus near-occlusion.

66. **(D)** A pressure gradient refers to the difference between two pressures, in this case, the pressure proximal and distal to the stenosis. As a stenosis increases from a 50% narrowing to a 90% narrowing, the distal pressure will decrease even more resulting in an increased difference between pressures.

67. **(C)** A paradoxical embolism is a rare condition where a clot from the venous system embolizes through a septal wall defect in the heart to the cerebral arteries causing a stroke.

68. **(D)** Amaurosis fugax is a temporary partial or complete blindness, typically in one eye. This symptom is often described as "a shade lowering down over the eye." The source of this symptom is often emboli through the ophthalmic artery from the ipsilateral ICA.

69. **(C)** Tunica media

70. **(A)** Tunica intima

71. **(B)** Tunica adventitia

72. **(C)** Approximately 70% to 80% of the blood from the CCA is received by the ICA.

73. **(A)** The VAs originate from the proximal portions of the right and left subclavian arteries and course along the posterior aspect of both sides of the neck through the foramen of the transverse processes of the cervical spine and eventually join together intracranially to form the basilar artery.

74. **(D)** This carotid waveform is indicative of a patient on an intraaortic balloon pump. The double systole from balloon inflation followed by reversal of flow from balloon deflation is typical for the waveform.

75. **(C)** The CCA is responsible for providing blood flow to both the ECA and the ICA. The ICA is responsible for providing blood flow to the anterior and middle portions of the brain and requires flow throughout the cardiac cycle; therefore, the CCA should normally have a moderate amount of diastolic flow. Absent or reduced diastolic flow within the CCA may suggest more distal disease.

76. **(C)** The image in Figure 2–63 shows a vascular mass at the area of the carotid bifurcation which is consistent with a diagnosis of a carotid body tumor. Carotid body tumors can be asymptomatic; however, they have been associated with difficulty swallowing when they become large.

77. **(C)** The findings in Figure 2–64 of a linear echogenic structure within the lumen of the artery with a history of trauma are consistent with a carotid dissection.

78. **(B)** The color flow image in Figure 2–65 represents the normal helical flow pattern from flow separation that commonly occurs within the carotid bulb.

79. **(D)** The ECA branches identified with color Doppler is an easy way to distinguish it from the ICA.

80. **(B)** A bruit is a noise that is produced by the vibrations of the surrounding tissues as the result of turbulent flow in the artery that is commonly heard with a hemodynamically significant stenosis.

81. **(C)** Vertigo is a nonlateralizing symptom related to the vertebrobasilar system.

82. **(B)** A 50% to 69% stenosis according to the published SRU consensus criteria is PSV 125-230 cm/s and EDV 40-100 cm/s.

83. **(B)** Laminar flow is the flow pattern that exists most commonly in the normal carotid vessels.

84. **(D)** High PRF settings will not cause aliasing in a normal vessel; however, they may cause the vessel to not completely fill with color. Tortuous vessels, stenosis, and low PRF settings all have the potential to cause aliasing.

85. **(C)** The right and left VAs join intracranially to form the basilar artery, which eventually bifurcates into the P_1 segments of the right and left posterior cerebral arteries.

86. **(C)** A PSV of 317 cm/s with an end-diastolic velocity of 142 cm/s and an ICA/CCA ratio of 4.2 is consistent with a greater than 70% ICA stenosis and would correlate with the CTA.

87. **(D)** The majority of patients with subclavian steal syndrome are asymptomatic.

88. **(A)** The normal flow within the ICA will have low-resistant monophasic flow throughout the cardiac cycle.

89. **(B)** The findings shown in Figure 2–67 are consistent with normal flow velocities for an ICA suggesting that the symptoms are related to an alternate cause.

90. **(C)** Dysphasia is difficulty speaking or impaired speech. Dysphagia is difficulty swallowing, hemiplegia is paralysis on one side of the body, and hemianopia is blindness in one half of the visual field.

91. **(A)** The basilar is not a branch of the ECA.

92. **(D)** FMD is a nonatherosclerotic disease that affects the mid to distal segments of a vessel and is commonly referred to as a string of beads because of its appearance.

93. **(A)** All of the items except for hypotension, or low blood pressure, increase a patient's risk of stroke.

94. **(D)** Absent diastolic flow is indicative of a distal obstruction. The ICA should always have diastolic flow, and its absence signifies distal obstruction or even brain edema or brain death.

95. **(C)** A typical carotid protocol includes grayscale, spectral, and color Doppler of the CCA, ICA, ECA, and vertebrals. Measurement of a stenosis with calipers is generally not performed as the stenosis criteria are based on velocity measurements.

96. **(D)** The plaque in Figure 2–68D is consistent with heterogeneous plaque with mixed echogenicity and a smooth surface.

97. **(B)** The plaque in Figure 2–68B is consistent with a very irregular surface which is highly suspicious for ulceration.

98. **(C)** The plaque in Figure 2–68C is consistent with homogeneous plaque with uniform low level echogenicity and a smooth surface.

99. **(A)** The plaque in Figure 2–68A is consistent with heterogeneous plaque with mixed echogenicity and an irregular surface.

100. **(C)** Aliasing is present in the color Doppler image in Figure 2–69 and is the result of turbulent blood flow caused by a tortuous vessel and not the result of a narrowing.

Suggested Readings

1. Pellerito JS, Polak JF. *Introduction to Vascular Ultrasound*. 7th ed. Philadelphia, PA: Elsevier; 2020.

2. Kupinski AM. *Diagnostic Medical Sonography: The Vascular System*. 2nd ed. Baltimore, MD: Wolters Kluwer; 2018.

3. Grant EG, Benson CB, Moneta GL, et al. Carotid artery stenosis: Gray-scale and Doppler ultrasound diagnosis – Society of Radiologist in Ultrasound Consensus Conference. *Radiology*. 2003;229:340–346.

4. Rumwell C, McPharlin M. *Vascular Technology: An Illustrated Review*. 5th ed. Pasadena, CA: Davies Publishing; 2017.

5. North American Symptomatic Carotid Endarterectomy Trial Collaborators. Beneficial effect of carotid endarterectomy in symptomatic patients with high-grade carotid stenosis. *N Engl J Med*. 1991;325:445–453.

6. Executive Committee for the Asymptomatic Carotid Atherosclerosis Study. Endarterectomy for asymptomatic carotid stenosis. *JAMA*. 1995;273:1421–1428.

7. Moneta GL, Edwards JM, Chitwood RW, et al. Correlation of North American Symptomatic Carotid Endarterectomy Trial (NASCET) angiographic definition of 70% to 99% internal carotid artery stenosis with duplex scanning. *J Vasc Surg*. 1993;17:152–159.

8. Zierler E. *Strandness's Duplex Scanning in Vascular Disorders*. 5th ed. Philadelphia, PA: Wolters Kluwer; 2015.

9. Braum RM, Bertino RE, Milbrandt J, et al. Ultrasound imaging of carotid artery stenosis: Application of the society of radiologist in ultrasound consensus criteria to a single institution clinical practice. *Ultrasound Q*. 2008;24:161–166.

10. Bluth E. Plaque morphology as a risk factor for stroke. *JAMA*. 2000;284:177.

11. El-Barghouty N, Nicolaides A, Bahal V, et al. The identification of high risk carotid plaque. *Eur J Vasc Endovasc Surg*. 1996;11:470–478.

12. Reiter M, Effenberger I, Sabeti S, et al. Increasing carotid plaque echolucency is predictive of cardiovascular events in high-risk patients. *Radiology*. 2008;248:1050–1055.

13. Grogan JK, Shaalan WE, Cheng H, et al. B-mode ultrasonographic characterization of carotid atherosclerosis plaques in symptomatic and asymptomatic patients. *J Vasc Surg*. 2005;42(3):435–441.

14. Hobson RW 2nd, Mackey WC, Ascher E, et al. Management of atherosclerotic carotid artery disease: Clinical practice guidelines of the Society for Vascular Surgery. *J Vasc Surg*. 2008;48(2):480–486.

15. Wood MM, Romine LE, Lee YK, et al. Spectral Doppler signature waveforms in ultrasonography: A review of normal and abnormal waveforms. *Ultrasound Q*. 2010;26(2):83–99.

16. Sullivan TM. Surveillance and follow-up after carotid angioplasty and stenting. In: Mansour MA, Labropoulos N, eds. *Vascular Diagnosis*. Philadelphia, PA: Elsevier Saunders; 2005:183–191.

17. Stroke Risk Factors. (n.d.). Available online at http://www.stroke-association.org. Accessed on September 15, 2014.

18. Lee DH, Gao FQ, Rankin RN, et al. Duplex and color Doppler flow sonography of occlusion and near occlusion of the carotid artery. *AJNR Am J Neuroradiol*. 1996;17:1267–1274.

19. Conrad MF, Michalczyk MJ, Opalacz A, et al. The natural history of asymptomatic severe carotid artery stenosis. *J Vasc Surg*. 2013;27(5):27S.

20. Kallmayer M, Tsantilas P, Zieger C, et al. Ultrasound surveillance after CAS and CEA: What's the evidence? *J Cardiovasc Surg (Torino)*. 2014;55(2 Suppl 1):33–41.

21. Salem MK, Bown MJ, Sayers RD, et al. Identification of patients with a histologically unstable carotid plaque using ultrasonic plaque image analysis. *Eur J Vasc Endovasc Surg*. 2014;48(2):118–125.

22. Intersocietal Accreditation Commission. IAC standards and guidelines. 2019. Available online at https://www.intersocietal.org/vascular/standards/IACVascularTestingStandards2019.pdf. Accessed on August 20, 2019.

23. Khoury MH, Gornik HL. Fibromuscular dysplasia (FMD). *Vasc. Med*. 2017;22(3):248–252.

24. Rohren EM, Kliewer MA, Carroll BA, et al. A spectrum of Doppler waveforms in the carotid and vertebral arteries. *Am J Roentgenol*. 2003;181(6):1695–1704.

3

Intracranial Cerebrovascular

CEREBROVASCULAR ANATOMY

Intracranial Anatomy

The majority of the cerebral arteries are classified with a number as well as a name. The number indicates a specific course or a point in which it branches. In general, the segments labeled with the number 1 are more centrally located in the brain while the segments labeled with the number 2 are located more peripheral (Fig. 3–1).

Anterior Cerebrovascular Anatomy

The intracranial anterior circulation is composed of the following arteries:

- Middle cerebral arteries (MCAs)
- Anterior cerebral arteries (ACAs)
- Terminal internal carotid arteries (tICAs)

Once the intracranial ICA enters the subarachnoid space, it terminates (tICA) at the bifurcation of the MCA and ACA. The MCA continues laterally toward the surface of the brain as the main M_1 branch. As the MCA continues to course laterally, it eventually splits into the M_2 segments in the insular area of the brain. There is typically a right MCA and a left MCA that are symmetrical in nature. The ACA begins as the A_1 segment coursing medially for a short distance until passing the anterior communicating artery (ACoA) where it becomes the A_2 segment. There are typically a right and left ACA as well; however, they are often asymmetrical in nature, differing from the MCAs.

Posterior Cerebrovascular Anatomy

The intracranial posterior circulation is composed of the following arteries:

- Vertebral arteries (VAs)
- Basilar artery (BA)
- Posterior cerebral arteries (PCAs)

The VAs enter the foramen magnum and cross the subarachnoid space, eventually joining together to form the BA. The BA continues cephalad until it terminates with the bifurcation of the right and left PCAs. The initial segment that arises from the basilar proximal to the takeoff of the posterior communicating artery (PCoA) is known as the P_1 segment. The PCA becomes the P_2 segment distal to the PCoA as it courses posteriorly around the cerebral peduncle.

Communicating Arteries

The arteries that are responsible for connecting the different segments of the cerebrovascular system are known as communicating arteries. These communicating arteries can become collateral pathways in the presence of significant extracranial cerebrovascular disease. The communicating arteries consist of the following arteries:

- ACoA—There is one ACoA that connects the right and left ACAs.
- PCoA—There is a right PCoA and a left PCoA that connect the posterior circulation to the anterior circulation.

Circle of Willis

The circle of Willis is a connection of small vessels that lie at the base of the brain, which includes portions of the anterior and posterior circulation. The average sizes of these cerebral arteries range from 2 to 4 mm with the entire circle being no larger than the size of a quarter. The arteries that make up the circle of Willis include:

- ACoA
- A_1 segments of both ACAs
- Both terminal ICAs (tICAs)
- Both PCoAs
- P_1 segments of both PCAs

The ACoA and the A_1 segments of both ACAs make up the anterior portion of the circle while both PCoAs and the P_1

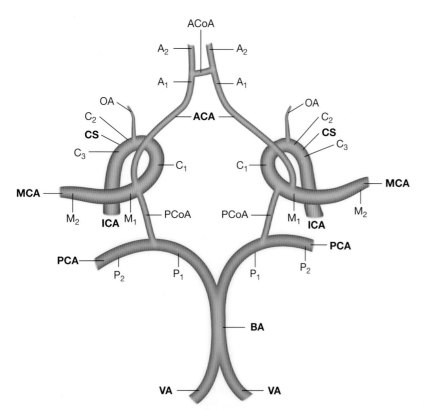

FIGURE 3–1. Illustration of cerebral arteries with their different segments.

segments make up the posterior portion of the circle. The anterior and posterior portions are joined together on each side by both tICAs completing the circle (Fig. 3–2). Anatomical variants are very common with only about 20% of people having a complete circle of Willis. A common variant is the absence of one of the communicating arteries such as the ACoA or the PCoA. This can become clinically significant in a situation where the communicating arteries serve as collateral pathways in the presence of extracranial internal carotid artery (ICA) disease. This will be discussed in more detail later in this chapter.

Carotid Siphon and Periorbital Vascular Anatomy

The distal ICA enters the base of the skull to become the intracranial ICA. As the ICA courses cephalad, it has been known to take a tortuous path typically in a "U"-shaped pattern (Fig. 3–3). This tortuous portion of the intracranial ICA is known as the carotid siphon (CS). The siphon is separated into three segments along its tortuous path. The three segments of the CS are:

- Parasellar—The most inferior segment.
- Genu—The middle segment.
- Supraclinoid—The most superior segment.

These segments can be differentiated with transcranial Doppler (TCD) by their different directions of flow in relationship to the TCD probe. This will be discussed in further detail later in this chapter.

The first intracranial branch of the ICA, originating at the area of the CS, is the ophthalmic artery (OA). The OA and its branches are responsible for providing blood flow to the eye in a normal patient; however, the branches of the OA communicate with the various branches of the ECA and can serve as collateral

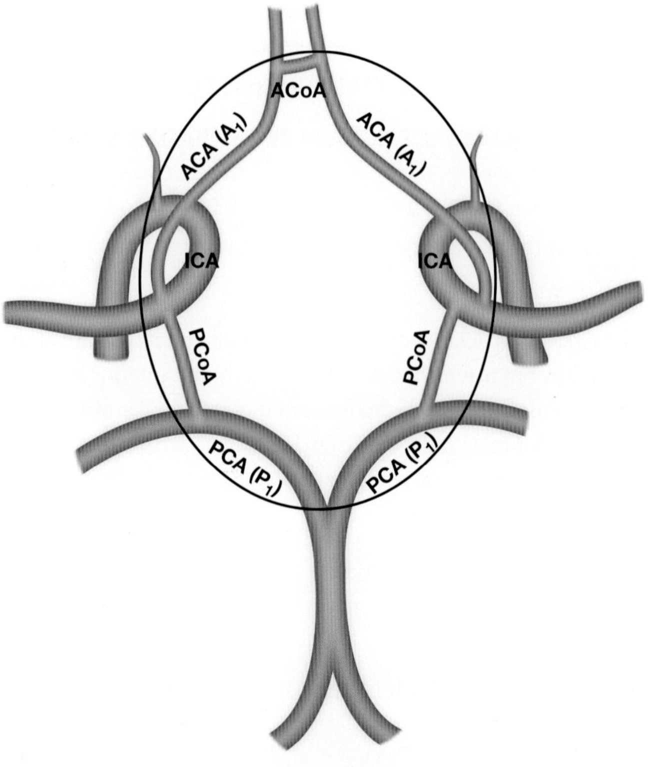

FIGURE 3–2. Illustration of the circle of Willis.

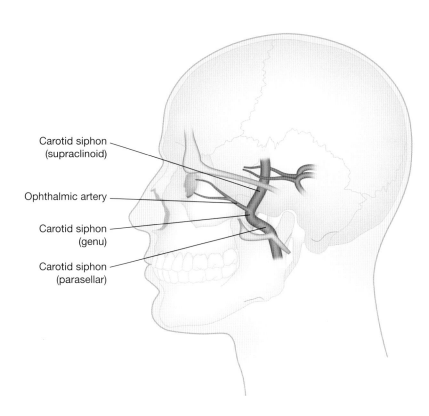

Carotid siphon
(supraclinoid)

Ophthalmic artery

Carotid siphon
(genu)

Carotid siphon
(parasellar)

FIGURE 3–3. Illustration of the carotid siphon and the ophthalmic artery.

pathways in the presence of significant ipsilateral ICA disease. The branches of the OA are:

- Supraorbital artery—Branches directly from the OA and communicates with the superficial temporal artery branch of the ECA.

- Frontal artery—Branches directly from the OA and communicates with several branches of the ECA.

- Nasal artery—Branches from the frontal artery and eventually becomes the angular artery. It communicates with the facial artery branch of the ECA.

TRANSCRANIAL DOPPLER

Types

There are two types of TCD in use today as diagnostic tools. The first is standard TCD. This is considered a blind but direct test because there is no imaging involved; however, you are directly insonating the vessels of interest and obtaining hemodynamic information. The second type is TCD imaging or TCDI. This method uses duplex to obtain an image with color Doppler as well as hemodynamic information. Both methods use low-frequency (1.8-3.6 MHz) pulsed range gated transducers with appropriate power levels (10-100 mW/cm^2) in order to penetrate the skull. When imaging through the transorbital window, the power should be decreased despite the absence of known bioeffects with ultrasound. The angle of insonation is usually assumed to be zero degrees when performing any form of TCD, although there are charts for angle-corrected TCDI. When

performing TCD, the velocity measurements are typically evaluated as the time-average mean velocity (TAMV) rather than peak systolic velocity (PSV)

Breakout box: When insonating the arteries posterior to the eye, due to the risk of heating the Food and Drug Administration (FDA) recommends equipment approved for ophthalmic scanning and MI ≤ 0.23 and TI ≤ 1.0.

Clinical Applications

The following are the most common applications of TCD:

- Evaluation of intracranial disease such as stenosis, occlusion, and arteriovenous malformation.

- Monitoring for vasospasm in patients with subarachnoid hemorrhage (SAH).

- Assessing for collateral pathways in the presence of extracranial cerebrovascular disease.

- Intraoperative monitoring.

- Evaluation of the vertebral/basilar system.

- Evaluation for suspected brain death.

- Stroke prediction in children with sickle cell disease (SCD).

Patient Position

The patient is positioned supine for the majority of the examination and is expected to remain still and avoid any type of motion. TCD examinations require very subtle movements due to the small size of the vessels so even the slightest bit of motion can make the examination more difficult. In order to access the vertebrobasilar system, it is also possible to have the patient roll on to the right or left side and tuck their chin to their chest. The key is to try and keep the patient as comfortable as possible to avoid movement.

Technique

Equipment

Standard dedicated TCD units utilize a pulsed, range gated transducer with a frequency of 2 MHz. These dedicated units are nonimaging units and are used to obtain hemodynamic information only such as PSV, end-diastolic velocity (EDV), and TAMV. They can also determine flow direction as well as the depth of the blood vessels.

TCDI examinations utilize a standard imaging ultrasound unit with a broadband phased array transducer with a frequency between 1.8 and 3.6 MHz. These standard ultrasound units typically have software packages that will allow them to display all the same parameters as the dedicated TCD units, so the diagnostic criteria for interpretation are the same.

Transcranial Windows

Both TCD and TCDI utilize the same areas in order to insonate the cerebral arteries. These areas are known as the transcranial or ultrasonic windows (Fig. 3–4). The following are the four transcranial windows:

- Transtemporal
- Transorbital
- Suboccipital
- Submandibular

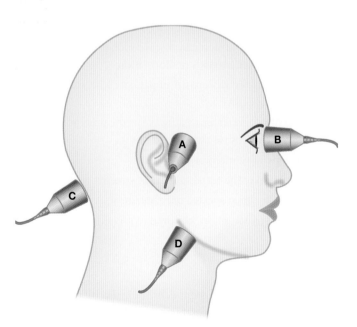

FIGURE 3–4. The four transcranial windows. **(A)** Transtemporal, **(B)** transorbital, **(C)** suboccipital, **(D)** submandibular.

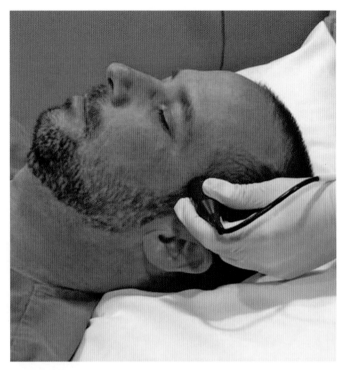

FIGURE 3–5. Transtemporal approach.

The transtemporal window is located by placing the probe on the temporal bone superior to the zygomatic arch and anterior to the tragus (Fig. 3–5). The thickness of the temporal bone can vary significantly among patients. For this reason, not every patient will have an optimal transtemporal window. The following arteries are generally surveyed through the transtemporal window:

- MCA
- ACA
- PCA
- MCA/ACA bifurcation
- tICA

The transorbital window is located by placing the probe on the eyelid insonating through the frontal bone, optic canal, and superior orbital fissure (Fig. 3–6). The following arteries are generally surveyed through the transorbital window:

- CS
- OA

The suboccipital window is located by placing the probe on the back of the neck and angling upward toward the head insonating through the foremen magnum (Fig. 3–7). The following arteries are generally surveyed through the suboccipital window:

- Right and left VAs
- BA

The submandibular window is located by placing the probe at the angle of the mandible and angling upward toward the

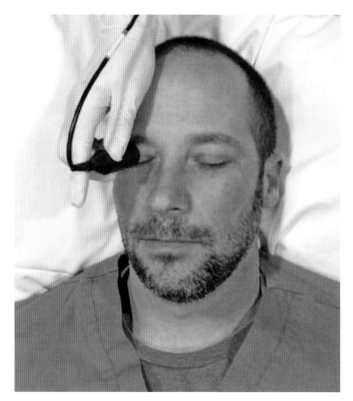

FIGURE 3-6. Transorbital approach.

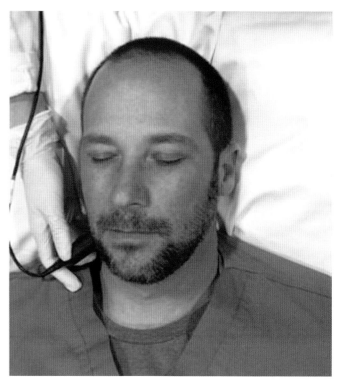

FIGURE 3-8. Submandibular approach.

head (Fig. 3–8). This approach is different from the others in that it is not used to insonate an intracranial vessel. It is used to insonate the extracranial ICA just before it enters the skull. This approach is typically used to obtain the ICA velocity for

the calculation of the MCA/ICA ratio when evaluating a patient for vasospasm. MCA/ICA ratio is a ratio use to distinguish the difference between vasospasm and hyperemia which will be discussed in further detail later in this chapter.

Standard Protocol (TCD)

Standard TCD examinations include insonating the cerebrovascular arteries with PW Doppler waveforms obtained from the ICAs, MCAs, ACAs, PCAs, OAs, CS, VAs, and BAs. Standard TCD uses a blind but direct approach as described earlier in this chapter, meaning that there is no image to reference. For that reason, the technologist must rely on other parameters to identify the different cerebral vessels. The parameters used to identify the specific cerebral vessels are:

- Direction of flow—This refers to the direction of flow in relationship to the probe. This can also be helpful in determining which segment of the vessel you are in for certain vessels. For example, with the probe placed on the transtemporal window, the P_1 segment of the PCA will have flow going toward the probe while the P_2 segment will have flow going away from the probe.

- Transcranial windows—Each transcranial window will only allow insonation of specific vessels.

- Depth—This refers to the depth at which the sample volume is placed. Each vessel has a depth range at which it typically lies intracranially.

- Spatial relationship between the arteries—This refers to the fact that a vessel can be sampled in incremental steps

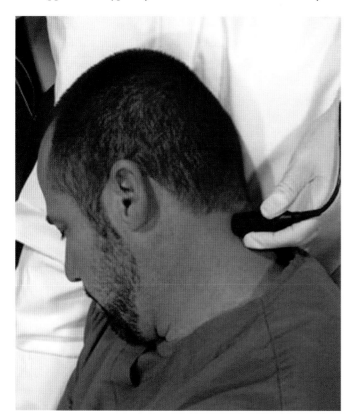

FIGURE 3-7. Suboccipital approach.

TABLE 3–1 • Typical Criteria for Identifying the Cerebral Arteries During a TCD Examination Through Each Transcranial Window

TCD Window	Vessel	Direction of Flow in Relationship to Transducer	Sample Volume Depth	TCD Normal Mean Velocity (cm/s)
Transtemporal	MCA	M_1—toward M_2—away	30–60 mm	55 ± 12
Transtemporal	tICA	Toward and/or away	60–70 mm	39 ± 9
Transtemporal	ACA	Away	60–75 mm	50 ± 11
Transtemporal	PCA	P_1—toward P_2—away	60–75 mm	40 ± 10
Transorbital	OA	Toward	35–55 mm	21 ± 5
Transorbital	CS	Toward, bidirectional, away	65–80 mm	41–47 ± 14
Suboccipital	VA	Away	60–90 mm	38 ± 10
Suboccipital	BA	Away	70–120 mm	41 ± 10
Submandibular	ICA	Away	35–80 mm	30 ± 9

without major changes in waveform and velocity until the point that it changes to another vessel. For example, the MCA can be traced incrementally at different depths without change until you reach the MCA/ACA bifurcation, at which point you will see a change in flow direction.

- TAMV—As a general rule for (TAMV), the MCA > ACA > PCA = BA = VA. There are published ranges of average mean flow velocities that can be used as a guideline; however, there are many physiologic factors that can affect flow velocities of the cerebral arteries. This general rule is often the better approach making each patient their own normal baseline.

See Table 3–1.

Transtemporal Window. Standard TCD examinations typically begin with the probe placed on the temporal bone from a posterior approach angling anterior and superior through the transtemporal window. If a suitable window is obtained, the arteries that can be identified are the MCAs, ACAs, tICAs, and PCAs. The examination generally begins with the sample volume set at a depth of about 50-55 mm and the first waveform identified is most often the MCA. The waveform will demonstrate flow toward the probe (Fig. 3–9). The sample volume is then tracked in incremental steps more superficially while tracing the MCA from M_1 segment to M_2 segment. This helps prove the identity of the MCA and serves as the main road map

for the transtemporal window. The average mean flow velocity for the MCA is 55 ± 12 cm/s. The MCA is then tracked by moving the sample volume depth to about 55-65 mm. At this depth is where the bifurcation of the tICA into the MCA/ACA is often identified. At this level, the waveform will demonstrate flow in both directions toward (MCA) and away (ACA) from the probe (Fig. 3–10). From the level of the MCA/ACA bifurcation, the sample volume depth can be increased further to a depth of approximately 60-80 mm to identify the ACA. The ACA waveform will demonstrate flow going away from the probe toward the front of the patient's head (Fig. 3–11). The average mean flow velocity for the ACA is 50 ± 11 cm/s. The tICA can be identified by returning the sample volume depth back to the level of the bifurcation (55–65 mm) and angling the probe slightly inferior. The tICA will be identified as a waveform demonstrating flow toward the probe (Fig. 3–12). The average mean flow velocity for the tICA is 39 ± 9 cm/s. From this same level of the MCA/ACA bifurcation, the sample volume depth is increased to a depth of about 60-70 mm and the probe is rotated posteriorly and inferiorly to locate the PCA. The P_1 segment is typically the first portion identified and displayed as a waveform with flow going toward the probe. As the posterior rotation is continued, the P_2 segment is eventually reached and is then displayed as a waveform with flow going away from the probe (Fig. 3–13). The average mean flow velocity for the PCA is 39 ± 10 cm/s.

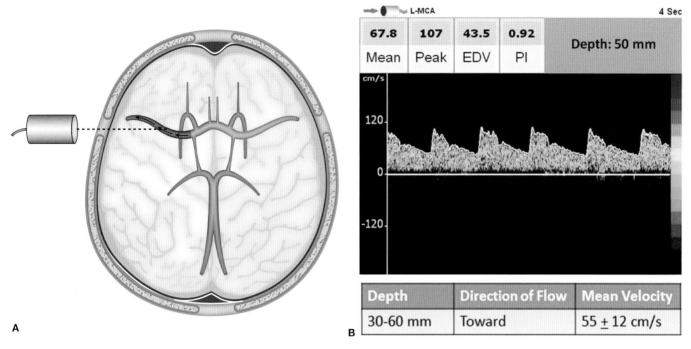

FIGURE 3–9. **(A)** The middle cerebral artery (MCA) is obtained through the transtemporal window. **(B)** Demonstrates a normal low-resistant MCA waveform with flow toward the probe.

Suboccipital Window. To insonate the VAs and the BA during a standard TCD examination, the suboccipital window is used. The probe is most commonly placed in the center of the posterior neck angled up toward the head in the direction of the foramen magnum and the sample volume is set at a depth of approximately 60 mm. The probe is then slightly angled either to the right or the left to identify the right and left VAs. Once both VAs are identified, each of them should be tracked in incremental steps from a depth of 55 mm to about 90 mm. The VA waveforms should demonstrate flow away from the probe toward the head (Fig. 3–14A). The average mean flow velocity for the VA is 38 ± 10 cm/s. The VAs join intracranially to form

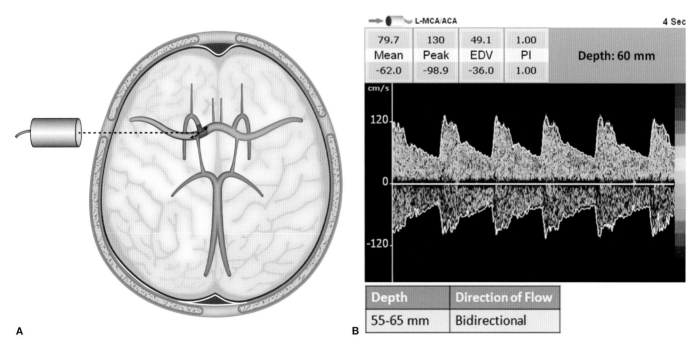

FIGURE 3–10. **(A)** The middle cerebral artery/anterior cerebral artery (MCA/ACA) bifurcation is obtained through the transtemporal window as the MCA is tracked deeper to a depth of about 55-65 mm. **(B)** Demonstrates normal bidirectional waveforms representing the MCA above the baseline and the ACA below the baseline.

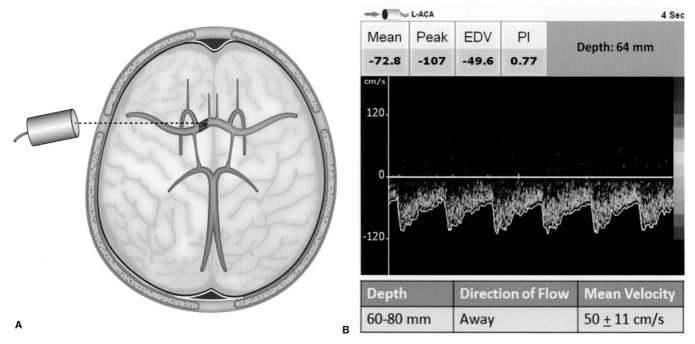

FIGURE 3–11. (A) The anterior cerebral artery (ACA) is obtained through the transtemporal window by angling anteriorly. **(B)** Demonstrates a normal low-resistant ACA waveform with flow away from the probe.

a single vessel known as the BA. It is often difficult to determine the exact level at which this transition occurs; however, it is typically at a depth of approximately 89-90 mm. The BA waveform will also demonstrate flow going away from the probe toward the head (Fig. 3–14B). The average mean flow velocity for the BA is 41 ± 10 cm/s.

Transorbital Window. It is possible to insonate the OAs and CSs through the transorbital window by having the patient close their eyes and placing the probe on the eyelid using a small amount of acoustic gel. The probe is angled just slightly toward the patient's midline. The OA is typically identified with the sample volume set at a depth of approximately 40-60 mm.

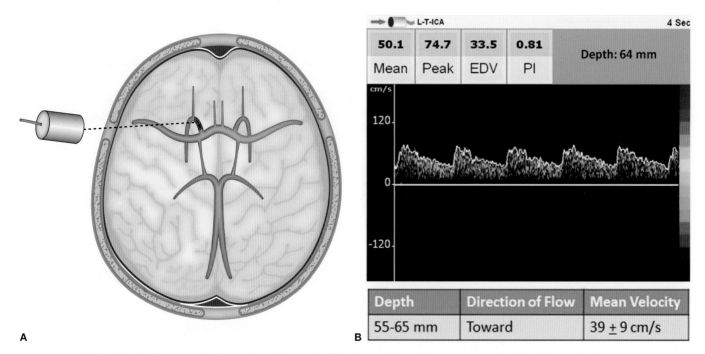

FIGURE 3–12. (A) The terminal internal carotid artery (ICA) is obtained through the transtemporal window by locating the middle cerebral artery/anterior cerebral artery (MCA/ICA) bifurcation and angling inferiorly. **(B)** Demonstrates a normal low-resistant ICA waveform with flow toward the probe.

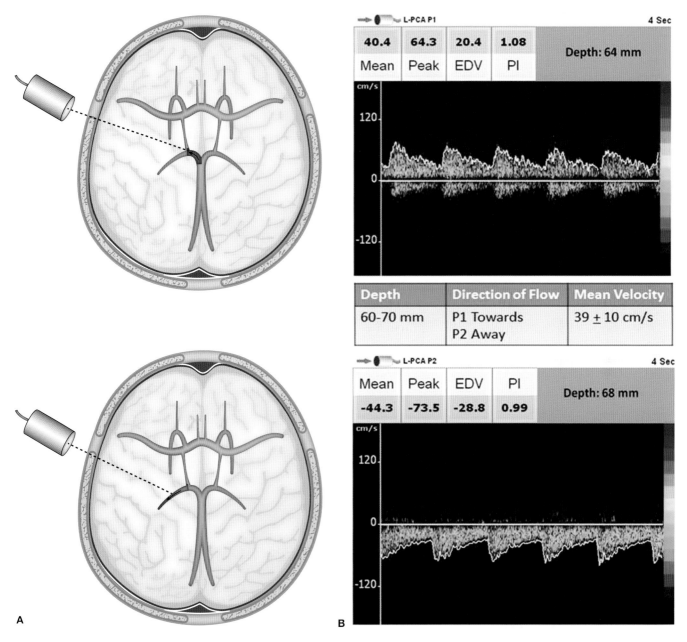

FIGURE 3–13. (A) The posterior cerebral artery (PCA) is obtained through the transtemporal window by angling posteriorly. **(B)** Demonstrates a normal low-resistant PCA (P₁) waveform with flow toward the probe and a normal low-resistant PCA (P₂) waveform with flow away from the probe.

The OA waveform should have flow going toward the transducer since it is the main source of blood supply to the eye. It will also have a high resistance signal compared to the other intracranial arteries because it is not supplying blood flow to the brain in a normal patient (Fig. 3–15). The average mean flow velocity for the OA is 21 ± 5 cm/s. When the sample volume is increased to a depth of approximately 60-70 mm the CS can be identified. Because of its tortuous nature the direction of flow will be determined by which segment of the CS is being insonated. The parasellar segment waveform will demonstrate flow toward the probe, the genu segment waveform will demonstrate bidirectional flow, and the supraclinoid

segment waveform will demonstrate flow away from the probe (Fig. 3–15). The average mean flow velocity for the CS is 41 to 47 ± 5 cm/s and varies depending on which segment you are insonating.

Submandibular Window. This window is used to insonate the extracranial ICA and is typically used to calculate the MCA/ICA ratio in patients with suspected SAH. The probe is placed at the angle of the mandible and is angled up toward the patient's head with the sample volume set at a depth of approximately 35-80 mm. The ICA waveform will demonstrate flow away from the probe toward the patient's head (Fig. 3–16).

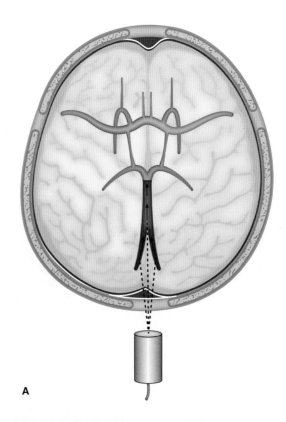

A

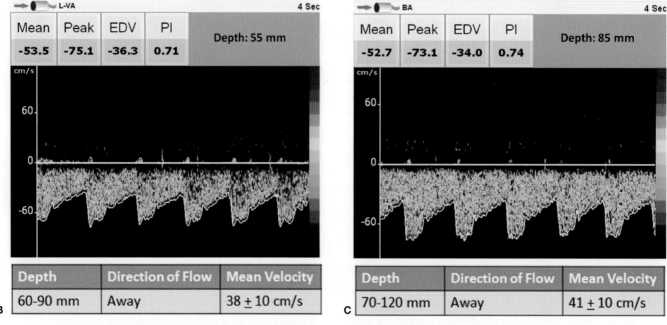

B

C

FIGURE 3–14. **(A)** The vertebral artery (VA) and basilar artery (BA) are obtained through the suboccipital window by angling up toward the patient's head. **(B)** Demonstrates a normal low-resistant VA waveform with flow away from the probe. **(C)** Demonstrates a normal low-resistant BA waveform with flow away from the probe.

Standard Protocol (TCDI)

The protocol for a TCDI examination is identical to that of a standard TCD examination. The main advantage that TCDI has over standard TCD is that it offers an easier and more reliable method to identify the vessels with the addition of duplex imaging. In addition, it allows for visualization of structural anatomy.

Normal waveform directions and average mean flow velocities are similar for both examinations. The use of color Doppler with TCDI determines direction of blood flow while PW Doppler is used to determine the TAMV.

Transtemporal Window. In a patient with an adequate temporal window with the transducer placed on the temporal bone,

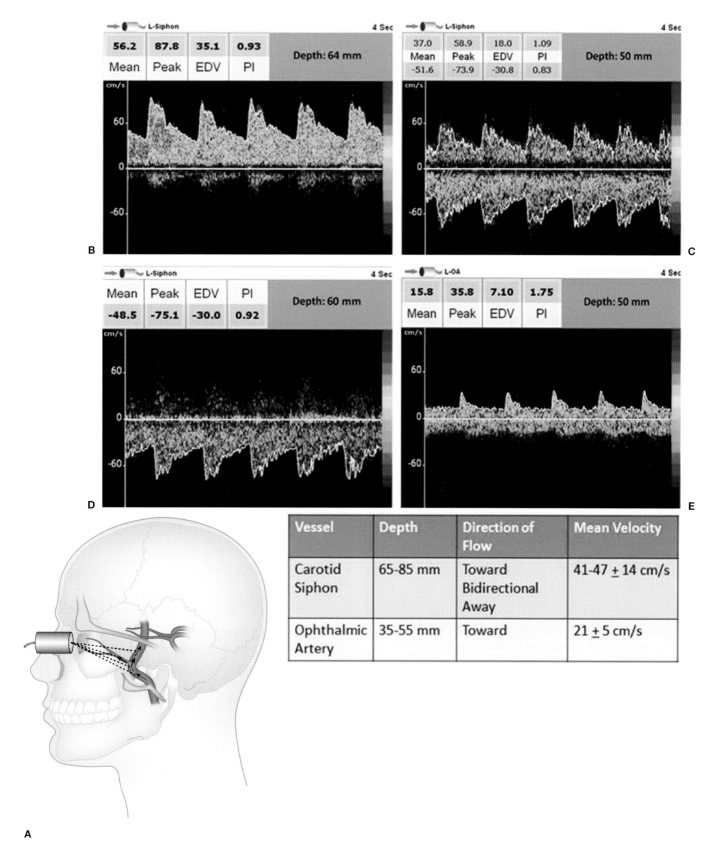

FIGURE 3–15. **(A)** The ophthalmic artery (OA) and carotid siphon (CS) are obtained through the transorbital window. **(B)** Demonstrates a normal low-resistant CS waveform from the parasellar segment with flow toward the probe. **(C)** Demonstrates a normal low-resistant CS waveform from the genu segment with bidirectional flow. **(D)** Demonstrates a normal low-resistant CS waveform from the supraclinoid segment with flow away from the probe. **(E)** Demonstrates a normal high-resistant OA waveform with flow toward the probe.

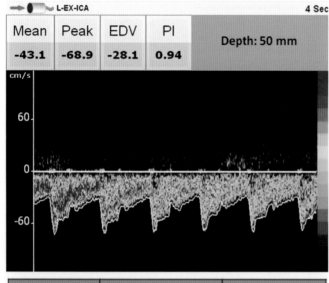

Mean	Peak	EDV	PI
-43.1	-68.9	-28.1	0.94

Depth: 50 mm

Depth	Direction of Flow	Mean Velocity
35-80 mm	Away	30 ± 9 cm/s

FIGURE 3–16. Demonstrates a normal low-resistant extracranial internal carotid artery (ICA) waveform with flow away from the probe from the submandibular window.

the 2D image will reveal certain anatomical landmarks such as the sphenoid wings, petrous ridges, anterior clinoid processes, and cerebral peduncles (Fig. 3–17). With color and PW Doppler, the MCA, tICA, ACA, and PCA should be identified through the transtemporal window.

Suboccipital Window. With the transducer placed in the center of the posterior neck, the 2D landmark used to identify the suboccipital window is the foramen magnum (Fig. 3–18). With color and PW Doppler, the VAs and BAs should be identified through the suboccipital window.

Transorbital Window. With the transducer placed on the eyelid, the 2D landmark visualized with this approach is the orbit itself with the optic nerve posterior to the eye which appears as shadowing (Fig. 3–19). Using color and PW Doppler, the OAs and CSs should be identified through the transorbital window. The transorbital window also allows for the measurement of the sheath of the optical nerve, which is used to monitor intracranial pressures.

Submandibular Window. The submandibular window is an approach more commonly utilized with standard TCD examinations and used to calculate the MCI/ICA ratio. There is no

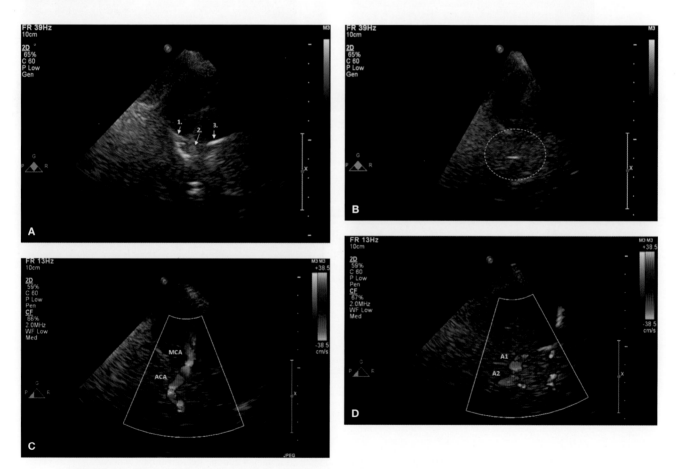

FIGURE 3–17. (A) Transtemporal window demonstrating 2D grayscale boney landmarks shown as echogenic linear structures. (1) Sphenoid wing. (2) Anterior clinoid process. (3) Petrous ridge. **(B)** Transtemporal window demonstrating the 2D grayscale parenchymal landmarks of the cerebral peduncles (*circled*). **(C)** Transtemporal window demonstrating a color Doppler image of the middle cerebral artery (MCA) (*red*) with flow toward the transducer and the anterior cerebral artery (ACA) (*blue*) with flow away from the transducer. **(D)** Transtemporal window demonstrating a color Doppler image of the A₂ segment of the ACA (*blue*) with flow away from the transducer.

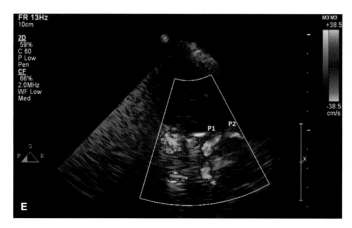

E

FIGURE 3–17. (*Continued*) **(E)** Transtemporal window demonstrating a color Doppler image of the posterior cerebral artery (PCA) with the P$_1$ segment (*red*) with flow toward the transducer and the P$_2$ segment (*blue*) with flow away from the transducer.

data for usage during a TCDI; therefore, it is often not part of the examinations.

Limitations

The limitations of TCD and TCDI examinations include:

- Inadequate temporal windows
- Recent eye surgery is a contraindication to performing an examination using the transorbital approach
- Misidentification of vessels (not typically an issue with TCDI)
- Too much patient motion

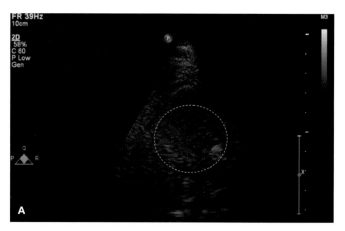

A

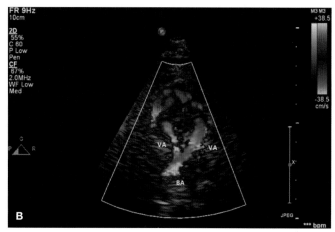

B

FIGURE 3–18. **(A)** Suboccipital window demonstrating the foramen magnum (*circled*). **(B)** Suboccipital window demonstrating a color Doppler image of the vertebral arteries and basilar artery (*blue*) with flow away from the transducer.

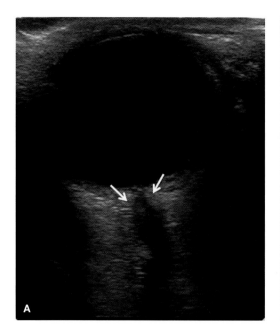

A

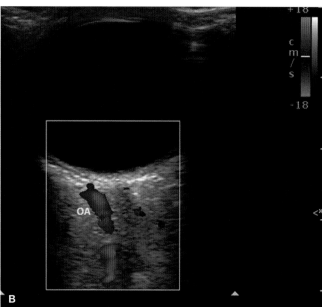

B

FIGURE 3–19. **(A)** Transorbital window demonstrating the optic nerve shadow (*arrows*). **(B)** Transorbital window demonstrating a color Doppler image of the ophthalmic artery (*red*) with flow toward the transducer.

Interpretation of Results

Normal Findings

Normal findings for both TCD and TCDI examinations will demonstrate cerebral waveforms with flow in the correct direction for each of the arteries as described earlier in this chapter. Typically, the mean flow velocities of the cerebral arteries will remain consistent at or around their standard averages without any focal increase. As mentioned earlier, there are physiologic factors that can globally affect mean flow velocities so it is important to remember that the standard average velocities are just a guide and that global increases may be just hyperemia as a result of normal factors.

Stenosis and Occlusion

Stenosis of the intracranial cerebral arteries can be identified with TCD by characteristic PW Doppler waveform changes. Those changes are:

- A focal increase in velocity at the suspected area of stenosis
- Poststenotic turbulence
- Poststenotic velocity drop

In general with both TCD and TCDI, a greater than 30% increase in velocity compared to a normal contralateral vessel segment suggests the presence of an intracranial stenosis (Fig. 3–20) and an increase of 50% or more is definitive. There are some absolute velocity criteria available; however, they can sometimes be unreliable due to physiologic changes. The most commonly used velocity criteria use angle–corrected PSV thresholds published by Baumgartner in 1999. Table 3–2 shows the PSV thresholds that indicate a more than 50% stenosis in each vessel. Stenosis can occur in any of the cerebral arteries due to atherosclerosis as well as other noninflammatory diseases that are less common. Common areas for stenosis to occur intracranially include the MCA and CS.

An intracranial occlusion is typically detected by the absence of flow in a particular artery at the estimated depth with the presence of flow in all of the adjacent arteries. Standard TCD can be somewhat limited when evaluating for a cerebral artery occlusion since you cannot actually visualize the vessels. This is one of the advantages TCDI has over standard TCD. The most common cerebral artery to occlude resulting in stroke is the MCA. With standard TCD, the presence of an MCA occlusion can be inferred when the other cerebral arteries demonstrate flow without the ability to demonstrate flow in the MCA. In 2001, Demchuk et al.

Vessel	PSV Threshold (cm/s)
MCA	≥ 220
ACA	≥ 155
PCA	≥ 145
BA	≥ 140
VA	≥ 120

TABLE 3–2 • PSV Angle-Corrected Thresholds indicating a ≥ 50% Intracranial Stenosis with TCDI

proposed the Thrombolysis in Brain Ischemia (TIBI) criteria for classifying MCA flow status with TCD before and after thrombolysis treatment. The scale runs from 0 (occlusion) to 5 (normal). Evaluation of the TIBI score before and after thrombolysis was found to correlate with the degree of stroke and clinical outcome.

Collateral Flow

In the presence of extracranial hemodynamically significant disease, the brain often will compensate for lack of flow to a particular portion of the brain by providing collateral flow from another area. Transcranial examinations can be used to determine if collateral flow is present and can often determine which alternate area is providing that collateral flow. In general, arteries that serve as the conduit for collateral flow will have a global increase in velocity and this is one of the findings that make it possible for TCD to determine that collateral flow is occurring. The three main collateral pathways that can be identified with TCD are:

- Crossover flow through the ACoA
- Posterior to anterior flow through the PCoA
- ECA to ICA flow through the OA

Anterior Communicating Artery. This type of collateral flow is known as "crossover" flow because it is shunting blood from one hemisphere to the contralateral hemisphere either right to left or left to right depending on which side has the extracranial disease. The findings that are associated with this type of collateral flow are:

- The presence of hemodynamically significant carotid disease
- Increased velocities in the contralateral ACA
- Reversed flow direction and increased velocities in the ipsilateral ACA
- Increased turbulent flow in the ACoA when identified (typically with TCDI)

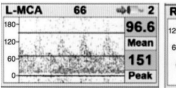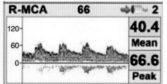

FIGURE 3–20. Left middle cerebral artery (MCA) stenosis showing more than 50% increase in velocity compared to contralateral MCA.

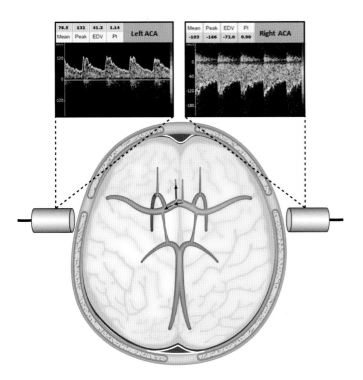

FIGURE 3–21. Demonstrates findings suggesting the presence of crossover flow in a patient with a left extracranial internal carotid artery (ICA) occlusion. The two findings are increased velocity in the right anterior cerebral artery (ACA) providing the collateral flow contralateral to the occlusion as well as reversed flow in the left ACA ipsilateral to the occlusion.

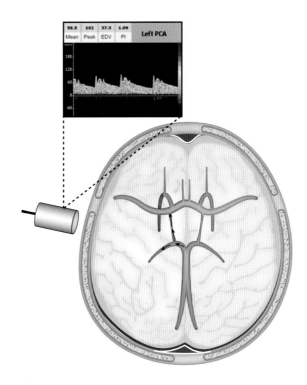

FIGURE 3–22. Demonstrates an elevated mean velocity in the left posterior cerebral artery suggesting the presence of collateral flow through the posterior communicating artery in a patient with a left extracranial internal carotid artery (ICA) occlusion.

The increase in velocity in the contralateral ACA is caused by the increased flow volume required to perfuse the contralateral hemisphere. The reversal of flow direction in the ipsilateral ACA is the effect of the flow now being supplied from the contralateral side. Normally the ACA waveform demonstrates flow going away from the probe resting on the temporal bone, but in the case of crossover flow, the waveform demonstrates flow coming toward the probe (Fig. 3–21).

Posterior Communicating Artery. When this type of collateral flow is present, blood is being shunted from the posterior circulation to the anterior circulation through the PCoA. The findings that are associated with collateral flow through the PCoA are:

- The presence of hemodynamically significant carotid disease
- Increased velocities in the ipsilateral PCA (P_1 segment)
- P_1/P_2 velocity ratio more than 1.5 in the ipsilateral PCA
- Visualization of the PCoA (TCDI)
- Increased velocities within the BA

Similar to the increase in velocity that is present in the contralateral ACA with crossover flow, the increase in velocity in the ipsilateral PCA is caused by increased flow volume (Fig. 3–22).

Ophthalmic Artery. This type of collateral flow is possible due to the communication of the ECA branches with the branches of

the OA. Because of this communication, blood can be shunted from the ECA to the ICA. The findings that are associated with this type of collateral flow are:

- The presence of hemodynamically significant carotid disease
- Reversed flow direction in the ipsilateral OA
- Increase in velocity and decrease in pulsatility in the ipsilateral OA

The OA normally provides blood flow to the eye and its normal flow direction is toward the probe resting on the patient's eyelid. When the ECA is providing collateral flow via the OA, it reverses its direction demonstrating flow away from the probe and toward the head to provide blood flow to the brain. When the OA provides blood flow to the brain, the waveform also changes from being high resistance to low resistance (Fig. 3–23).

Vasospasm

Vasospasm is a delayed complication associated with a SAH where the cerebral arteries contract causing narrowing that reduces blood flow to the brain. This reduction in blood flow can lead to ischemic neurologic deficits and even death. Vasospasm is typically aggressively treated with medical therapy and often with intervention such as angioplasty. Vasospasm is mainly seen in the larger cerebral arteries and usually starts around 3-4 days following the SAH. The maximum degree of vasospasm usually occurs between days 7 and 14. The hemodynamic effect of

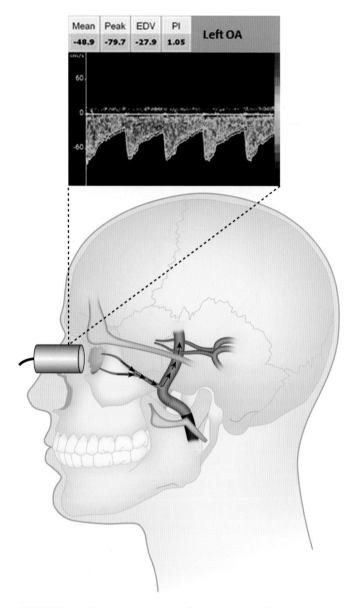

Mean	Peak	EDV	PI	Left OA
-48.9	-79.7	-27.9	1.05	

FIGURE 3–23. Demonstrates reversed flow in the ophthalmic artery as well as a change to a low-resistance waveform on the ipsilateral side of an internal carotid artery occlusion which are consistent findings indicating collateral flow from the external carotid artery branches through the ophthalmic artery.

vasospasm is increased velocities in the affected artery. If no vasospasm is detected by TCD by days 7-8 after SAH, clinically significant vasospasm can be ruled out.

TCD can be used to monitor these patients daily by recording the mean velocities of each cerebral vessel to determine if vasospasm is occurring and to what degree. In general, the higher the velocity the higher the degree of vasospasm and the greater the chance for neurologic deficits. These patients will often have higher than normal velocities as a result of hyperemia due to the medical treatments they are receiving. It is important not to mistake hyperemia for vasospasm. In order to avoid this issue, most laboratories utilize the MCA/ICA ratio, also known as the hemispheric or Lindegaard ratio. It is calculated by taking the highest MCA velocity and dividing it by the extracranial ICA velocity obtained from the submandibular window (Fig. 3–24). In general, if the MCA/ICA ratio is over 3 that is consistent with vasospasm. Under 3 would be considered hyperemia. Table 3–3 shows typical vasospasm criteria for some of the cerebral arteries. A common therapy used to prevent and treat vasospasm is a combination of induced hypertension, hypervolemia, and hemodilution known as the triple "H" therapy.

Brain Death

Brain death is a clinical diagnosis, and although TCD cannot 100% confirm a diagnosis of brain death, TCD can be used to aid in the diagnosis. Clinically, the diagnosis of brain death is made when cerebral circulation has stopped. A direct evaluation of cerebral circulatory arrest can be made with conventional angiography. Similarly, nuclear medicine can be used to document absence of blood flow to the brain. Sometimes, the patient is too ill to travel to radiology, and TCD is ideal in that it can be performed portably. Two clinical tests used to test for brain death are confirmation of the absence of reflexes and the apnea test. With the apnea test, the patient's ventilator is turned off but the patient is still given 100% oxygen. When the CO_2 level builds up, respiratory motion should be visualized. If not, the brain stem is not functioning. The brain maintains a steady perfusion due to cerebral autoregulation, which is how the brain maintains a steady blood flow even in the presence of hypotension. This autoregulation may be interrupted by SAH, hypoxia, encephalopathy, CVA, tumor, and infectious causes. When the perfusion pressure decreases, the cerebral arterioles dilate to increase flow. Excess CO_2 in the bloodstream causes dilatation of the cerebral vessels. Low CO_2, called hypocapnia, causes vasoconstriction of these vessels.

TCD can be used to look for intracranial blood flow, but only evaluates the central intracranial circulation. If the patient has a limited window, the absence of flow may be suggestive of brain death, or it may be a bad window. For this reason, TCD is used to rule out brain death by finding normal flow, or suggesting the presence of brain death with absence of flow or abnormal spectral waveforms. The classic to-and-fro spectral waveform typically appears as a short sharp peak followed by either a short reversal of diastolic flow or no diastolic flow at all (Fig. 3–25). TCD alone cannot make the determination of brain death; however, it can offer valuable information to help the clinical decision making.

Intraoperative Monitoring

TCD is sometimes used to monitor cerebral blood flow during surgery. What makes TCD a favorable choice is that it is noninvasive and can be done rather easily. Common procedures that have employed TCD as a monitoring tool are carotid

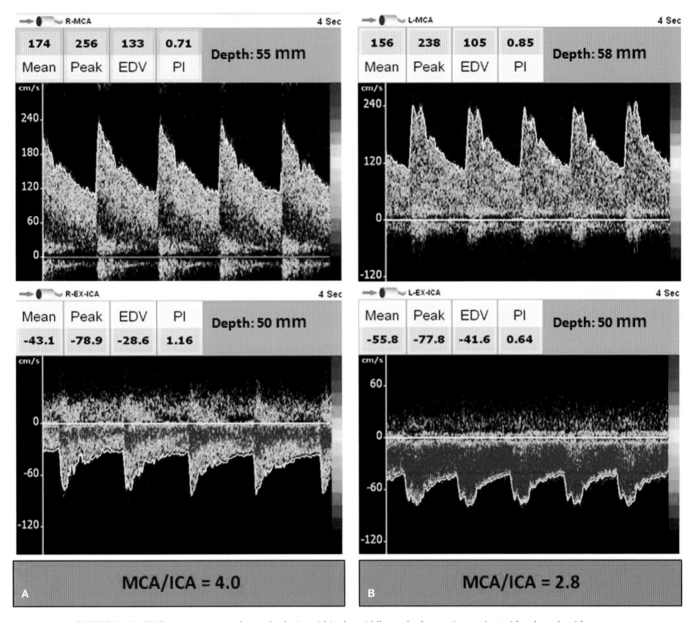

FIGURE 3–24. (A) Demonstrates an elevated velocity within the middle cerebral artery in a patient with subarachnoid hemorrhage (SAH) with a middle cerebral artery/anterior cerebral artery (MCA/ICA) ratio of 4.0 consistent with vasospasm. **(B)** Also demonstrates an elevated velocity within the middle cerebral artery in a patient with SAH; however, the MCA/ICA ratio is only 2.8 which is consistent with just hyperemia. This is a prime example of patients both with elevated MCA velocities using the MCA/ICA ratio to distinguish between hyperemia and vasospasm.

endarterectomy and open heart surgery. Typically, the MCA is insonated at a depth of about 50 mm and either monitored throughout the procedure or at specific times with high-frequency. TCD intraoperative monitoring is used to detect abnormalities during surgery such as microembolization (Fig. 3-26), hypoperfusion, and hyperperfusion.

Sickle Cell Monitoring

Children with SCD have an 11% increased risk of death from stroke before age 18 due to the abnormally shaped cells in the small blood vessels of the brain. TCD can be used to calculate the risk of stroke in these patients, which may initiate blood transfusions as treatment. Table 3–4 provides the velocities for normal and abnormal TCD when evaluating for SCD. These values come from a clinical study called Stroke Prevention Trial in Sickle Cell Anemia (STOP).

The head size in the pediatric population is going to be different than in the adult population, so adjustments must be made accordingly. Table 3–5 shows vessel depth in relation to head diameter.

TABLE 3–3 • Velocity and Ratio Criteria for Vasospasm in the Cerebral Arteries

Vessel	Mean Velocity (cm/s)	MCA/ICA Ratio	Interpretation
MCA	< 120 ≥ 120 ≥ 140 ≥ 200	< 3 3–4 5–6 ≥ 6	Hyperemia Mild vasospasm Moderate vasospasm Severe vasospasm
ACA	≥ 100 ≥ 120–140 ≥ 140–200 ≥ 200	N/A	Possible vasospasm or hyperemia Probable mild vasospasm or hyperemia Moderate vasospasm Severe vasospasm
VA/BA	≤ 60 ≥ 60–80 ≥ 80–140 ≥ 140	N/A	No evidence of vasospasm Possible vasospasm or hyperemia Probable moderate vasospasm or hyperemia Severe vasospasm or hyperemia

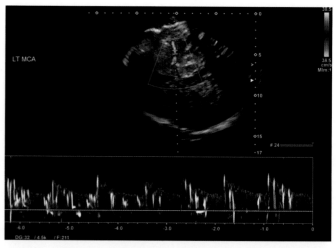

FIGURE 3–26. Transcranial Doppler of middle cerebral artery (MCA) showing microbubble artifact in the spectral waveform.

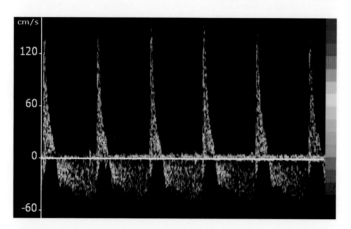

FIGURE 3–25. Transcranial Doppler (TCD) waveform with to-and-fro flow demonstrating a sharp peak followed by reversal of diastolic flow that is present in a patient with suspected circulatory arrest otherwise known as "brain death."

TABLE 3–4 • Normal and Abnormal Values of Pediatric TCD for Evaluation of Sickle Cell Disease Based on the STOP Criteria

Vessels imaged: MCA, terminal ICA, MCA/ACA bifurcation, ACA, PCA, basilar artery
Velocity values are the time-averaged mean of the maximum velocity (TAMM)

Normal	< 170 cm/s
Conditional	170–199 cm/s
Abnormal	≥ 200 cm/s

Source: Nichols FT, Jones AM, Adams RJ. Stroke prevention in sickle cell disease (STOP) study guidelines for transcranial Doppler testing. *J Neuroimaging.* 2001;11(4):354–362.

TABLE 3–5 • Vessel Depth and Head Diameter in TCD

Head Diameter (cm)	MCA Distal	MCA Proximal	MCA/ACA Bifurcation	ACA	PCA	Top of Basilar Artery
12 cm	30–36	30–54	50–54	50–58	40–60	60
13 cm	30–36	30–58	52–62	52–62	42–66	65
14 cm	34–40	34–62	56–68	56–68	46–70	70
15 cm	40–46	40–66	56–72	56–72	50–70	75

Source: Nichols FT, Jones AM, Adams RJ. Stroke prevention in sickle cell disease (STOP) study guidelines for transcranial Doppler testing. *J Neuroimaging.* 2001;11(4):354–362.

Questions

1. Which vessels can be insonated through the transtemporal window?

   (A) MCA, ACA, PCA, tICA, ACoA, PCoA

   (B) MCA, ACA, CS, ACoA, PCoA

   (C) CS, OA, tICA, MCA

   (D) VA, BA, PCA, PCoA, ACoA

2. Which of the following parameters can be used to identify a specific intracranial artery during a TCD examination?

   (A) PSV

   (B) Direction of blood flow at insonation depth

   (C) Waveform shape

   (D) Vessel diameter

3. What direction (in relation to the transducer) is the blood flow in the OA when it is being used as a collateral pathway from the external carotid artery to the ICA?

   (A) Toward

   (B) Away from

   (C) Bidirectional

   (D) Alternating

4. Which numbers for the MCA are consistent with severe vasospasm?

   (A) Mean velocity: more than 180 cm/s and MCA/ICA: 3.0

   (B) Mean velocity: more than 180 cm/s and MCA/ICA: 4.0

   (C) Mean velocity: more than 200 cm/s and MCA/ICA: 3.0

   (D) Mean velocity: more than 200 cm/s and MCA/ICA: 6.0

5. While performing a TCD examination through the temporal windows on a patient with right-sided paralysis, you obtain normal velocities throughout the left ACA and left PCA and are unable to obtain a good signal from the left MCA. What is the most likely diagnosis?

   (A) The patient has a focal stenosis of the left ACA

   (B) The patient has collateral flow through the left ACA

   (C) The patient has a left MCA occlusion

   (D) The patient does not have a good left temporal window

6. A focal increase in the mean velocity from 65 to 185 cm/s at a depth of 50 mm insonating through the transtemporal window is obtained. What is the most likely diagnosis?

   (A) Hemodynamically significant stenosis of the ACA

   (B) Severe vasospasm of the ACA

   (C) Severe vasospasm of the MCA

   (D) Hemodynamically significant stenosis of the MCA

7. Which of the following vessels can be insonated through the suboccipital window?

   (A) MCA

   (B) PCoA

   (C) BA

   (D) PCA

8. The largest intracranial branch originating from the ICA is the

   (A) MCA

   (B) OA

   (C) ACA

   (D) PCA

Questions 9 through 16: Match the structures in Figure 3–27 with the names of the arteries in Column B.

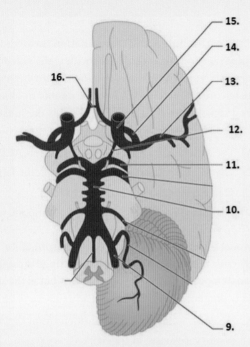

FIGURE 3–27. (Reproduced, with permission, from Waxman SG. *Clinical Neuroanatomy,* 29th ed. New York, NY; 2020; Figure 12–2. Copyright © McGraw Hill.)

COLUMN A	COLUMN B
9. _____	(A) MCA
10. _____	(B) PCoA
11. _____	(C) VA
12. _____	(D) ACA
13. _____	(E) BA
14. _____	(F) ACoA
15. _____	(G) ICA
16. _____	(H) PCA

17. **The BA gives rise to which of the following arteries?**

(A) Posterior communicating artery

(B) VAs

(C) ICAs

(D) PCAs

18. **With the TCD probe placed on the transtemporal window angled posteriorly at a depth of 67 mm, a waveform is obtained with a flow direction that is away from the probe with a mean flow velocity of 36 cm/s. Which vessel is most likely being insonated?**

(A) M_2 segment of the MCA

(B) P_1 segment of the PCA

(C) P_2 segment of the PCA

(D) M_3 segment of the MCA

19. **The normal TCD waveform in Figure 3–28 was obtained from the transorbital approach. Which vessel is most likely being insonated?**

(A) MCA

(B) ACA

(C) OA

(D) CS

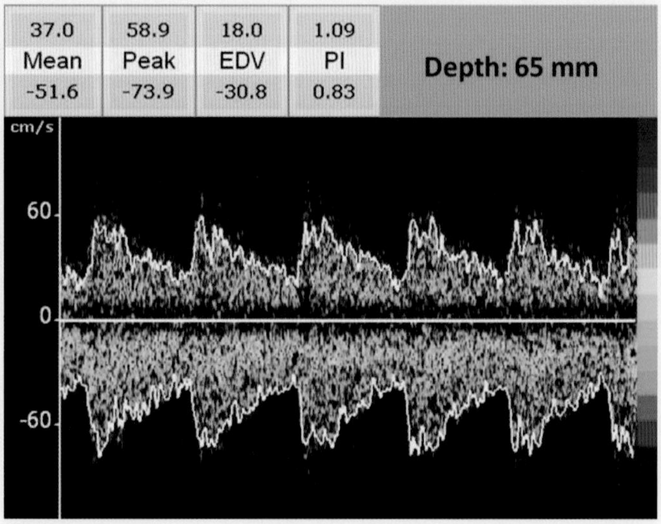

37.0	58.9	18.0	1.09	
Mean	Peak	EDV	PI	Depth: 65 mm
-51.6	-73.9	-30.8	0.83	

FIGURE 3–28.

Questions 20 through 23: Match the following color Doppler image with the names of the correct intracranial arteries in Figure 3–29.

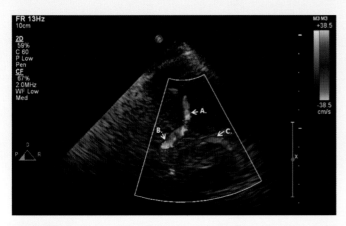

FIGURE 3–29.

20. ACA _____

21. MCA _____

22. PCA _____

23. The normal waveform shown in Figure 3–30 was obtained through the suboccipital window at a depth of 65 mm during a TCD examination. What is this vessel's identity?

(A) MCA

(B) BA

(C) VA

(D) CS

24. The angle of insonation during a TCD examination is assumed to be

(A) 60 degrees

(B) 90 degrees

(C) 45 degrees

(D) 0 degree

Questions 25 through 32: Match the cerebral arteries in column A with the normal direction of flow in relationship to the TCD probe in column B (flow directions in column B can be used more than once).

COLUMN A	COLUMN B
25. ACA _____	(A) Flow toward probe
26. PCA (P_1 segment) _____	(B) Flow away from probe
27. MCA _____	(C) Bidirectional flow
28. BA _____	
29. OA _____	
30. tICA _____	
31. VA _____	
32. CS (genu segment) _____	

33. Which of the following transcranial windows is used to obtain the extracranial ICA used to calculate the MCA/ICA ratio in patients with suspected vasospasm?

(A) Submandibular window

(B) Transtemporal window

(C) Suboccipital window

(D) Transorbital window

34. Which is the following is a sign of collateral flow through the ACoA that can exist when there is significant extracranial cerebrovascular disease?

(A) Reversed flow within the ACA on the ipsilateral side of the disease

(B) Increased velocities within the MCA on the ipsilateral side of the disease

(C) Decreased velocities within the ACA on the contralateral side of the disease

(D) Reversal of flow in the MCAs bilaterally

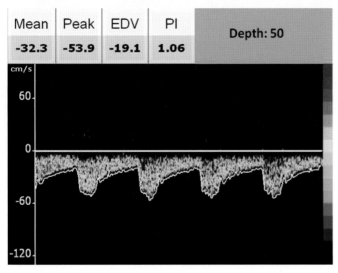

Mean	Peak	EDV	PI	Depth: 50
-32.3	-53.9	-19.1	1.06	

FIGURE 3–30.

35. The waveform seen in Figure 3–31 was obtained through the right transorbital approach at a depth of 42 mm in a patient with a known right extracranial ICA occlusion. What vessel is most likely being insonated and what does the waveform indicate?

    (A) CS with normal flow dynamics

    (B) OA with normal flow dynamics

    (C) OA with retrograde low-resistance collateral flow

    (D) CS with retrograde low-resistance collateral flow

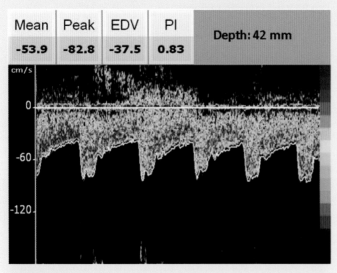

FIGURE 3–31.

36. Hyperemia is a typical response to patients being treated post SAH that results in which of the following?

    (A) Lower cerebral artery velocities

    (B) Higher cerebral artery velocities

    (C) No change to the cerebral artery velocities

    (D) No flow within the cerebral arteries

37. Vasospasm is a common condition that occurs in patients with SAH that typically occurs during which time period?

    (A) 1-3 days following the SAH

    (B) 4-7 days following the SAH

    (C) 7-14 days following the SAH

    (D) 14-25 days following the SAH

38. The posterior cerebral circulation is composed of which of the following vessels?

    (A) PCAs

    (B) MCAs

    (C) ACoA

    (D) tICA

39. The ICA bifurcates intracranially into which two vessels?

    (A) MCAs and ACAs

    (B) MCAs and PCAs

    (C) ACAs and PCAs

    (D) ACAs and PCoAs

40. Which of the following transducers can be used to perform transcranial examinations?

    (A) High-frequency pulsed-wave transducer

    (B) Low-frequency pulsed-wave transducer

    (C) Low-frequency continuous wave transducer

    (D) High-frequency linear array transducer

41. With the TCD probe placed on the suboccipital window, a vessel is insonated at a depth of 90 mm with an average mean flow velocity of 50 cm/s. Which vessel does this most likely represent?

    (A) BA

    (B) VA

    (C) PCA

    (D) PCoA

42. The most reliable way to distinguish the difference between hyperemia and vasospasm is with the use of which parameter?

    (A) PSV

    (B) TAMV

    (C) MCA/ICA ratio

    (D) EDV

43. Which of the following is TRUE about blind TCD examinations?

    (A) All patients have visibility through the transtemporal window

    (B) The suboccipital window allows visualization of the PCAs

    (C) It may be possible to obtain flow information from the contralateral transtemporal window

    (D) High acoustic power levels should be used when insonating the OAs due to the depth of the vessels

44. The MCA/ICA ratio that identifies the presence of vasospasm rather than just hyperemia is

    (A) MCA/ICA ratio more than 6

    (B) MCA/ICA ratio more than 2

    (C) MCA/ICA ratio more than 4

    (D) MCA/ICA ratio more than 3

45. **During a TCD examination, all of the below findings are consistent with a hemodynamically significant stenosis EXCEPT**

    (A) A focal increase in velocity

    (B) Global increase in mean flow velocity

    (C) Velocity drop distal to elevated velocity

    (D) Localized turbulence

46. **The waveform in Figure 3–32 was obtained through the transtemporal window at a depth of 62 mm. What is most likely the identification of this area?**

    (A) MCA

    (B) ACA

    (C) tICA

    (D) MCA/ACA bifurcation

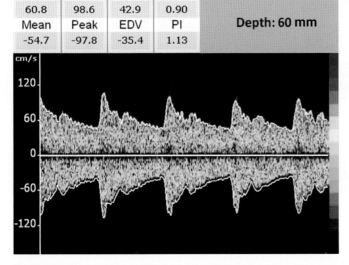

FIGURE 3–32.

47. **The waveforms of the MCA in Figure 3–33 were obtained through the transtemporal window at a depth of 55 mm and 60 mm. What do these findings suggest?**

    (A) Normal flow dynamics of the MCA

    (B) Mild vasospasm of the MCA

    (C) Hemodynamically significant stenosis of the MCA

    (D) Moderate vasospasm of the MCA

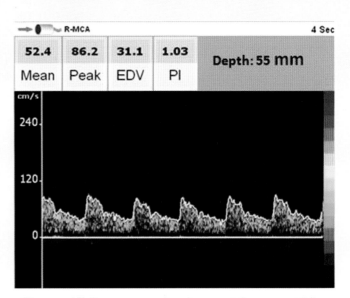

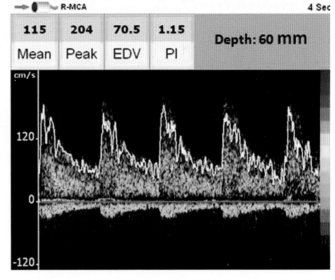

FIGURE 3–33.

48. The waveform in Figure 3–34 was obtained through the transtemporal window with the probe angled anteriorly at a depth of 65 mm. What does this finding suggest?

(A) Reversed flow within the ACA

(B) Reversed flow within the MCA

(C) Normal flow dynamic of the ACA

(D) Hemodynamically significant stenosis of the MCA

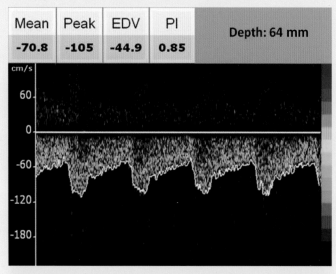

FIGURE 3–34.

49. A patient with a left ICA occlusion returns to your laboratory for a TCD examination that is unremarkable with the exception of an elevated TAMV of 105 cm/s within the left PCA. What do these findings most likely suggest?

(A) A hemodynamically significant stenosis of the left PCA

(B) Collateral flow from the external carotid artery to the ICA

(C) Collateral crossover flow from the right cerebral hemisphere

(D) Collateral flow through the PCoA

50. Which cerebral artery has the highest incidence of occlusion resulting in a cerebrovascular accident?

(A) MCA

(B) ACA

(C) PCA

(D) BA

Answers and Explanations

1. **(A)** MCA, ACA, PCA, tICA, ACoA, and PCoA can all be insonated through the transtemporal window during a TCD examination.

2. **(B)** All of the cerebral arteries have average insonation depths, normal flow directions, and average mean flow velocities that can help identify each artery during a TCD examination. Only certain arteries can be visualized through each of the ultrasonic windows, which also help to identify the arteries.

3. **(B)** The normal direction of flow in the OA through the transorbital approach is toward the probe as it provides blood flow to the eye. When the OA is providing collateral flow to the brain, it will have a reversed flow direction which is away from the probe that is resting on the orbit through the transorbital approach.

4. **(D)** A mean velocity more than 200 cm/s and an MCA/ICA 6.0 or more are consistent with severe vasospasm.

5. **(C)** Hemiparalysis is a lateralizing symptom that affects the contralateral side of the body. Right-sided paralysis would indicate that there is a problem with perfusion to the brain's left hemisphere. When the ACAs and PCAs are able to be insonated and the MCA is not, this is suspicious for an MCA occlusion.

6. **(D)** The average depth of the MCA is 55-65 mm with an average mean velocity of 55 cm/s ± 12. A focal increase to 185 cm/s at a depth of 50 mm is consistent with a hemodynamically significant stenosis within the MCA.

7. **(C)** Both of the VAs as well as the basilar artery can be insonated through the suboccipital window. The PCAs cannot be visualized through this window.

8. **(A)** The largest intracranial branch originating from the ICA is the MCA.

9. **(C)** VA

10. **(E)** BA

11. **(H)** PCA

12. **(B)** PCoA

13. **(A)** MCA

14. **(D)** ACA

15. **(G)** ICA

16. **(F)** ACoA

17. **(D)** The BA gives rise to the right and left PCAs.

18. **(C)** The PCA can be insonated with the TCD probe angled posteriorly from the transtemporal window at an average depth of 60-70 mm with an average mean velocity of 39 cm/s ± 10. The P_1 segment will have flow that is toward the probe while the P_2 segment will have flow that is away from the probe.

19. **(D)** The genu segment of the CS will have bidirectional flow that has a low-resistance type waveform for a normal patient.

20. **(B)** ACA

21. **(A)** MCA

22. **(C)** PCA

23. **(C)** The VA can be insonated from the suboccipital window at an average depth of 55-90 mm with an average mean velocity of 38 cm/s ± 10 with flow going away from the probe.

24. **(D)** The angle of insonance during a TCD examination is always assumed to be 0 degrees.

25. **(B)** ACA normally has flow going away from the probe.

26. **(A)** P_1 segment of the PCA normally has flow going toward the probe.

27. **(A)** MCA normally has flow going toward the probe.

28. **(B)** BA normally has flow going away from the probe.

29. **(A)** OA normally has flow going toward the probe.

30. **(A)** tICA normally has flow going toward the probe.

31. **(B)** VA normally has flow going away from the probe.

32. **(C)** CS (genu segment) normally has bidirectional flow.

33. **(A)** The submandibular window is used to obtain the extracranial ICA velocity that is used to calculate the MCA/ICA ratio in patients with suspected vasospasm.

34. **(A)** When there is collateral flow through the ACoA in the presence of extracranial disease, the two main findings on TCD are a global increase in velocity within the ACA contralateral to the disease and reversed flow within the ACA ipsilateral to the disease.

35. **(C)** The waveform in Figure 3–31 represents the changes to flow direction and resistance that occur when the OA is providing collateral flow. The OA will reverse its flow direction from toward the probe to away from the probe and change to a more low-resistance waveform as it is now providing blood flow to the brain.

36. **(B)** Hyperemia is a typical response to patients being treated post SAH that results in elevated cerebral artery velocities.

37. **(C)** It is rare for vasospasm to occur early after a subarachnoid hemorrhage. Typically, the maximum degree of vasospasm occurs between 7 and 14 days post SAH.

38. **(A)** The VAs join intracranially to form the BA that bifurcates into the PCAs. These vessels are components of the posterior cerebral circulation.

39. **(A)** The ICA bifurcates intracranially into the MCAs and ACAs.

40. **(B)** A pulsed-wave, low-frequency transducer is needed for TCD examinations.

41. **(A)** The BA can be insonated from the suboccipital window at an average depth of 89-90 mm with an average mean velocity of 41 cm/s ± 10 with flow going away from the probe.

42. **(C)** MCA/ICA ratio is the most reliable way to distinguish between hyperemia and vasospasm in patients with SAH.

43. **(C)** Some patients have an inadequate transtemporal window. It may be possible to use the contralateral transtemporal window to complete the examination.

44. **(D)** An MCA/ICA ratio more than 3 indicates vasospasm over hyperemia.

45. **(B)** All of the following are findings associated with a stenosis of the cerebral arteries except for a global increase in velocity which usually indicates hyperemia or collateralized flow.

46. **(D)** The waveform in Figure 3–32 represents the MCA/ACA bifurcation that can be insonated from the transtemporal window at an average depth of 55-65 mm with bidirectional flow representing the ACA as flow away from the probe and the MCA as flow toward the probe.

47. **(C)** There is a focal increase in mean flow velocity within the MCA that is more than double which is consistent with a hemodynamically significant stenosis.

48. **(C)** The waveform in Figure 3–34 represents a normal ACA that can be insonated from the transtemporal window at an average depth of 60-80 mm with an average mean velocity of 50 cm/s ± 11.

49. **(D)** The main finding present on a TCD examination when there is collateral flow through the PCoA in the presence of extracranial disease is a global increase in velocity of the PCA on the ipsilateral side of the disease.

50. **(A)** The MCA has the highest incidence of occlusion resulting in a cerebrovascular accident.

Suggested Readings

1. Pellerito JS, Polak JF. *Introduction to Vascular Ultrasound.* 7th ed. Philadelphia, PA: Elsevier; 2020.

2. Kupinski AM. *Diagnostic Medical Sonography: The Vascular System,* 2nd ed. Baltimore, MD: Wolters Kluwer; 2017.

3. Katz ML, Alexandrov AV. *A Practical Guide to Transcranial Doppler Examination.* 1st ed. Littleton, CO: Summer Publishing, LLC; 2003.

4. Rumwell C, McPharlin M. *Vascular Technology: An Illustrated Review.* 5th ed. Pasadena, CA: Davies Publishing; 2017.

5. Aaslid R. *Transcranial Doppler Sonography.* New York, NY: Springer-Verlag/Wien; 1986.

6. Newell D, Aaslid R. *Transcranial Doppler.* New York, NY: Raven Press; 1992.

7. Lindegaard KF, Nornes H, Bakke SJ, et al. Cerebral vasospasm diagnosis by means of angiography and blood velocity measurements. *Acta Neurochir(Wien).* 1989;100(1–2):12–24.

8. Lindegaard KF. The role of transcranial Doppler in the management of patients with subarachnoid haemorrhage: a review. *Acta Neurochir Suppl.* 1999;72:59–71.

9. Aaslid R, Huber R, Nornes H. Evaluation of cerebrovascular spasm with transcranial Doppler ultrasound. *J Neurosurg.* 1984;60(1):37–41.

10. Fujioka KA, Nonoshita-Karr L. The effects of extracranial arterial occlusive disease. *J Vas Technol.* 2000;24(1):27–32.

11. Sloan MA, Alexandrov AV, Tegeler CH, et al. Therapeutics and Technology Assessment Subcommittee of the American Academy of Neurology. Assessment: transcranial Doppler ultrasonography: report of the Therapeutics and Technology Assessment Subcommittee of the American Academy of Neurology. *Neurology.* 2004;62(9):1468–1481.

12. Felberg RA, Christou I, Demchuck AM, et al. Screening for intracranial stenosis with transcranial Doppler: the accuracy of mean flow velocity thresholds. *J Neuroimaging.* 2002;12(9):9–14.

13. Baumgartner RW, Mattle HP, Schroth G. Assessment of ≥ 60% and 50% intracranial stenosis by transcranial color-coded duplex sonography. *Stroke.* 1999;30:87.

14. AIUM.org. Safety in diagnostic ultrasound educational activities using nonpregnant participants. Available online at https://www.aium.org/officialStatements/76https://www.aium.org/officialStatements/76. Accessed on May 23, 2020.

15. Nichols FT, Jones AM, et al. Stroke prevention in sickle cell disease (STOP) study guidelines for transcranial Doppler testing. *J Neuroimaging.* 2001;11(4):354–362.

4

Peripheral Arterial

PERIPHERAL ARTERIAL ANATOMY

Vessel Anatomy

The peripheral arteries are similar to the cerebrovascular arteries in that they contain a high intraluminal pressure and their role is to bring oxygenated blood from the heart to the surrounding tissues and structures. The blood flow is created by the pumping action of the heart. These arteries are also composed of the same three layers as the cerebrovascular arteries. These three layers, as mentioned earlier in Chapter 2, are the innermost layer (tunica intima), middle layer (tunica media), and outermost layer (tunica adventitia).

Lower Extremities

The abdominal aorta bifurcates in the pelvic region to become the right and left common iliac arteries. The common iliac arteries then bifurcate into the internal and external iliac arteries. The internal iliac arteries supply blood flow to the pelvic organs. The internal iliac arteries are also sometimes referred to as the hypogastric arteries. The external iliac arteries continue distally to supply blood flow to the lower extremities. As the external iliac arteries continue distally, they become the common femoral arteries (CFAs) just below the inguinal ligament. The CFA continues distally for a short distance and then bifurcates into the superficial femoral and profunda femoris arteries (PFAs) (Fig. 4–1). The PFA, also known as the deep femoral artery, courses posterior and lateral to the superficial femoral artery (SFA) as it descends in the thigh. Because of its posterior course, the PFA is typically only seen with ultrasound at its origin from the CFA. The superficial femoral continues distally as well and passes through the adductor canal. As the SFA passes through the adductor canal into the popliteal fossa, it becomes the popliteal artery. The popliteal artery continues distally for a short distance before bifurcating into the anterior tibial artery

(ATA) and tibioperoneal trunk (Fig. 4–1). The tibioperoneal trunk also continues for a short distance before it bifurcates into the posterior tibial and peroneal arteries. The ATA continues distally in the anterior compartment of the lower leg until it courses anterior to the ankle to become the dorsalis pedis artery (DPA). The posterior tibial artery (PTA) courses distally in the posterior compartment of the lower leg until it courses posterior to the medial malleolus, bifurcating into the medial and lateral plantar arteries. The peroneal artery courses distally along the medial aspect deep within the lower leg and eventually branches into multiple segments which communicate with the posterior and ATAs. The plantar arteries and DPAs lead to the plantar arch which gives off the metatarsal and digital arteries.

Upper Extremities

The aortic arch has three main branches, as mentioned in Chapter 2. The first and largest of the branches is the brachiocephalic, also known as the innominate artery. The brachiocephalic artery bifurcates into the right common carotid artery and the right subclavian artery. The second branch of the aortic arch is the left common carotid artery followed by the third branch which is the left subclavian artery. The vertebral arteries branch from the subclavian arteries shortly after the origin to provide blood flow to the brain. There are several other branches from the subclavian that provide blood flow to the thoracic region. The subclavian artery courses lateral posterior to the clavicle until it passes the outer border of the first rib where it becomes the axillary artery (Fig. 4–2). The axillary artery continues distally for a short distance and becomes the brachial artery. The brachial artery continues distally until just below the antecubital fossa where it bifurcates into the ulnar and radial arteries. The ulnar artery continues distally along the medial aspect of the forearm until it crosses to the ulnar side of the wrist where it becomes the superficial palmar arch, which is completed by a branch of the radial artery.

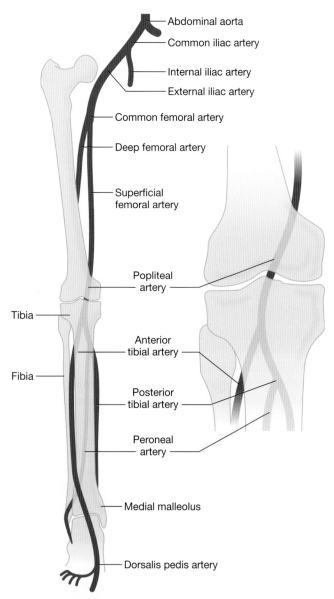

FIGURE 4–1. Illustration of lower extremity arteries. (Reproduced, with permission, from Tintinalli JE, Ma OJ, Yealy DM, et al. *Tintinalli's Emergency Medicine: A Comprehensive Study Guide,* 9th ed. New York, NY; 2020; Figure 44–4. Copyright © McGraw Hill.)

The radial artery courses distally along the lateral aspect of the forearm until it crosses to the lateral side of the wrist, toward the dorsum, and eventually joins the deep palmar branch of the ulnar artery to form the deep palmar arch. The deep and superficial palmar arches give rise to the digital arteries (Fig. 4–3).

PATHOLOGY OF THE PERIPHERAL ARTERIAL SYSTEM

Atherosclerosis Obliterans

Atherosclerosis (ASO) is the most common pathology and cause of obstruction in arteries. It describes a variety of conditions such as intimal thickening and the accumulation of plaque.

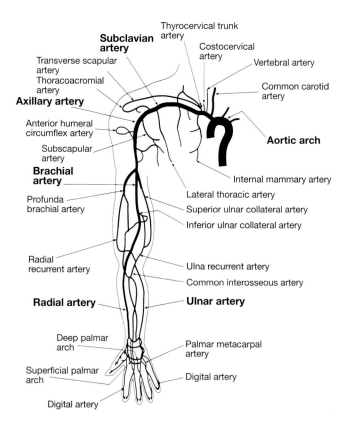

FIGURE 4–2. Illustration of the upper extremity arteries. (Reproduced, with permission, from Odwin CS, Fleischer AC. *Lange Review: Ultrasonography Examination,* 4th ed. New York, NY; 2012; Figure 14–6. Copyright © McGraw Hill.)

It most commonly affects the intimal and medial layers of the arteries and can lead to stenosis or occlusion. One of the most common sites for ASO to occur, other than the carotid system, is in the lower extremities. Common areas of ASO within the lower extremities include the distal superficial femoral-popliteal area as well as aortoiliac region and the popliteal trifurcation.

Thromboangiitis Obliterans

Thromboangiitis obliterans (TAO), also known as "Buerger's disease," is a type of arteritis that is caused by inflammation of the arterial walls which leads to thrombosis of the vessels. It is typically found in younger males and is associated with heavy cigarette smoking. It usually affects the distal arteries of the hands and feet but can be seen in conjunction with ASO of the larger arteries as well. It is often associated with other collagen vascular disorders.

Embolism

An embolism, as described earlier related to the cerebrovascular system, is a solid, liquid, or gas that can affect the peripheral arterial system by becoming lodged in the small arteries of the hands and feet. The most common type of embolus is plaque that breaks off and travels through the blood vessels. The source of emboli can be any area where plaque is present. Emboli to the hands or feet can result in ischemic changes to the fingers

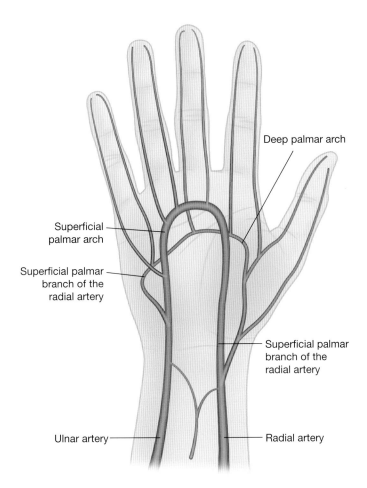

FIGURE 4–3. Illustration of the upper extremity hand arteries.

and the toes. Blue toe syndrome, in which the tips of the toes turn blue, is often the result of emboli.

Peripheral Aneurysm

An aneurysm is defined as a dilatation of the arterial walls. A peripheral aneurysm is typically a focal dilatation that is greater than 1.5x the size of the most proximal artery segment. Peripheral arterial aneurysms are relatively rare. The most common areas for them to occur are the popliteal, common femoral, or SFAs. Unlike abdominal aortic aneurysms, where the greatest clinical concern is the risk of rupture, with peripheral aneurysms the greatest clinical concern is emboli. The flow dynamic within the aneurysm leads to the formation of thrombus, in many cases making the aneurysm a source for embolization.

Pseudoaneurysm

A pseudoaneurysm is created by a hole in the artery wall that allows blood to flow out of the vessel into a confined area of surrounding tissue. Pseudoaneurysms, or false aneurysms, derive their name from the fact that unlike "true" aneurysms, which are outpouchings involving all three layers of the blood vessel wall, the pseudoaneurysm has no endothelial wall. The hole in

the artery is often iatrogenic, meaning the result of a procedure in which a catheter punctures the arterial wall, such as cardiac catheterization. If the hole fails to seal postprocedure, a pseudoaneurysm may form. The channel created from the hole in the artery to the patent portion of the pocket of flow is known as the "neck" of the pseudoaneurysm. The size of the neck may help predict success in nonsurgical treatments. Pseudoaneurysms often thrombose resulting in a hematoma. If they do not thrombose on their own, they can be treated with manual compression, thrombin injection, or surgical repair. Other rarer causes of pseudoaneurysms are infection and complications from intravenous drug abuse (IVDA).

Dissection

A dissection, as mentioned earlier in Chapter 2, is a tear in the intimal layer of an artery resulting in an intimal flap within the vessel lumen, often causing a false lumen. A dissection is most commonly caused by some type of trauma or severe hypertension. Invasive procedures performed on the lower extremity arteries can also be the cause of dissection.

Popliteal Entrapment

Popliteal artery entrapment syndrome is thought to be caused by compression of the popliteal artery by the head of the gastrocnemius muscle. It is usually seen in younger males and can be unilateral or bilateral. Over time, with continued compression of the popliteal artery, it can lead to thrombosis or atherosclerotic changes. Noninvasive testing for popliteal entrapment includes performing ankle-brachial indices and pulse volume recordings (PVRs) at rest and with plantar flexion and passive dorsiflexion (Figs. 4–4 and 4–5). With popliteal entrapment, there will an obvious reduction in pressures and waveforms during the maneuvers.

Compartment Syndrome

Compartment syndrome is a condition caused by extreme swelling within the osteofascial compartments of a limb. The swelling may become so severe that it may inhibit perfusion to that portion of the arm or leg, resulting in ischemia from extrinsic compression. Compartment syndrome is typically a clinical diagnosis with findings such as pain, numbness, weakness, and at later stages, absent or weak pulses. Common causes include revascularization after a prolonged ischemic event, and trauma causing bleeding within a compartment. The treatment for compartment syndrome is typically a fasciotomy, in which the skin and tissues of the affected compartment are surgically flayed open and left open to air until the swelling decreases. This radical procedure decreases the extrinsic pressure on the vessels and permits flow.

Thoracic Outlet Syndrome

Thoracic outlet syndrome (TOS) is a condition caused by compression of the subclavian artery, subclavian vein, or brachial

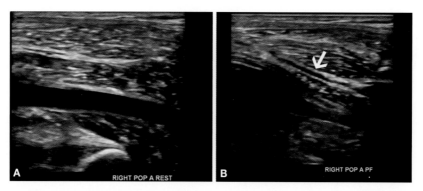

FIGURE 4–4 Grayscale of popliteal artery entrapment. **(A)** Popliteal artery at rest is widely patent. **(B)** Popliteal artery with plantar flexion reveals markedly reduced arterial diameter (arrow).

plexus by an extra cervical rib or thoracic musculature. The compression can involve the artery, vein, nerve, or a combination of the three with the majority affecting just the nerve. TOS is position dependent, meaning that the compression only occurs with the arm in a certain position. TOS is four times more common in women and usually affects people between 20 and 40 years of age. Treatments include thoracic and shoulder exercises and/or surgical removal of an extra cervical rib and muscle alteration.

Raynaud's Syndrome

Raynaud's syndrome is a vasospastic disorder in which the digital arteries of the fingers and/or toes go into spasm as a result of exposure to cold temperatures or high emotional conditions. Raynaud's syndrome can cause intermittent or permanent ischemia to the fingers and toes. Patients may experience either primary or secondary Raynaud's conditions. Primary Raynaud's (often called Raynaud's disease) typically results in intermittent symptoms and is considered idiopathic. With primary Raynaud's disease, the patient's digits change color when exposed to cold temperatures. Initially, they turn white followed by blue and then eventually turn red during the rewarming period.

Therefore, Raynaud's is sometimes referred to as a "patriotic disease" (Fig. 4–6). Secondary Raynaud's is the result of another disease process, such as scleroderma, and results in permanent symptoms. Secondary Raynaud's, sometimes called Raynaud's phenomenon, is also seen in combination with underlying obstructive disease. There are often ischemic changes, and tissue loss may occur with long-standing secondary Raynaud's disease.

Takayasu's Arteritis

Takayasu's arteritis is a relatively rare type of arteritis that affects the aortic arch and its large branches such as the brachiocephalic, common carotid, and subclavian arteries. The disease is most common in females under 40 and is more common in Asia.

Coarctation of Aorta

Coarctation of the aorta is a congenital condition that involves narrowing of the thoracic aorta. This condition may cause decreased blood flow to several areas of the body, including vital organs in the abdomen such as the kidneys as well as other areas like the lower extremities. It can cause hypertension and/or leg ischemia and the treatment is usually surgical repair.

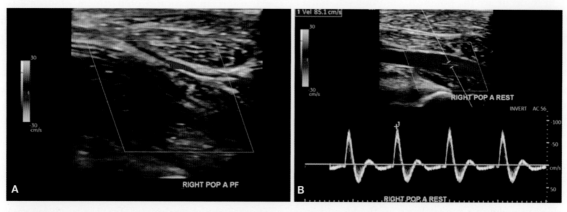

FIGURE 4–5 **(A)** Color Doppler of popliteal artery during plantar flexion with popliteal entrapment shows markedly reduced vessel size and little to no color flow. **(B)** Same popliteal artery at rest showing normal color and spectral flow.

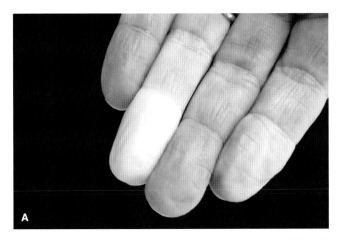

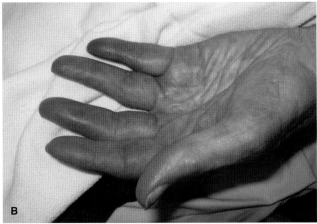

FIGURE 4–6. Primary Raynaud's. **(A)** Peripheral upper extremity digit turns white with cold or stress, followed by red and/or **(B)** blue coloration.

PATIENT ASSESSMENT AND INTEGRATION OF DATA

Risk Factors

One of the biggest risk factors that contributes to peripheral arterial disease, but is uncontrollable, is age. As a person's age increases, so does the likelihood of developing ASO. Other risk factors that contribute to the development of peripheral arterial disease are:

- Hypertension—Has been thought to contribute to the ASO process by producing excess strain on the walls of the arteries.
- Diabetes mellitus—Increases the likelihood of developing ASO. In the lower extremities, it can cause the medial layer of the arteries to become calcified. This is commonly referred to as arteriosclerosis, or "hardening of the arteries." Diabetics also have higher incidence of foot and toe lesions and often have difficulty with healing of these wounds, frequently resulting in infections and amputations.
- Hyperlipidemia—Also referred to as "high cholesterol," results in high lipid levels [low-density lipoproteins (LDL), triglycerides] in the blood which lead to an increase in ASO.
- Tobacco use—Damages the endothelial lining of blood vessels and contributes to ASO.

Signs and Symptoms

Chronic Occlusive Disease

The symptoms associated with chronic occlusive disease are very specific in nature and are very good indicators that vascular disease is present. The main symptoms that suggest that vascular disease is present are:

- Claudication—Defined as exercise-induced pain that is relieved by rest, it is caused by lack of adequate blood supply to an exercised limb. Claudication is considered a reproducible symptom, meaning that the patients can typically walk the same distance each instance before experiencing symptoms. In other words, a patient with "one block claudication" can consistently walk one block before having pain and needing to do rest. When the pain subsides, the patient can walk another block before resting again, and so on. Claudication symptoms can occur at various levels, such as the buttock, thighs, or calves, which usually indicates the probable level of disease. For example, buttock symptoms would indicate possible aortoiliac disease while thigh symptoms might suggest iliac or femoral disease and calf symptoms point to femoral-popliteal disease. In general, the more severe the peripheral arterial disease, the more severe the symptoms and the quicker they present with exercise.
- Ischemic rest pain—Associated with severe peripheral arterial disease, rest pain presents as severe pain in the most distal portion of the limb (usually the foot, toes, or heel) when the patient is at rest. The symptoms usually occur at night, in bed, when the patient's legs are at the level of the heart. The symptoms are typically relieved by the patient placing their legs in a dependent position, allowing gravity to facilitate return of blood flow to the feet. If the patient complains of leg pain in bed, which is only relieved by sitting up and dropping the legs down, that is a sign of ischemic rest pain. With ischemic rest pain, while supine, the patient's lower legs and feet are often pale. After the patient drops their legs down, they fill with blood and turn red, a common phenomenon referred to as "dependent rubor."

Acute Occlusive Disease

Acute symptoms are often the result of an acute event such as a spontaneous occlusion caused by thrombosis or an embolism. These types of events are considered limb threatening and should be treated emergently. The symptoms associated with acute occlusive disease are known as the six Ps. The six Ps include:

- Pain—Pain to the limb or foot. Usually, ischemic rest pain.
- Paralysis—Loss of muscular function to the limb. One of the signs of irreversible ischemia.
- Paresthesia —Sensation of numbness or tingling. Another sign of irreversible ischemia.
- Pallor—Pale color to the skin due to lack of blood flow to the limb.

- Pulselessness—No palpable pulses obtained.
- Poikilothermia—The inability to regulate one's body temperature. Limb is cold to the touch.

Clinical Assessment

The clinical assessment of patients with suspected peripheral arterial disease typically starts with evaluating the probability of ASO based on risks, symptoms, and physical findings. During this assessment, the technologist will ask questions regarding risk factors, and a physical examination will be performed. The physical examination should include an inspection of the limb for specific signs suggesting peripheral arterial disease such as skin changes, lack of hair growth, ulcerations, and tissue loss or gangrene. Skin color changes depend on the condition of the limb. Skin color changes can vary from pallor due to lack of blood supply, cyanotic (bluish discoloration) due to deoxygenated hemoglobin, or rubor (reddish discoloration) due to damaged dilated vessels. Other less specific findings such as a lack of hair growth can be a sign of peripheral arterial disease. Ulcerations caused by arterial disease are often isolated to the tibial area near the ankle. They are usually deep and very painful as compared to ulcerations caused by venous disease. They may also demonstrate difficulty healing in the presence of severe arterial insufficiency and may require revascularization in order to heal. In situations where there is little to no blood supply to the lower limb, there may be signs of necrosis and tissue loss which often results in a total or partial amputation of the foot or limb.

SEGMENTAL SYSTOLIC PRESSURES

Patient Positioning

Patients for segmental pressure studies should be changed into gown, leaving on only the underwear below the waist. Ideally, the room will be relatively warm to avoid vasoconstriction. The patient should be placed in a supine position with the extremities at around the same level as the heart to reduce the effects of hydrostatic pressure. The legs should be fully extended and in a relaxed position. The arms should be relaxed by each side. The

head may be slightly elevated for comfort. It is important to note that patients should be instructed to rest in the supine position for a minimum of 20 minutes before beginning the examination. This is to avoid inaccurate results due to reduced blood flow caused by exercise in a diseased limb.

Technique

Once the patient is in the proper position and has rested for the appropriate amount of time, the study begins by placing blood pressure cuffs at different levels of the arms and legs. There are different sized cuffs for the different areas of the limb. It is important to always use the most appropriately sized cuff to avoid a common artifact known as "cuff artifact." Cuff artifact is caused when the underlying limb is either too large or too small for the cuff size being used. In order to avoid cuff artifact, the cuff width must be ≥ 20% larger than the diameter of the underlying limb. If the cuff is too wide for the limb, it can result in a falsely low pressure reading. On the other hand, if the cuff is not wide enough for the limb, a falsely elevated pressure reading will result. The latter is more common in the lower extremities.

There are cuffs typically used for each level of the limb which will be appropriate for the majority of patients. Cuff sizes may also vary depending on the technique used. In the lower extremities, there is the option of using a three- or four-cuff technique. The three-cuff technique utilizes one larger thigh cuff, as opposed to the four-cuff technique which utilizes two smaller thigh cuffs. Both techniques utilize two cuffs below the knee, with one at the level of the calf and the other at the ankle (Fig. 4–7). There are specialized cuffs for the digits. The advantage to the three-cuff technique is that the thigh pressure reading is typically more accurate. This technique eliminates the cuff artifact that is often seen with the four-cuff technique due to the size of an average thigh. The cuff artifact that is often seen with the four-cuff technique usually results in a high thigh pressure reading that is 30 mm Hg higher than the highest brachial pressure. The advantage of the four-cuff technique is that it provides the ability to determine high and low thigh pressure readings, which can further differentiate the level of disease. The typical sized cuffs for the lower extremities are:

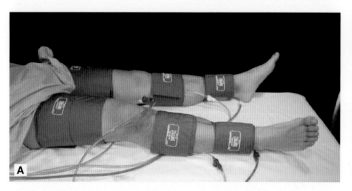
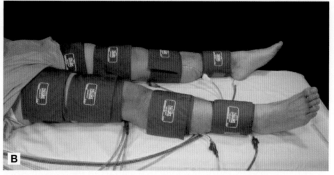

FIGURE 4–7. **(A)** Demonstrates the proper positioning and sizing of the lower extremity blood pressure cuffs using the three-cuff technique. **(B)** Demonstrates the proper positioning and sizing of the lower extremity blood pressure cuffs using the four-cuff technique. (Reproduced, with permission, from Odwin CS, Fleischer AC. *Lange Review: Ultrasonography Examination,* 4th ed. New York, NY; 2012; Figure 14–21. Copyright © McGraw Hill.)

- 12-cm cuff for high thigh and low thigh (four-cuff technique)
- 17- to 19-cm cuff for thigh (three-cuff technique)
- 10-cm cuff for calf and ankle

For upper extremity examinations, there are also typically sized cuffs for the different levels of the limb that will be appropriate for the majority of patients. Upper extremity examinations typically employ the use of three cuffs per arm at the levels of the upper arm, forearm, and wrist (Fig. 4–8). There are also specialized cuffs for the digits. The typical sized cuffs for the upper extremities are:

- 12-cm cuff for the upper arm
- 10-cm cuff for the forearm
- 5- to 10-cm cuff for the wrist

A lower extremity study typically starts with bilateral brachial systolic pressure measurements obtained using an 8- to 10-MHz continuous wave (CW) Doppler probe over the brachial artery. The highest of the two brachial pressures will be used later to calculate the pressure indices. All of the systolic pressure measurements are obtained by finding an audible Doppler signal from a reference artery, and then achieving full cessation of flow by inflating the cuff above the last audible signal. The cuff is then slowly deflated until the first audible signal returns,

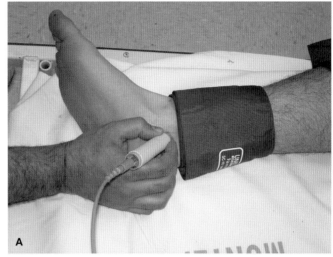

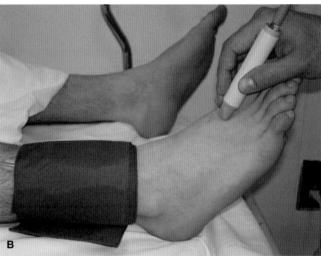

FIGURE 4–9. Demonstrates the proper technique for evaluation of the posterior tibial and dorsalis pedis arteries. **(A)** The posterior tibial is located medial and distal to the medial malleolus with the continuous wave (CW) Doppler probe at a 45-degree angle. **(B)** The dorsalis pedis is located on the anterior surface of the foot with the CW Doppler probe at a 45-degree angle. (Reproduced, with permission, from Odwin CS, Fleischer AC. *Lange Review: Ultrasonography Examination*, 4th ed. New York, NY; 2012; Figure 14–17. Copyright © McGraw Hill.)

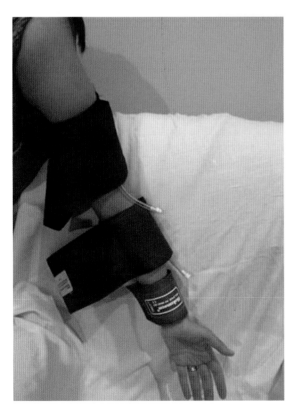

FIGURE 4–8. Demonstrates the proper positioning and sizing of the upper extremity blood pressure cuffs for a systolic segmental pressure and pulse volume recording study.

indicating the systolic pressure reading. Segmental systolic pressures are obtained and recorded, one leg at a time, starting at the ankle and working upward to the thigh one level at a time.

At the ankle level two pressures are obtained, one at the DPA and the other at the PTA (Fig. 4–9). Typically, the higher of the two pressures obtained is used as the reference artery for the remainder of the segmental pressures starting at the calf level. Usually, one systolic pressure reading is obtained at the calf and thigh levels. There are some protocols that require two pressures at the calf level (DPA and PTA). This is to further differentiate which vessels contain disease. It is important to note that at the higher levels in the leg (thighs), the pressure readings obtained are of the vessels which lie underneath the cuff and not the pressure of the reference artery used to obtain the audible Doppler signal.

Ankle Brachial Indices (ABI)					
Right	**mm Hg**	**Index**	**Left**	**mm Hg**	**Index**
Brachial	132		Brachial	139	
Ankle (Posterior tibial artery)	145	1.04	Ankle (Posterior tibial artery)	148	1.06
Ankle (Dorsalis pedis artery)	150	1.07	Ankle (Dorsalis pedis artery)	142	1.02
ABI:		**1.07**	**ABI:**		**1.06**

FIGURE 4–10. An example of how a normal ankle-brachial index is calculated by taking the higher of the two ankle pressures [posterior tibial artery (PTA) and dorsalis pedis artery (DPA)] and dividing that by the higher of the two brachial pressures.

Pressure indices are ratios that are calculated for each systolic pressure obtained at the different segments of the limb. These indices are a way of comparing the lower extremity pressures to the body's systemic blood pressure. They are calculated by taking the limb pressures and dividing them by the higher brachial pressure. The concept of pressure indices relates back to the Bernoulli principle which describes a drop in pressure distal to significant disease. This concept is described in more detail in Chapter 1. The most widely utilized of these indices is the ankle-brachial index (ABI). The ABI ratio should be calculated for both PTAs as well as both DPAs. When referring to an individual's ABI value, the higher of the two (DPA or PTA) is reported for each ankle. An example of how an ABI is calculated is shown in Figure 4–10.

The limitation of the ABI measurement is that it does not allow for determination of a level of disease. The segmental systolic pressures are utilized to attempt to further define the different levels of disease. In general, there should not be more than a 30 mm Hg drop in pressure between any two adjacent cuffs. A pressure drop more than 30 mm Hg would indicate significant disease proximal to the cuff with the lower pressure. A limitation to segmental pressures sometimes occurs when multiple levels of disease exists. This can occur when the proximal diseased segments cause a significant reduction in pressure to the distal segments which may have additional disease present and can result in a less than 30 mm Hg drop, thus masking the disease in the distal segment.

An upper extremity examination is conducted in the same fashion as a lower extremity examination. Both brachial artery systolic pressures are typically obtained first, with the higher of the two used to calculate the pressure indices. Pressures at the wrist are obtained for both the radial and ulnar arteries with each being used to obtain an audible Doppler signal via CW transducer. Usually, the higher of the two pressures is used as a reference artery to obtain the systolic pressure at the forearm. The ratios are calculated in the same matter as in the lower extremities. Similar to the lower extremity examination, segmental systolic pressures are evaluated for significant pressure gradients. In general, there should not be more than a 20 mm Hg pressure difference between any two adjacent cuffs. Also, when evaluating the upper extremities, the brachial pressures are compared to each other and there should also be less than a 20 mm Hg difference between the two upper extremities.

Limitations

The following are all considered limitations of segmental systolic pressure testing:

- Site-specific disease—Segmental systolic pressures cannot determine a specific type or location of a lesion; however, they can determine the general level of disease that is present. For example, pressure testing cannot diagnose a 75% stenosis in the external iliac artery; however, it can determine that aortoiliac disease is likely present.

- Cuff artifact—As described earlier, cuff artifact occurs when the cuff used is either too large or too small for the limb being tested. Cuffs that are too large will result in a falsely lower pressure reading that can lead to a false-positive reading. Cuffs that are too small, the more common type of the two, will result in a falsely elevated pressure reading that can result in a false-negative reading. Having a thorough understanding of this concept will reduce the chances of inaccurate interpretation.

- Calcified vessels—When patients have calcified vessels, falsely elevated pressure readings of noncompressible vessels result, which can lead to a false-negative reading. In these cases, the interpreter should rely more heavily on toe pressure readings, as these vessels are not affected by calcification. Both of these issues will be discussed in more detail later in this chapter. This is a common problem in diabetic patients because their arteries have a higher incidence of calcification.

- Multilevel disease—When multiple levels of disease exist, it is often times difficult to accurately interpret segmental systolic pressures. This is because there may not be a significant pressure gradient at the second level of disease. When significant proximal disease is present, it may mask the more distal disease in this fashion resulting in false negative results. It is important to note that these limitations such as cuff artifact, calcified vessels, and multilevel disease are limitations specific to segmental pressures and do not have the same effect on PVR waveforms. For this reason, we should rely more heavily on the waveform for accuracy when these limitations exist.

Interpretation of Results

The interpretation criteria for lower extremity pressure testing can vary between institutions. In general, the lower extremity limb pressures should be equal to or higher when compared to the highest brachial pressure; however, some criteria will consider a slight drop in pressure of 10 mm Hg when compared to the highest brachial as normal. Conversely, if the pressure reading in the limb is much higher than the highest brachial, it is considered falsely elevated and this is most likely due to calcified vessels or cuff artifact. Even though interpretation criteria can vary, Table 4–1 demonstrates widely utilized criteria for ABIs that can be used as a reference. There is no actual equivalent to the ABI when it comes to interpretation of upper extremity examinations. The general rule still applies that the wrist and forearm pressures should be equal to or higher than the higher brachial pressure.

When it comes to the interpretation of the segmental systolic limb pressures of the extremities, the following

TABLE 4–1 • (A) Common Resting Ankle-Brachial Indices Criteria for Severity of Peripheral Arterial Disease. (B) Represents a Common Modification to the Standard Criteria That Further Categorizes Abnormal Into Mild-to-Moderate and Severe Disease

A.

ABI	Interpretation
1–1.4	Normal
0.91–0.99	Borderline
< 0.90	Abnormal
> 1.4	Noncompressible

B.

Common Modifications to Criteria	
ABI	**Interpretation**
1–1.4	Normal
0.91–0.99	Borderline
0.41–0.90	Mild-to-moderate PAD
< 0.40	Severe PAD
> 1.4	Noncompressible

interpretive criteria is often utilized to consider the examination normal:

- 30 mm Hg or less difference between any two adjacent lower limb segment systolic pressures
- High thigh systolic pressure reading 30 mm Hg or more above the higher brachial systolic pressure (only applies to the four-cuff technique with 12-cm cuffs)
- 17- to 19-cm single thigh cuff systolic pressure reading equal to the higher brachial systolic pressure (only applies to the three-cuff technique)
- 20 mm Hg or less difference between any two adjacent upper limb segment systolic pressures
- 20 mm Hg or less difference between brachial systolic pressures

See Figure 4–11 showing normal segmental pressure examinations of the lower and upper extremities.

When there is a pressure gradient between two adjacent segments, the level of disease can be identified with the exception of the high thigh pressure, which does not have an adjacent cuff for comparison. In general, when the high thigh pressure is less than 30 mm Hg when compared to the higher brachial pressure, it indicates aortoiliac disease. A pressure gradient 30 mm Hg or more between the thigh and the calf indicates femoral-popliteal disease, and between the calf and the ankle indicates tibial disease (Fig. 4–12).

EXERCISE TESTING

Technique

Exercise testing is commonly performed on patients with claudication type symptoms when their resting studies are normal or close to normal. It can also be used to determine the severity of the effect of known vascular disease on an exercised limb. Protocols may vary slightly between institutions but usually consist of preexercise ABIs followed by walking on a treadmill at a speed of around 1.5-2 mph at an incline grade of 10%. The exercise is usually performed for a maximum of 5 minutes or until the symptoms become intolerable. Toe ups or other types of specialized exercise equipment can be used if the patient cannot walk on a treadmill. Once the exercise is stopped, the patient's postexercise ABIs are obtained immediately following and then every 2 minutes until they return to preexercise levels. When performing postexercise ABIs, it is only necessary to obtain a postpressure reading from the higher brachial pressure at rest.

Interpretation of Results

Exercise testing can be used to evaluate the severity of disease as well as whether there are single or multiple levels of disease. The normal response to exercise is an increase in pressure and

VPR

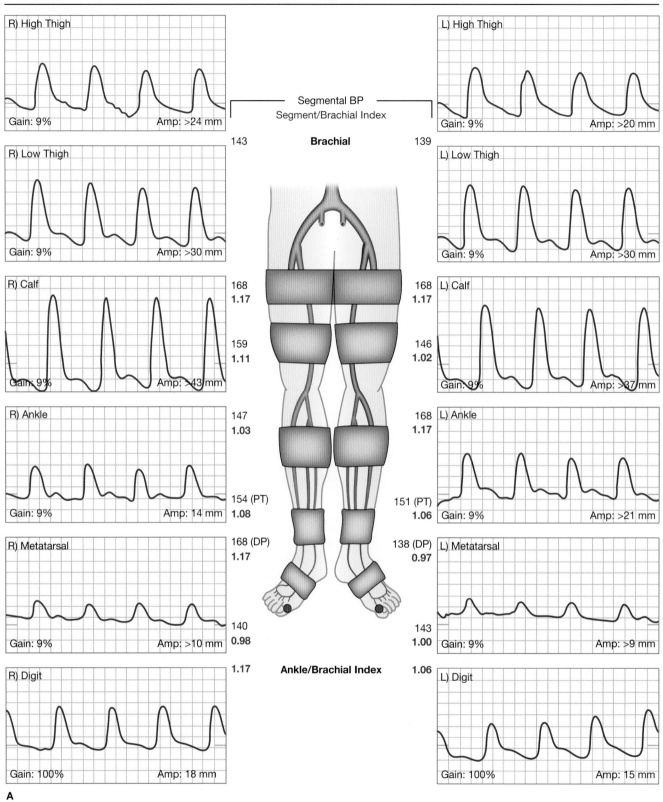

R) High Thigh
Gain: 9%   Amp: >24 mm

L) High Thigh
Gain: 9%   Amp: >20 mm

Segmental BP
Segment/Brachial Index

143   **Brachial**   139

R) Low Thigh
Gain: 9%   Amp: >30 mm

L) Low Thigh
Gain: 9%   Amp: >30 mm

R) Calf
Gain: 9%   Amp: >43 mm
168
1.17

L) Calf
Gain: 9%   Amp: >37 mm
168
1.17

159
1.11

146
1.02

R) Ankle
147
1.03

L) Ankle
168
1.17

154 (PT)
1.08

151 (PT)
1.06
Gain: 9%   Amp: >21 mm

R) Metatarsal
Gain: 9%   Amp: >10 mm
168 (DP)
1.17

138 (DP)
0.97
L) Metatarsal

140
0.98

143
1.00
Gain: 9%   Amp: >9 mm

1.17   **Ankle/Brachial Index**   **1.06**

R) Digit
Gain: 100%   Amp: 18 mm

L) Digit
Gain: 100%   Amp: 15 mm

A

FIGURE 4–11. **(A)** Shows a completely normal systolic segmental pressure and pulse volume recording study of the lower extremities.

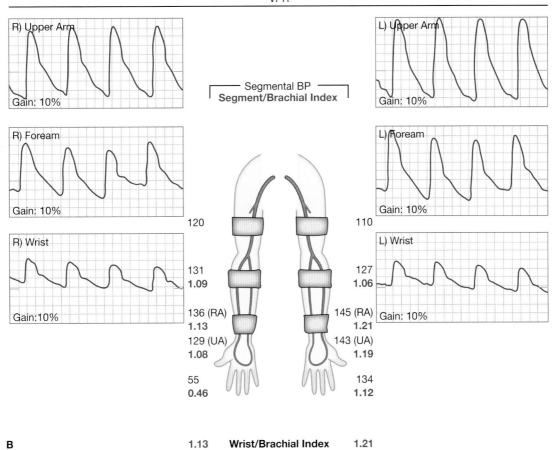

VPR

Segmental BP
Segment/Brachial Index

| R) Upper Arm | L) Upper Arm |
| Gain: 10% | Gain: 10% |

| R) Foream | L) foream |
| Gain: 10% | Gain: 10% |

120   110

| R) Wrist | L) Wrist |

131   127
1.09   **1.06**

136 (RA)   145 (RA)
1.13   **1.21**
| Gain:10% | Gain: 10% |
129 (UA)   143 (UA)
1.08   **1.19**

55   134
0.46   **1.12**

B   **1.13**   **Wrist/Brachial Index**   **1.21**

FIGURE 4–11. (*Continued*) **(B)** Shows a completely normal systolic segmental pressure and pulse volume recording study of the upper extremities.

ANALOG DOPPLER WAVEFORMS

Technique

Analog Doppler waveforms are obtained using the same 8- to 10-MHz CW Doppler probe used for obtaining the audible signal during segmental limb pressures. The analog Doppler waveforms are obtained from each specific site by placing acoustic gel on the CW Doppler probe and placing it on the area of interest. The CW Doppler probe should be angled approximately 45 degrees from

ABI readings. When the pressures drop below resting levels, it confirms that some degree of vascular disease is present. The larger the drop in pressure, the more severe the disease is. There is additional information that can be obtained related to the amount of time it takes for the postexercise pressure to recover. The length of recovery can suggest whether there is single level or multilevel disease. If the postexercise pressure returns to the preexercise level in less than 5 minutes, that indicates single level disease. When the recovery time is greater than 10 minutes, that indicates that multilevel disease is present.

Segmental BP					
Right	**mmHg**	**Index**	**Left**	**mmHg**	**Index**
Brachial	152	Index	Brachial	150	Index
High Thigh	201	1.32	High Thigh	178	1.17
Low Thigh	176	1.16	Low Thigh	194	1.28
Calf	136	0.89	Calf	131	0.86
Ankle (PT)	106	0.70	Ankle (PT)	106	0.70
Ankle (DP)	115	0.76	Ankle (DP)	107	0.70

← 40 mm Hg ▼ (Right, between Low Thigh and Calf)
← 30 mm Hg ▼ (Right, between Calf and Ankle)
← 40 mm Hg ▼ (Left, between Low Thigh and Calf)
← 30 mm Hg ▼ (Left, between Calf and Ankle)

FIGURE 4–12. Demonstrates abnormal systolic segmental pressures. Both sides show a significant (>30 mm Hg) pressure drop between the lower thigh and calf (femoral-popliteal disease) as well as between the calf and ankle (tibial disease). This would be considered multilevel disease bilaterally.

the surface of the skin to obtain a strong Doppler shift. Analog Doppler waveforms will be displayed either on the monitor or strip printer and should be stored for further analysis. For the lower extremities, the following Doppler waveforms are obtained:

- CFA
- SFA
- Popliteal artery
- PTA
- DPA

For examination of the upper extremities, the following waveforms are obtained:

- Subclavian artery
- Brachial artery
- Radial artery
- Ulnar artery

Interpretation of Results

The analysis of analog Doppler waveforms is usually of a qualitative nature in which the shape of the waveform determines if disease is present as well as its severity. CW Doppler waveforms can also be used to calculate quantitative measures such as pulsatility index; however, these measurements are usually reserved for PW spectral Doppler waveforms. Normal analog Doppler waveforms of the extremities are high-resistance waveforms that have bidirectional flow due to resistance in the distal arterial beds. The waveforms normally demonstrate a multiphasic shape with a rapid upstroke, rapid downstroke, short flow reversal toward the end of systole, and a return to forward flow. At times, the return to forward flow is lost, resulting in a bidirectional waveform. This is very common in older patients and the lack of resumed forward flow is due to the loss of elasticity of vessel walls (Fig. 4–13). When disease progresses to a certain point, resistance begins to decrease, and the CW Doppler waveforms will display monophasic forward flow. A unidirectional biphasic waveform usually suggests that mild disease is present

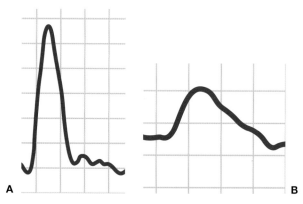

FIGURE 4–14. Analog Doppler waveforms. **(A)** Biphasic unidirectional. **(B)** Monophasic. Both have unidirectional flow and are consistent with the presence of peripheral arterial disease.

while monophasic waveforms suggest moderate to severe disease (Fig. 4–14). A monophasic waveform obtained at a specific site in an extremity typically indicates that there is disease proximal to this area; however, sometimes it can indicate more distal disease as well. Figure 4–15 shows an example of an analog Doppler waveform examination.

Controversies in Ultrasound

Up until recently, there has been a long-standing controversy regarding the terminology of monophasic, biphasic, and triphasic. Waveform terminology has been debated in vascular conferences and the published literature for decades. In 2020, a group of vascular professionals published an article: Interpretation of Peripheral Arterial and Venous Doppler Waveforms: A Consensus Statement from the Society for Vascular Medicine and Society for Vascular Ultrasound. This consensus officially defines waveforms by their morphology. The terms "triphasic" and "monophasic" have been replaced with "multiphasic." Multiphasic implies a waveform that crosses the baseline, now called the "zero-flow baseline," and "monophasic" implies a waveform that has forward flow throughout systole and diastole. The article also further defines "high-resistance" and "low-resistance" flow patterns. Unfortunately, this article came out during the editing process of this book, and the changes could not be reflected throughout. You are strongly encouraged to obtain a copy of this article from the *Journal of Vascular Ultrasound* or *Vascular Medicine*. Information can be found at the end of the chapter under "Suggested Reading."

PLETHYSMOGRAPHY—PULSE VOLUME RECORDINGS

Patient Positioning Up

PVRs are commonly performed in conjunction with segmental systolic pressures, so the positioning and patient preparation is the same.

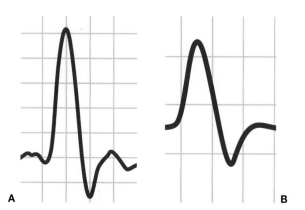

FIGURE 4–13. Analog Doppler waveforms. **(A)** Triphasic. **(B)** Biphasic bidirectional. Both have bidirectional flow and are consistent with normal peripheral artery flow.

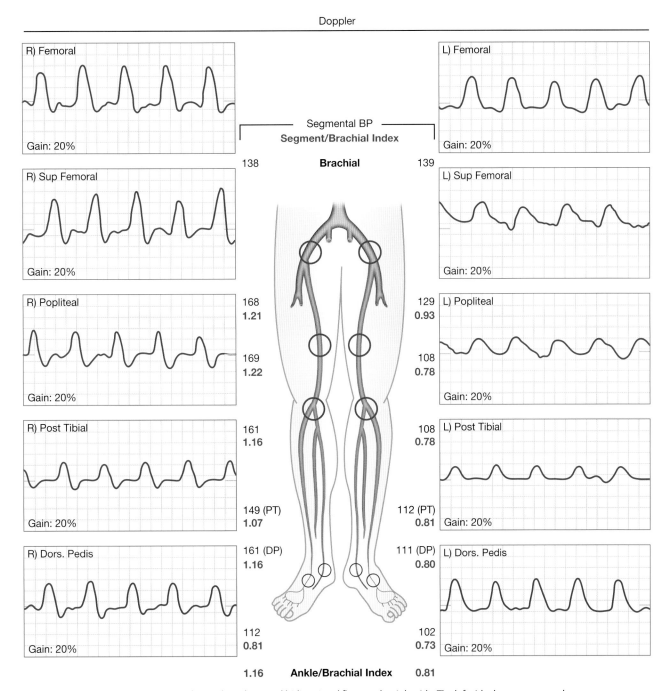

FIGURE 4-15. Analog Doppler study with normal bidirectional flow on the right side. The left side demonstrates a change to unidirectional and dampened flow throughout suggesting the presence of inflow disease of the iliac artery. The waveform becomes even more dampened at the level of the calf suggesting disease at the femoral-popliteal level as well.

Technique

PVRs are performed using the same cuffs as the segmental pressures so the PVR waveforms are acquired at the same levels, which include readings at one or two thigh levels, one calf, and one ankle level. Some lower extremity protocols include another reading at the metatarsal level. PVR waveforms represent the entire amount of perfusion through the underlying segment of the limb including collateral flow. Some of the limitations that exist with segmental pressures, such as cuff artifact

and calcified vessels, do not apply to PVR waveforms as they are not affected.

The cuffs are inflated one level at a time to a pressure that obstructs venous outflow and allows only arterial inflow to be measured. This is usually approximately 55-65 mm Hg. Through each full cardiac cycle, a volume of blood passes through the limb, producing a change in volume underneath each cuff. That change in volume is displayed as a waveform on the computer screen of the system. At each level, a waveform is stored for analysis.

Lower extremity examinations are typically initiated by obtaining a waveform at the calf level with the gain adjusted to allow the full waveform to be displayed. Once the gain is set, it should not be adjusted for the remainder of the examination so that the amplitude (size) of the waveforms can be compared to one another. The reason the calf waveform is obtained first is because in a normal patient the calf amplitude is usually the highest of the waveforms. It is important to note that this rule does not apply at the digit level where the gain is typically much higher due to the smaller change in volume that occurs in the small vessels. This will be discussed in more detail later in this chapter.

Upper extremity examinations are conducted in a similar fashion using the same cuffs as the segmental pressures to obtain PVR waveforms. The forearm waveform is typically obtained first and the gain is adjusted and set, then the remainder of the waveforms are obtained.

Limitations

Similar to segmental pressure readings, PVR waveforms cannot determine a specific type or location of a lesion; however, they can determine the general level of disease that is present. PVR waveforms also cannot distinguish between collateral flow and regular flow, which can lead to underestimation of disease. It is important to note that PVR waveforms are not affected by cuff artifact or calcified vessels thus making them a more reliable method of assessing arterial flow than segmental pressures. These two tests are commonly used together to provide as much diagnostic information as possible.

Interpretation of Results

When evaluating PVR waveforms, it is possible to look at qualitative (shape of waveform) measures as well as quantitative (amplitude of waveforms) measures. There are other factors that can affect the amplitude of the waveform without affecting the shape of the waveform, so in general the qualitative measures are used for interpretation. The following categories are defined for the interpretation of PVR waveforms:

- Normal—Rapid upstroke, sharp peak, dicrotic notch present
- Mild PAD—Rapid upstroke, absent dicrotic notch with bowing downstroke
- Moderate PAD—Delayed upstroke and downstroke, absent dicrotic notch
- Severe PAD—Low to no amplitude, upstroke, and downstroke of equal timing

See Figure 4–16 for an example of each category.

Figure 4–17 shows an example of a patient with normal PVR waveforms and segmental systolic pressures on the left side. On the right, there is a decreased pressure in the low thigh cuff resulting in a more than 30 mm Hg pressure gradient with dampened PVR waveforms from the right calf down suggesting femoral-popliteal disease.

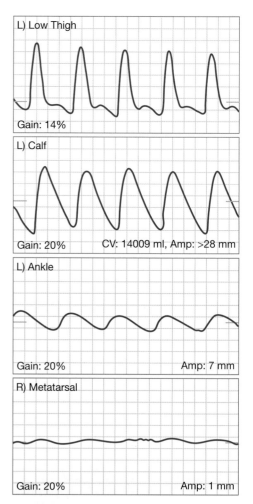

FIGURE 4–16. Categories of disease characterized by pulse volume recording waveforms. From top to bottom: Normal, mild peripheral arterial disease (PAD), moderate PAD, severe PAD.

DIGITAL PLETHYSMOGRAPHY

Technique

Digital plethysmography can be utilized to obtain waveforms that represent blood flow as well as systolic pressure measurements. Air cuff PVRs or photoplethysmography (PPG) sensors can be used to obtain digital waveforms. PPG is the most widely used method for assessing the digits due to its convenience and ease of use. The PPG sensor transmits infrared light into the body and detects differences in the reflected light as blood flows through an area, displaying the reflections as a waveform. The PPG sensor is held in contact with the skin using double-sided tape, straps, or clips designed for this purpose. The waveform shape mimics that of a normal PVR waveform with a rapid upstroke, sharp peak, and dicrotic notch (Fig. 4–18). PPG waveforms of the digits are commonly performed in conjunction with PVR waveforms and segmental pressures on the lower and upper extremities. The specific digits from which waveforms are obtained are typically determined by protocol and indication. For example, with a standard lower extremity examination, it is common to only obtain PPG waveforms and pressures of the great toe (first digit) as part of a routine protocol.

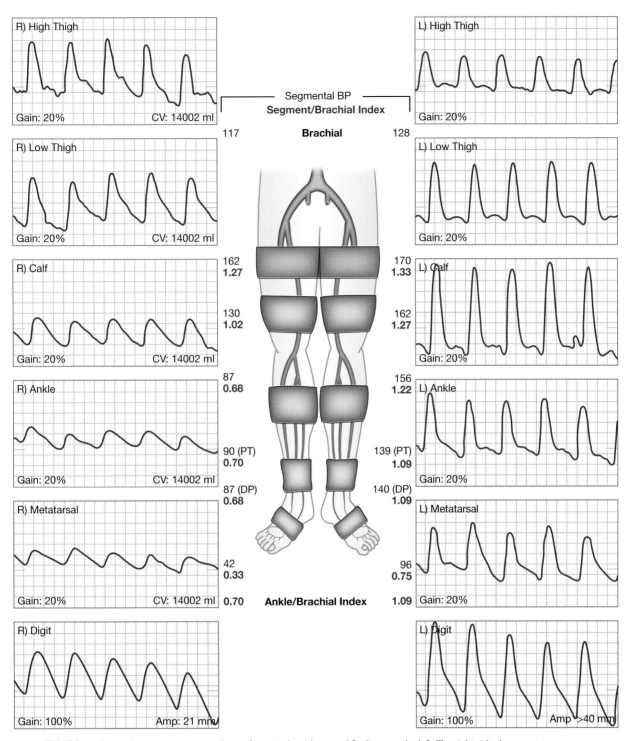

FIGURE 4–17. Noninvasive pressure and waveform study with normal findings on the left. The right side demonstrates a significant (>30 mm Hg) decrease in pressures between the high thigh and low thigh as well as between the low thigh and calf resulting in abnormally low pressure indices. The findings correlate with the dampened PVR waveforms suggesting the presence of femoral-popliteal disease.

It is also possible to obtain systolic pressure readings from the digits using a PPG sensor. A special sized cuff (usually 2–3 cm) is placed at the base of the digit with the PPG sensor at the tip. Once a PPG waveform is established, the cuff is inflated until flow ceases, the cuff is then slowly deflated until the first return pulse is seen and recorded as the systolic pressure.

Limitations

Limitations of digital plethysmography testing include:

- Cold temperatures—Cold temperatures can cause vasoconstriction of the digital vessels resulting in falsely abnormal findings. This limitation can be avoided by assuring the patient's hands or feet are kept at a warm temperature.

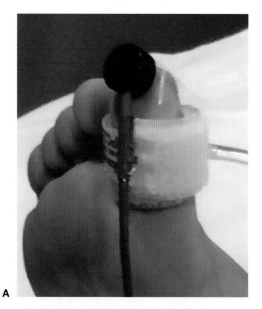

A

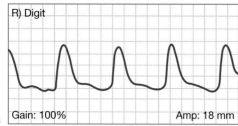

B

FIGURE 4–18. **(A)** Demonstrates the proper placement of the photoplethysmography (PPG) sensor and digital blood pressure for digital artery evaluation. **(B)** Represents a normal digital PPG waveform.

- Skin contact—The PPG sensor requires good contact with the skin surface to provide the best results. Lack of skin contact can diminish the waveforms and may also result in falsely abnormal findings.
- Ulcerations/tissue necrosis—Ulceration, tissue loss, or gangrene can prevent proper placement of the PPG sensor making it impossible to obtain pressures or waveforms from those particular digits.

Interpretation of Results

PPG waveform analysis is similar to the evaluation of PVR waveforms. A normal digital waveform obtained using a PPG sensor should have all the same characteristics as a normal PVR waveform including rapid upstroke, sharp peak, and dicrotic notch present. The categories of disease described earlier related to PVR waveforms also apply to digital PPG waveforms.

Digital waveforms can also be utilized to perform a modified Allen's test to evaluate the effect of harvesting the radial artery for surgery or for use of the radial artery in the creation of an arteriovenous fistula (AVF) for dialysis. With the PPG sensor placed on the second and third digits, one at a time, the radial artery is manually compressed at the level of the wrist and flow in the digits is monitored. If there is any noticeable reduction in

flow with the radial artery compressed, then it is likely that the hand will become symptomatic following surgery.

The digital pressure in the lower extremities can also be used to calculate a pressure index similar to the ABI. This index is known as the toe-brachial index, or TBI, and is calculated in the same manner as the ABI. The toe pressure is divided by the higher of the two brachial pressures to obtain the TBI on each side. A normal TBI value is 0.8 or more. Some criteria allow for a lower normal TBI value; however, 0.8 is a well-accepted standard in most vascular laboratories. TBIs can be especially useful when the ankle pressures are falsely elevated or noncompressible. In addition to evaluating the TBI, it is also important to evaluate the absolute pressure obtained from the toe. This can provide important information to the surgeon in terms of the ability of the limb to heal following surgery. Typically, a pressure of 50 mm Hg or more is sufficient for healing.

> **Note about: TBIs**
>
> TBIs are often referred to as the most accurate pressure ratios obtained during a lower extremity examination because the smaller digital vessels are usually spared from the calcification that can occur in the larger arteries. This is a common problem with diabetic patients. They can even be used as a substitute when exercise testing is performed on these patients for a more accurate assessment.

In the upper extremities, it is also possible to obtain digital pressures as well as calculate a digital-brachial index (DBI). DBIs are calculated in the same fashion as the ABIs and TBIs. A normal DBI for the upper extremity digits is 0.8 or more. Digital pressure can be used to determine if an AVF is causing ischemic symptoms by stealing blood flow from the hand. When performing digital pressures in patients with an AVF, the study should show reduced digital pressures that double when the fistula is compressed. Digital pressures that do not double with the fistula is compressed are consistent with an AVF steal and should be corrected to avoid further ischemia to the hand. Digital pressures and ratios can also be utilized to evaluate specific diseases of the upper extremities such as TOS and Raynaud's syndrome. The specific type of testing used for these diseases will be discussed in detail later in this chapter.

PERIPHERAL ARTERIAL DUPLEX

Patient Positioning

The patient positioning for a lower extremity arterial duplex examination is virtually the same as for a venous duplex examination. The patient is typically placed in the supine position with the leg of interest slightly bent at the knee and externally rotated (Fig. 4–19).

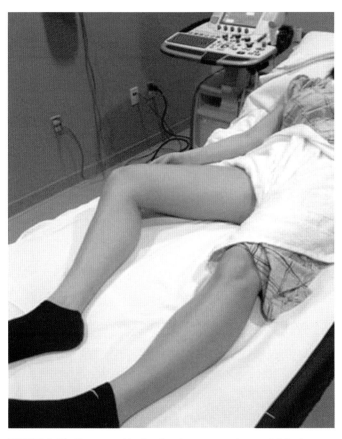

FIGURE 4–19. Proper positioning for a lower extremity arterial duplex examination with the patient supine and the limb externally rotated with the knee slightly bent.

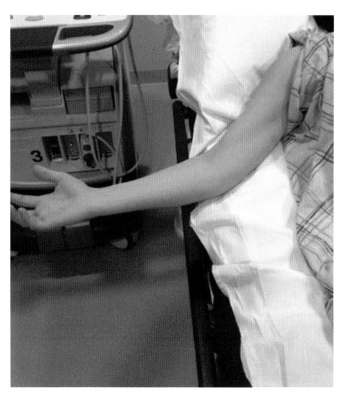

FIGURE 4–20. Proper positioning for an upper extremity arterial duplex examination with the patient supine and the limb externally rotated and abducted.

The same applies for the upper extremity arterial duplex when compared to the positioning for a venous duplex. The patient is typically placed in the supine position with the arm of interest slightly externally rotated and abducted (Fig. 4–20).

Technique

Lower Extremities

Protocols for peripheral arterial duplex can vary between institutions but most will include evaluation of the aortoiliac region and the full range of lower extremity arteries from the groin to the foot. They are also usually done in conjunction with ABIs or even full segmental pressures and PVRs. Duplex of the aortoiliac region will be discussed in Chapter 6.

Typically using a 5- to 7-MHz linear transducer, arterial duplex examinations utilize a combination of 2D grayscale imaging, color/power Doppler, and PW spectral Doppler to assess the lower extremity arteries. 2D grayscale imaging is used to visualize the vessel walls and identify any abnormalities such as atherosclerotic plaque or wall defects. Color Doppler can be used to identify any areas of narrowing within the artery and can also serve as a guide for the PW sample volume in order to obtain the highest velocities. The majority of the examination is performed in the longitudinal plane; however, transverse views can be used to identify certain pathologies such as aneurysms

or to further evaluate the degree of narrowing in the presence of plaque. PW Doppler waveforms should be obtained with peak systolic velocity (PSV) measurement from every major artery and the proximal, mid, and distal segments of longer arteries such as the SFA, PTA, ATA, and peroneal artery. When a stenosis is seen, additional PW Doppler waveforms should be obtained from the prestenotic region, at the region of the stenosis, and the poststenotic region. If an aneurysm is suspected, then anterior–posterior (AP) and transverse measurements should be obtained.

Following evaluation of the aortoiliac region, the examination should continue below the level of the inguinal ligament where the external iliac artery becomes the CFA and can be appreciated. The transducer is then moved distally to where the CFA bifurcates into the SFA and the PFA (Fig. 4–21). The PFA is usually only followed distally for a few centimeters before it dives deep into the thigh and can no longer be visualized. The SFA is followed distally along the medial aspect of the thigh for its entire course until it passes the adductor canal where it becomes the popliteal artery (Fig. 4–22). To visualize the popliteal artery, the transducer is rotated to the posterior area behind the knee known as the popliteal fossa. The popliteal artery is followed distally until it bifurcates into the ATA and the tibioperoneal trunk (Fig. 4–23). The ATA is then followed along the lateral aspect of the calf for its entire course to the dorsum of the foot where it becomes the DPA. The PTA is followed its

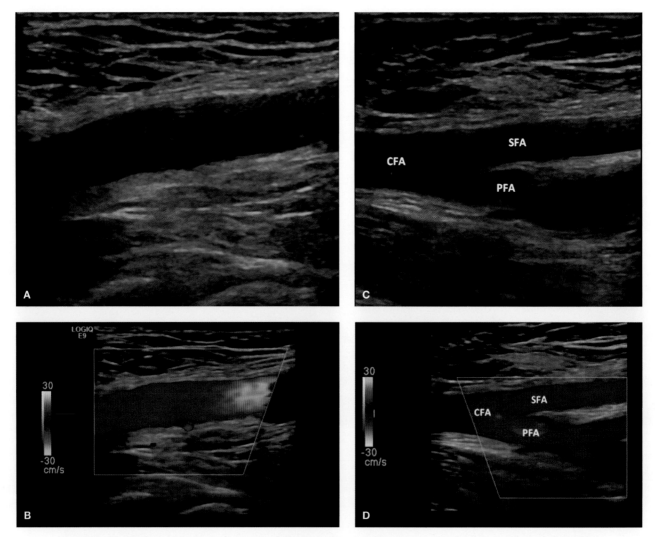

FIGURE 4–21. (A) 2D grayscale image of the common femoral artery. **(B)** Color Doppler image of the common femoral artery. **(C)** 2D grayscale image of the bifurcation into the superficial femoral and profunda femoris arteries. **(D)** Color Doppler image of the bifurcation into the superficial femoral and profunda femoris arteries.

entire length along the medial aspect of the calf down to the ankle. The peroneal artery can be visualized from a posterior medial approach and should also be followed distally for its entire course (Fig. 4–24).

Upper Extremities

An upper extremity duplex examination typically utilizes a 5- to 7-MHz linear array transducer to obtain images of the upper extremity arteries. The subclavian and axillary arteries can sometimes be deeper depending on the patient's body habitus and may require a lower frequency curvilinear transducer. Identical to the lower extremity, upper extremity duplex utilizes a combination of 2D grayscale imaging, color/power Doppler, and PW spectral Doppler to assess the upper extremity arteries. PW Doppler waveforms should be obtained with PSV measurements from every major artery and the proximal, mid, and distal segments of longer arteries such as the brachial artery, radial artery, and ulnar artery. In the presence of a stenosis, additional

PW Doppler waveforms should be obtained from the prestenotic region, at the area of the stenosis, and the poststenotic region. If an aneurysm is suspected, then the AP and transverse measurements should be obtained.

An upper extremity duplex examination typically starts with visualization of the subclavian artery from a supraclavicular approach in the area of the sternal notch. From the same approach, it may also be possible to visualize the brachiocephalic artery, which gives rise to the right subclavian artery on the right side. At times, it may only be possible to visualize the subclavian artery from the infraclavicular approach, making it difficult to evaluate the origin of the artery. The subclavian artery is then followed laterally past the first cervical rib where it becomes the axillary artery. The axillary artery is followed through the axilla where it eventually becomes the brachial artery. The brachial artery is followed along the medial aspect of the upper arm for its entire course to the antecubital fossa (Fig. 4–25). Just below the antecubital fossa, the brachial artery

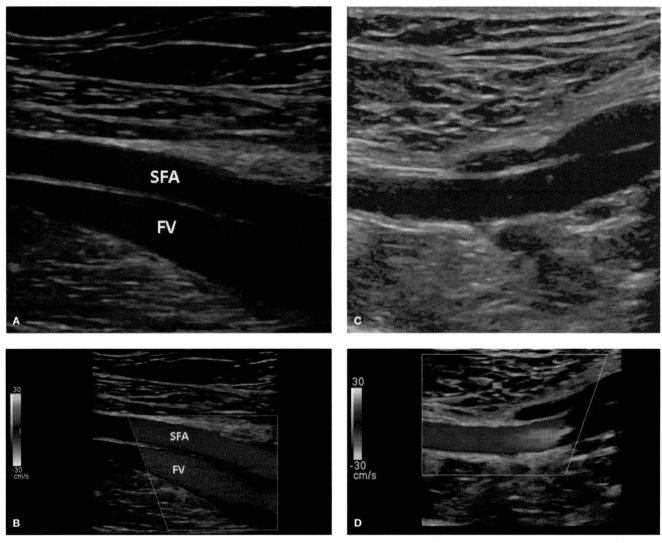

FIGURE 4–22. **(A)** 2D grayscale image of the superficial femoral artery and femoral vein. **(B)** Color Doppler image of the superficial femoral artery and femoral vein. **(C)** 2D grayscale image of the popliteal artery. **(D)** Color Doppler image of the popliteal artery.

bifurcates into the radial and ulnar arteries. The radial artery is followed along the lateral aspect of the forearm to the wrist. The ulnar artery is followed along the medial aspect of the forearm to the wrist (Fig. 4–26).

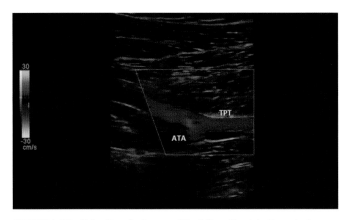

FIGURE 4–23. Color Doppler image of the bifurcation into the anterior tibial artery and tibioperoneal trunk.

Limitations

The limitations of arterial duplex of the extremities include:

- Body habitus—As with any ultrasound examination, lack of penetration due to a large body habitus can cause areas not to be visualized thus limiting the examination.
- Perfusion—Duplex ultrasound can diagnose a specific site of disease; however, it cannot assess the amount of perfusion to the lower extremity produced by collateral vessels. For this reason, arterial duplex is usually performed in combination with PVRs and pressure testing which can assess overall perfusion.
- Calcified plaque—May hide underlying disease due to distal shadowing.
- Access to anatomy—Dressings, braces, and intravenous (IV) lines are just some of the examples of items that can obstruct access to the anatomy being imaged. Any overlying jewelry should be removed.

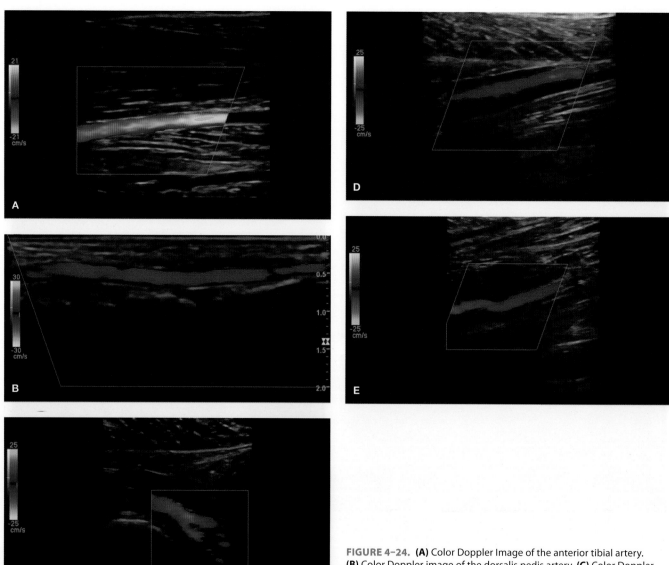

FIGURE 4–24. **(A)** Color Doppler Image of the anterior tibial artery. **(B)** Color Doppler image of the dorsalis pedis artery. **(C)** Color Doppler image of the bifurcation of the peroneal artery and posterior tibial artery. **(D)** Color Doppler image of the posterior tibial artery. **(E)** Color Doppler image of the peroneal artery.

- Technologist technique—Ultrasound is a modality that is very operator dependent and the results are only as accurate as the skill level of the sonographer performing the examination. Improper Doppler angle can cause over- or underestimation of disease; inability to properly identify the highest velocity within a stenosis can cause underestimation of disease, and inability to recognize changes in waveform characteristics can cause a missed diagnosis.

Interpretation of Results

B-Mode Findings

Normal B-mode grayscale images of the upper and lower extremity arteries should demonstrate smooth vessel walls with no evidence of thickening or plaque. The vessel should be free of internal echoes and vessel size should be unremarkable

(Fig. 4–27). Abnormal findings consist of intimal wall thickening as well as the presence of plaque. Plaque in the vessel will appear as either heterogeneous or homogeneous material invading the vessel lumen which can often show dense calcification with distal shadowing, making it difficult to visualize the underlying vessel lumen (Fig. 4–28). An occlusion is identified when the entire lumen is filled with this material. Color and power Doppler should also be used to identify a complete occlusion. The vessel size can also be assessed with grayscale imaging, typically in the transverse plane. A vessel is considered aneurysmal when there is a focal dilation greater than 50% the size of a normal segment (Fig. 4–29). Thrombus can often be appreciated along the side of the vessel walls within the aneurysm.

Color Doppler Findings

Normal color Doppler findings should show a laminar type flow pattern. In the presence of stenosis, color aliasing will occur and

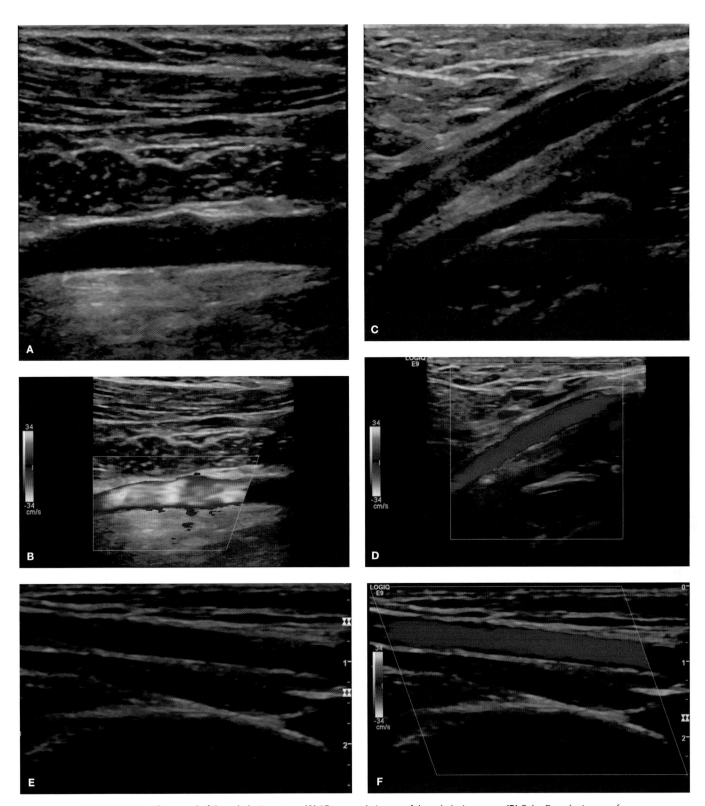

FIGURE 4–25. Ultrasound of the subclavian artery. **(A)** 2D grayscale image of the subclavian artery. **(B)** Color Doppler image of the subclavian artery. **(C)** 2D grayscale image of the axillary artery. **(D)** Color Doppler image of the axillary artery. **(E)** 2D grayscale image of the brachial artery. **(F)** Color Doppler image of the brachial artery.

color filling will only be visualized in the narrowed lumen of the artery. Color Doppler should be used as a guide for PW Doppler sample volume placement in order to measure the highest velocity through a stenotic lesion.

PW Doppler Findings

PW Doppler findings should be evaluated for changes in velocity as well as changes in contour as both may be affected by disease and can provide valuable information. A normal spectral

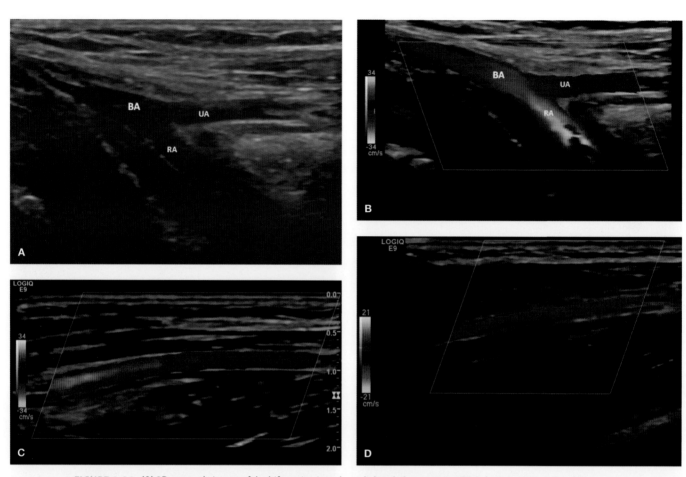

FIGURE 4–26. **(A)** 2D grayscale image of the bifurcation into the radial and ulnar arteries. **(B)** Color Doppler image of the bifurcation into the radial and ulnar arteries. **(C)** Color Doppler image of the radial artery. **(D)** Color Doppler image of the ulnar artery.

waveform obtained using PW Doppler of the upper and lower extremities should be high resistance with multiphasic laminar flow. This classic waveform should have a rapid upstroke, sharp peak, rapid downstroke, flow reversal caused by distal resistance, and flow returning above the baseline before the end of diastole. This last component of flow returning above the baseline is sometimes absent, resulting in a waveform that is still considered normal. The waveform should also display a clear spectral window underneath the peak systolic waveform, representing laminar flow (Fig. 4–30). Any time the distal resistance is lower, there will be obvious changes to the spectral waveform contour typically observed as monophasic flow. This scenario occurs postexercise or with significant arterial disease. The biggest difference between these two scenarios is that with significant disease, a delayed rise to peak systole will be appreciated that is not present in the postexercise waveform (Fig. 4–31). The following are other waveform changes that occur in the presence of significant arterial disease and are of importance:

- Spectral broadening—Spectral broadening occurs in the presence of turbulent flow, which is commonly seen at the exit point of a stenosis. This appears on a spectral waveform as a filling in of the spectral window underneath the peak systolic flow (Fig. 4–32).
- Poststenotic turbulence—A poststenotic turbulent (PST) waveform is seen just distal to a significant stenosis. This waveform demonstrates an ill-defined spectral border with spectral broadening and represents the turbulent flow following a significant stenosis (Fig. 4–33).

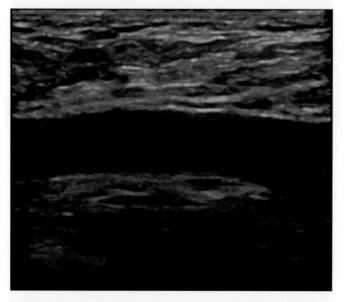

FIGURE 4–27. 2D grayscale image of a normal peripheral artery with no evidence of disease.

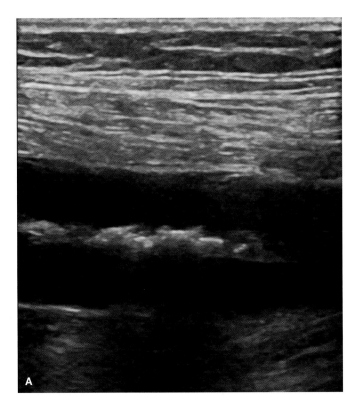

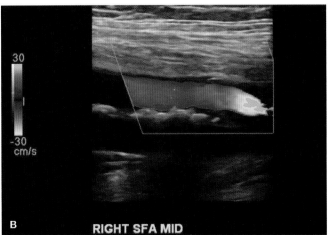

FIGURE 4–28. **(A)** 2D grayscale of a peripheral artery with the presence of calcified atherosclerotic plaque on the posterior wall with distal shadowing. **(B)** Color Doppler image showing the blood flow traveling through the narrowed lumen around the plaque.

- Preocclusive—A preocclusive waveform is seen just proximal to a complete or near complete occlusion. This waveform shows an abnormally high-resistance waveform with only forward flow in systole and no diastolic flow (Fig. 4–34).

PSV is the main factor used to determine the degree of stenosis in the extremities. There are some differences between the lower and upper extremities. For upper extremity duplex, there is no official criteria for the diagnosis of percent stenosis. A stenosis can be inferred by the presence of a focal increase in velocity (usually doubling compared to an adjacent segment proximal) followed by poststenotic turbulence and dampened flow more distally. While there are different diagnostic velocity criteria for

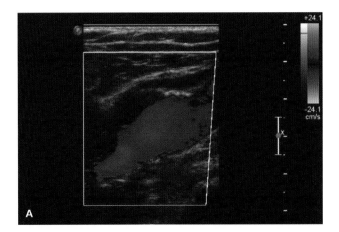

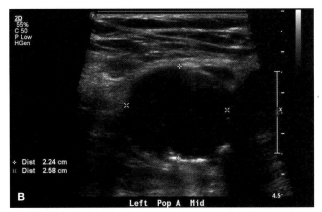

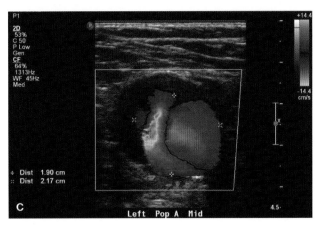

FIGURE 4–29. **(A)** Longitudinal Color Doppler image demonstrating a focal dilatation of the popliteal artery indicating a peripheral artery aneurysm. **(B)** Transverse 2D grayscale image of the same aneurysm demonstrating a maximum diameter of 2.58 cm. **(C)** Transverse Color Doppler image demonstrating a layer of intraluminal thrombus within the aneurysm with measurement of the true or patent lumen.

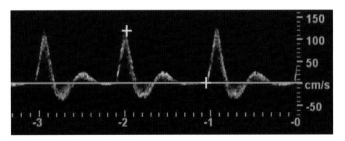

FIGURE 4–30. Bidirectional triphasic spectral PW Doppler waveform found in normal peripheral arteries.

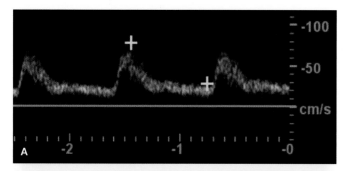

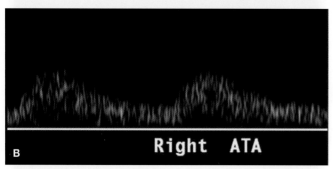

FIGURE 4–31. (A) Monophasic spectral PW Doppler waveform found in peripheral arteries when the distal arteriole beds dilate such as with exercise. **(B)** Monophasic spectral PW Doppler waveform that has a delayed rise to peak systolic known as "tardus parvus." This type of waveform suggests the presence of more proximal disease.

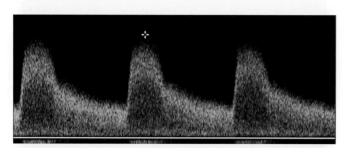

FIGURE 4–32. Monophasic spectral PW Doppler waveform that has filling in the spectral window a finding known as spectral broadening that is seen when turbulent flow is present.

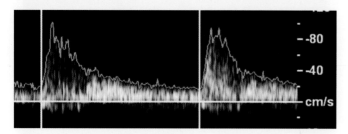

FIGURE 4–33. Spectral PW Doppler waveform that is found just distal to a stenosis known as a poststenotic turbulent waveform. This type of waveform exhibits spectral broadening, ill-defined spectral borders and reversal of flow.

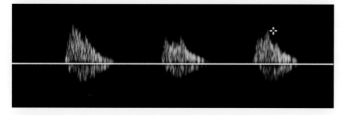

FIGURE 4–34. Monophasic spectral PW Doppler waveform with no diastolic flow is suggestive of a distal occlusion.

PSV ratio (V$_r$) = PSV at stenosis (V$_1$) / PSV proximal to stenosis (V$_2$)

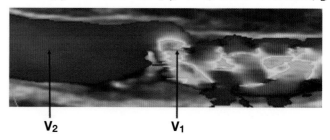

FIGURE 4–35. Demonstrates how to calculate the peak systolic velocity ratio when determining the percent stenosis.

the lower extremities, the use of the PSV ratio (V$_r$) is a widely accepted method for determining the percent stenosis. The peak systolic V$_r$ is calculated by taking the highest PSV through the stenosis and dividing it by the PSV obtained just proximal to the stenosis (Fig. 4–35). Table 4–2 shows the classification of arterial disease in the lower extremities using the PSV ratio.

OTHER ARTERIAL TESTING

Testing for Vasculogenic Impotence

Patient with significant occlusive disease in the aortoiliac area can have poor blood flow to the penis making it difficult or impossible to achieve an erection. This condition is known as vasculogenic impotence. Noninvasive testing can be performed in order to determine if lack of blood flow is the cause of the patient's impotence. There are both imaging and nonimaging techniques that can be used to evaluate blood flow to the penis.

Penile Pressures and Waveforms

Obtaining penile pressures and waveforms of the penis is a non-imaging technique utilized to determine if the blood flow to the penis is adequate. The examination uses a similar cuff technique as that used during the digital examination of the toes. The average cuff size used for penile examinations is 2.5 cm and cuffs can vary in length from 9 to 12 cm. Waveforms are obtained utilizing volume plethysmography (PVR) or PPG. The waveform analysis and categories of disease are the same as those used for the lower

TABLE 4–2 • Classifications of Arterial Disease Using Peak Systolic Velocity Ratio		
Description	**Percent Stenosis**	**PSV Ratio (V$_r$)**
Normal or mild	< 50%	< 2.2
Moderate	50–69%	> 2.0
Severe	70–99%	> 3.0
Occluded	Occluded	No flow

extremities. Penile systolic pressure can also be obtained in the same manner as the extremities using either an 8- to 10-MHz CW Doppler probe to obtain an audible signal or by utilizing the PPG waveform. This study is typically done in conjunction with a lower extremity pressure study. A penile-brachial index is then calculated in the same manner as an ABI. Typically, a PBI that is less than 0.65 is consistent with vasculogenic impotence. The following are the ranges seen with PBIs:

- Normal—0.75 or more
- Marginal—0.65 to 0.74
- Abnormal—less than 0.65

Penile Duplex

During a penile duplex examination, the penile vasculature is imaged in both the flaccid and the erect state. The erection is obtained using an injection of a specialized medication such as papaverine into the lateral aspect of the proximal shaft of the penis, causing vasodilation. The diameter size (AP × transverse) and PSVs are measured bilaterally for the cavernous arteries both pre- and postinjection. Protocols vary related to the amount of time waited to obtain postinjection measurements. There are also variations in the criteria used for the interpretation of the findings. The following are widely accepted interpretation criteria utilized in many laboratories:

- Normal preinjection findings—Cavernous arteries small in caliber. High-resistance spectral waveform with little to no diastolic flow.
- Normal postinjection findings—Cavernous arteries dilate in size (typically double). Waveform changes to a low-resistance waveform with increased diastolic flow. The PSV increases by at least 30 cm/s.

When the cavernous arteries display anything other than the above normal response to the injection, the examination is considered suspicious for vasculogenic impotence. It is important to note a possible complication that can occur following this examination is a painful sustained erection lasting longer than 3 hours. In this case, the patient should be instructed to contact his physician or go to the emergency room for treatment to reverse the effects of the injection.

Testing for Thoracic Outlet Syndrome

Technique

TOS, as described earlier in this chapter, is a condition caused by compression of the subclavian artery, subclavian vein, or brachial plexus by an extra cervical rib or thoracic musculature. This condition can be symptomatic or asymptomatic. The restriction to blood flow with TOS is position dependent. The most effective way to evaluate patients for TOS is with the use of digit PPG waveforms and pressures. Typically, one of the digits on each hand is selected and used for the entire examination. A resting study is always performed first with the patient's arms

resting in their lap while digit PPG waveforms and pressures are recorded. Testing is then repeated with the arms in a series of positions. The routine positions utilized for the examination can vary among institutions and can also be tailored to the individual patient depending on their symptoms. The goal is to place the arm in a position that is going to reproduce symptoms or reduce blood flow in the presence of TOS. The following positions are most commonly utilized:

- Military position with elbow pointing to the rear and arms almost upright with palms facing forward.
- Hands straight up 180 degrees.
- Arms straight out and abducted toward the rear.
- Adson maneuver with arms abducted out to sides (performed with head turned to each side).
- Costoclavicular maneuver with chest pushed forward and shoulders back.

See Figure 4–36 for an example of each position.

Interpretation of Results

For a study to be considered positive for TOS, the waveforms and pressures must be significantly reduced during one of the performed positional maneuvers and the maneuver must produce symptoms. It is important to maintain the positions long enough to produce symptoms (Fig. 4–37).

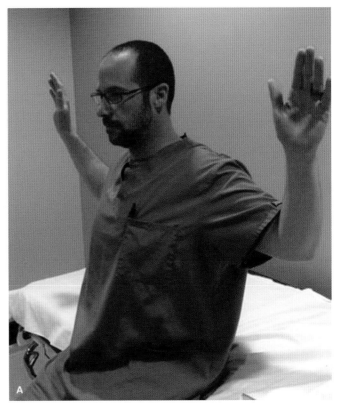

FIGURE 4–36. (A) Military position with elbow pointing to the rear and arms almost upright with palms facing forward.

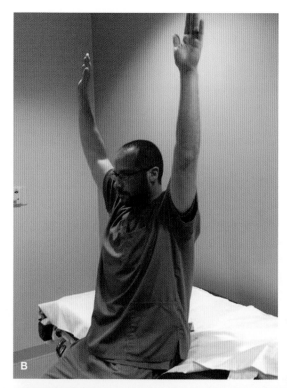
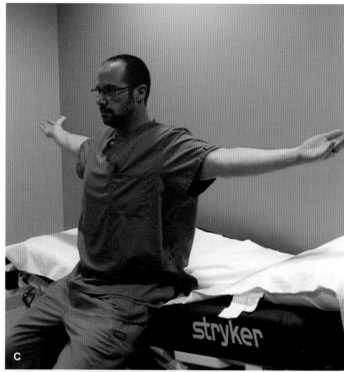
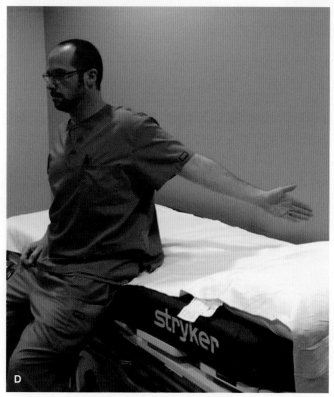
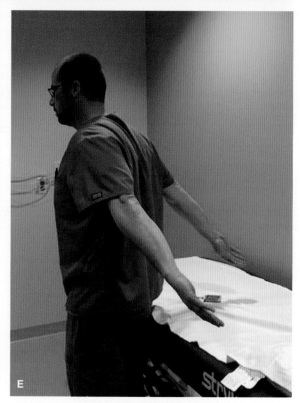

FIGURE 4–36. (*Continued*) **(B)** Hands straight up 180 degrees. **(C)** Arms straight out and abducted toward the rear. **(D)** Adson maneuver with arms abducted out to sides (performed with head turned to each side). **(E)** Costoclavicular maneuver with chest pushed forward and shoulders back.

Cold Immersion Testing

Technique

Cold immersion testing is performed primarily on patients with intermittent symptoms associated with primary Raynaud's syndrome of the hands or feet in an effort to reproduce the symptoms and confirm the diagnosis. Testing for primary Raynaud's disease is accomplished by first obtaining digital PPG waveforms and pressures at rest in a warm environment, then immersing the hands or feet in a basin of ice water for approximately 1-3 minutes. Once the hands or feet are removed

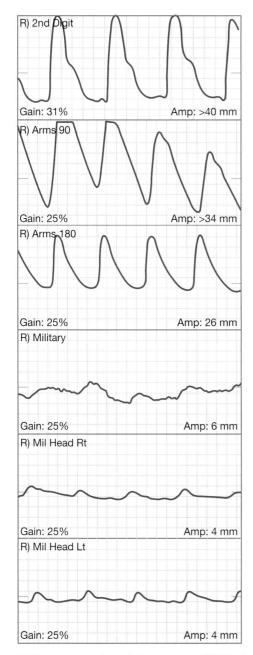

FIGURE 4–37. Demonstrates photoplethysmography (PPG) findings consistent with thoracic outlet syndrome. There is a reduction in flow during certain maneuvers as noted by the PPG waveforms.

from the water, they are quickly patted dry with a towel and the digital waveforms and pressures are obtained at 2 minutes, 5 minutes, and 10 minutes. Some labs add the additional step of measuring the finger temperature with an infrared temperature gun pre- and postcold immersion.

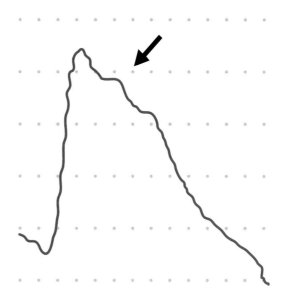

FIGURE 4–38. Peak pulsed waveform that is commonly seen in patients with primary Raynaud's syndrome. The *arrow* showing the dicrotic notch displaying higher than normal on the waveform.

Interpretation of Results

Resting digital pressures in a normal patient should be approximately 90% of the higher brachial pressure. The digital PPG waveforms should have the same normal characteristics as described earlier in this chapter or may display an abnormal "peaked pulse" on the systolic portion of the waveform (Fig. 4–38). This is a finding that is often seen on the resting waveforms of patients who have primary Raynaud's disease. The normal response to cold immersion is a drop in digital pressures with flattening of the PPG waveforms to some degree, with rapid recovery. In a patient with primary Raynaud's disease, the following findings are consistent with a positive diagnosis:

- Peaked pulse present on preimmersion PPG waveforms.
- Drop in systolic pressure of more than 16 mm Hg ± 3% postimmersion.
- Waveforms do not resume preimmersion shape within 5-10 minutes of being removed from ice water.

See Figure 4–39.

Duplex Evaluation of Lower Extremity Bypass Grafts

Types of Bypass Grafts

When significant peripheral arterial disease is present and requires intervention, there are two options for lower extremity

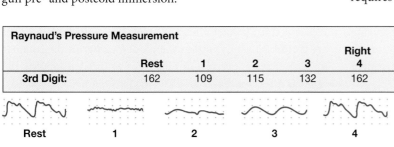

Raynaud's Pressure Measurement					Right
	Rest	1	2	3	4
3rd Digit:	162	109	115	132	162

Rest	1	2	3	4

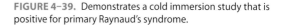

FIGURE 4–39. Demonstrates a cold immersion study that is positive for primary Raynaud's syndrome.

bypass grafts: the graft can either be synthetic (artificial) or an autogenous vein. Synthetic grafts such as polytetrafluoroethylene, also known as PTFE, are composed of a manufactured material and have a shorter life expectancy than their counterpart, the autogenous vein graft. Autogenous vein grafts are created using the patient's own vein. The veins that are commonly used are the great saphenous and small saphenous. If neither of these veins are an option, then the cephalic vein or basilic vein in the upper extremity are sometimes used. There are also different techniques used to perform autogenous vein grafts. The following are the different techniques utilized for vein grafts:

- In situ vein bypass graft—Performed using the great saphenous vein left in its normal anatomical location. The branches of the vein are ligated and the internal valves are removed with a valvulotome to allow blood to flow in the direction of the feet. The proximal end of the vein is anastomosed to the inflow artery and the distal end to the outflow artery.
- Reversed vein bypass graft—Performed by completely resecting the great saphenous or other autogenous vein and reversing its normal orientation before attaching it to the arteries. In this case, the anatomical distal end is attached to the proximal inflow artery and the anatomical proximal end is attached to the distal outflow artery. With this type of bypass, it is not necessary to remove the internal valves because in the reversed direction they do not prevent flow toward the feet.
- Orthograde vein bypass graft—Performed similarly to the reversed vein bypass graft by completely resecting the vein; however, with this technique, the vein is placed in its normal anatomical direction and valves are removed. This allows for the larger proximal portion of the vein to be attached to the proximal inflow artery and the smaller distal portion of the vein to be attached to the distal outflow artery.

Location of disease, availability of the veins, and necessity for the bypass are considered to determine which type of bypass graft is utilized.

Technique

Duplex surveillance of a lower extremity bypass is usually performed in conjunction with other physiologic testing such as ABIs and PVRs. Duplex is the preferred method of routine follow-up for lower extremity bypass graft evaluation due to its noninvasive nature. Postoperative graft surveillance duplex is typically performed every 3 months for the first year following surgery, every 6 months for the second year, and then once a year for the remaining life of the graft or patient. More frequent surveillance can be performed if symptoms are present.

Typically, a 10- to 12-MHz or 5- to 7-MHz linear transducer is used depending on the type and depth of the bypass graft. A 3- to 5-MHz curved transducer is utilized to assess aortoiliac

bypass grafts. Protocols may vary among institutions. Standard duplex surveillance of a lower extremity bypass includes 2D grayscale images, color Doppler images, and PW spectral Doppler waveforms with PSV measurements from the following areas:

- Inflow artery
- Proximal anastomosis
- Proximal bypass graft
- Mid-bypass graft
- Distal bypass graft
- Distal anastomosis
- Outflow artery

See Figure 4–40.

Additional images and spectral waveforms should be obtained from any areas of pathology. Similar to a stenosis seen on any duplex examination, PW spectral Doppler waveforms should be recorded from the prestenotic region, at the region of the stenosis, and in the poststenotic region. With in situ vein bypass grafts, evaluation to identify any missed branches that may have resulted in an AVF should be performed. This is accomplished by following the bypass graft in the transverse plane for its entire length. Close attention should also be paid to valve areas as well as anastomosis sites with autogenous vein grafts as they can be common locations for stenosis to occur.

Interpretation of Results

Normal Findings. Findings consistent with a normal duplex surveillance of a lower extremity bypass graft are smooth vessel walls with no evidence of thickening or intraluminal material and smooth laminar type color flow represented using color Doppler. It is important to note that a finding of some retrograde flow through the native artery proximal to the distal anastomosis is considered a normal finding and actually may be beneficial to the patient in some cases (Fig. 4–41). PW spectral Doppler waveforms should be high-resistance triphasic or biphasic type waveforms identical to those seen in the native lower extremity arteries in most cases. It is also common for these waveforms to take on a more low-resistance shape with diastolic flow throughout the cardiac cycle. This finding is commonly seen early on following the surgery. In general, the PSV throughout the bypass graft should not change dramatically from segment to segment.

Abnormal Findings. Abnormal grayscale, color Doppler, and PW spectral Doppler findings associated with bypass grafts are identical to the findings mentioned earlier in this chapter for native artery duplex findings. A stenosis will appear the same as a focal increase in PSV (>100%) followed by poststenotic turbulence just distal to the stenosis and reduced PSV with delayed rise to peak systole further distal to the stenosis (Fig. 4–42). The biggest difference is that most of the stenoses found within bypass grafts are the result of myointimal hyperplasia as opposed to atherosclerotic plaque.

In situ vein bypass grafts have a potential complication of an AVF. This occurs when a perforator branch of the great saphenous vein is not ligated during surgery. Once the vein is arterialized, it allows arterial flow to cross over into the deep venous system. The findings in this situation will consist of a large visible branch originating from the bypass graft that has very turbulent color Doppler flow. The PW spectral Doppler waveform will be a high-volume low-resistance waveform with high peak systolic and end-diastolic velocities similar to the waveform seen in a dialysis access graft (Fig. 4–43).

Duplex Evaluation of Hemodialysis Access

Hemodialysis access is a surgically created arteriovenous connection put in place to provide a more permanent site for cannulation during hemodialysis. It can be created in the form of an autogenous AVF where one end of a superficial vein is anastomosed to an artery or as a synthetic arteriovenous graft (AVG) where one end of the graft is anastomosed to an artery with the other end anastomosed to a vein. Due to the decreased rate of complications, AVFs are preferred over AVGs. Hemodialysis access dysfunction usually occurs from efferent venous stenosis.

The preferred order of hemodialysis access graft is forearm fistula→ upper arm fistula→ forearm graft→ upper arm graft→ thigh graft.

Autogenous AVFs are typically preferred over artificial grafts because they have a lower rate of infection, stenosis, and pseudoaneurysms. The cephalic vein is usually the vein of choice due to its location. Creating a fistula using the basilic vein usually requires the vein to be transposed from the medial aspect of the arm to the lateral before being attached to the artery because of its medial location. The Brescia–Cimino fistula remains the most common first choice for hemodialysis access.

The most common AV fistulas are (Fig. 4–44):

- Cephalic vein to radial artery (Brescia–Cimino fistula)
- Basilic vein to radial artery
- Cephalic vein to brachial artery
- Basilic vein to brachial artery

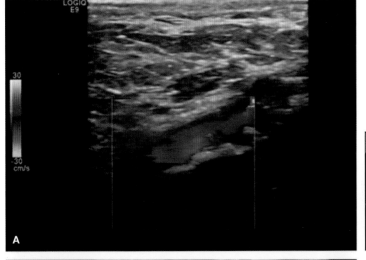
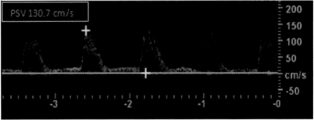
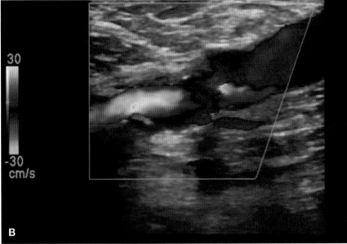
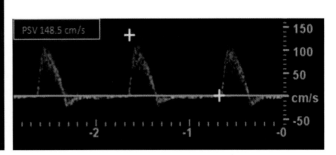

FIGURE 4–40. Typical scanning protocol and findings consistent with a normal bypass graft surveillance. **(A)** Color Doppler and PW Doppler images of the inflow artery. **(B)** Color Doppler and PW Doppler images of the proximal anastomosis.

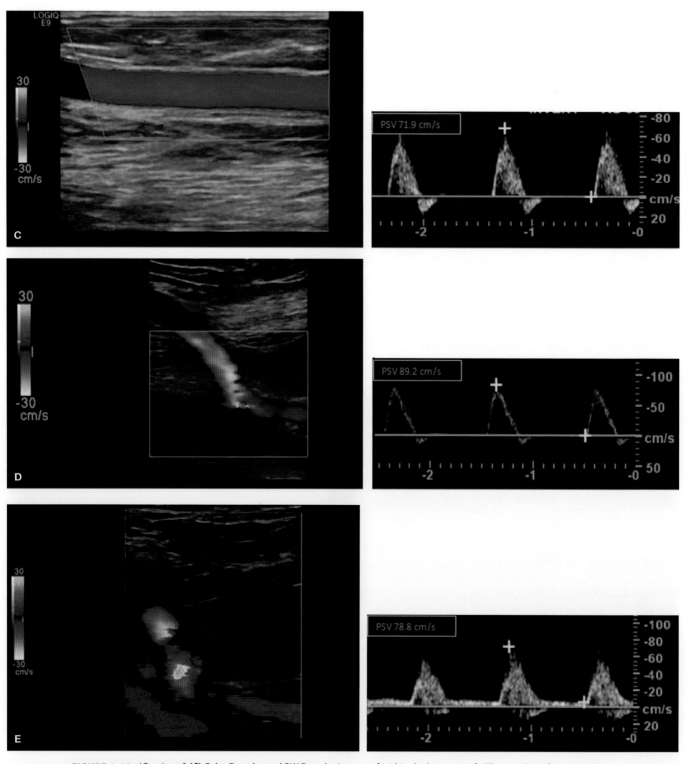

FIGURE 4–40. (*Continued*) **(C)** Color Doppler and PW Doppler images of within the bypass graft (The number of images taken within the bypass graft will vary depending on the length of the bypass). **(D)** Color Doppler and PW Doppler images of the distal anastomosis. **(E)** Color Doppler and PW Doppler images of the outflow artery.

Some labs use the Rule of 6s, although these parameters are not conservative enough for some physicians:

- External vessel diameter more than 6 mm
- Fistula is equal to or less than 6 mm deep
- Blood flow rate exceeds 600 mL/min

Other labs use external vessel diameter more than 4 mm, fistula less than or equal to 5 mm deep, and blood flow exceeding 500 mL/min.

The majority of hemodialysis access grafts are created in the upper extremities, starting with the distal vessels (Fig. 4–45). If possible, the graft should be placed in the

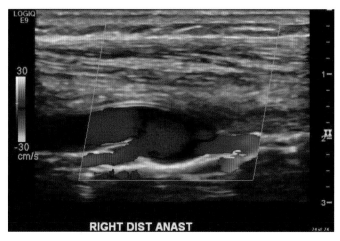

FIGURE 4–41. Color Doppler image of the distal anastomosis of a lower extremity bypass graft showing retrograde flow proximal to the distal anastomosis which is a normal finding.

nondominant arm. Occasionally, when all other options have been exhausted the access graft can be created in the lower extremity groin region.

The following is a list of the most common type of hemodialysis access grafts:

- Brachial artery to brachial vein graft (forearm loop)
- Axillary artery to axillary vein (upper arm loop)
- Upper arm straight graft

Technique

A 7- to 12-MHz linear transducer is used to evaluate the hemodialysis access. Minimal probe pressure is essential, so extra gel may be needed for adequate visualization. Standard duplex surveillance of a hemodialysis access includes 2D grayscale images, color Doppler images, and PW spectral Doppler waveforms with PSV measurements and volume flow measurements. There are some differences in the protocols for fistulas and grafts. For instance, there is only one anastomosis (arterial) with fistulas while there are two anastomoses (arterial and venous) with grafts. Table 4–3 shows the standard protocols for each. The volume flow is typically calculated by the ultrasound machine and requires obtaining a diameter measurement to make the area calculation, while the PW spectral Doppler measures the time averaged mean velocity. These two parameters are required to calculate the volume flow (Fig. 4–46). The formula for volume flow is shown in Table 4–3. As with every other duplex examination, when a stenosis is identified, PW spectral Doppler waveforms should be obtained from the prestenotic region, within the stenosis itself, and in the poststenotic region. An AVF can be considered mature and ready for dialysis use when it is at least 4 mm in size (internal diameter) with a volume flow more than 500 mL/min and no evidence of narrowing. Maturity of the fistula takes about 8-12 weeks post procedure.

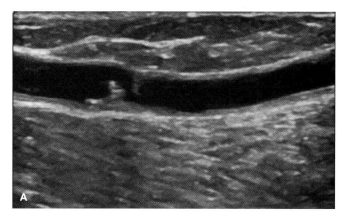

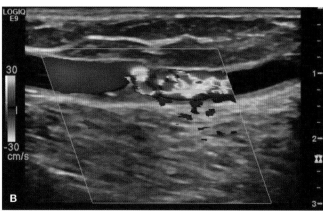

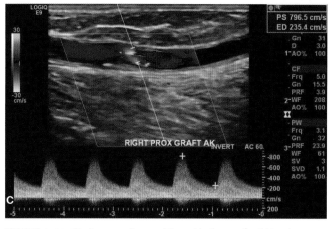

FIGURE 4–42. Findings consistent with a critical stenosis within a lower extremity bypass graft. **(A)** 2D grayscale image showing debris within the lumen of the bypass graft. **(B)** Color Doppler image of that same area demonstrating color aliasing with high velocity flow jet. **(C)** Spectral PW Doppler waveform at the area of the stenosis showing elevated peak systolic and end-diastolic velocities.

Interpretation of Results

Findings consistent with a normal hemodialysis access include:

- Vessels as well as fistula or graft are free of internal echoes.
- PSV measurements between 150 and 300 cm/s.
- Low-resistance waveforms with high diastolic flow.
- Intact fistula or graft walls.
- High volume flow (>500 mL/min).

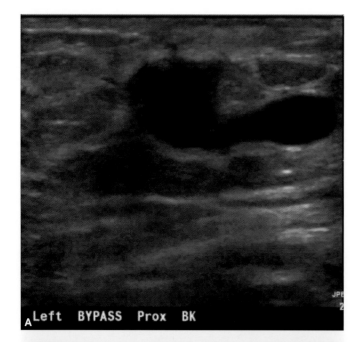

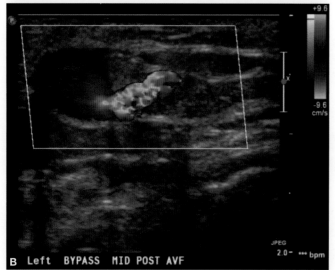

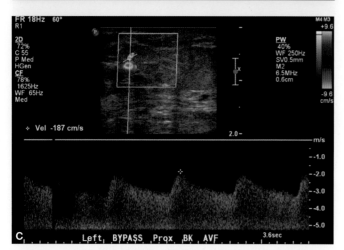

FIGURE 4–43. **(A)** Transverse 2D grayscale image of a lower extremity in situ vein bypass graft showing a missed accessory branch resulting in an arteriovenous fistula. **(B)** Same missed branch with color Doppler demonstrating color aliasing. **(C)** PW spectral Doppler waveform with classic arteriovenous fistula waveform in within the branch.

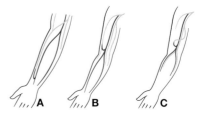

FIGURE 4–44. Arteriovenous fistulas for dialysis access. **(A)** Cephalic vein to radial artery. **(B)** Cephalic vein to brachial artery. **(C)** Basilic vein to brachial artery.

Findings consistent with diseased hemodialysis access include:

- Internal thrombus noted with no flow.
- A focal increase in PSV more than 100% indicating a hemodynamically significant stenosis within the fistula or graft (>100% increase in PSV is equal to a V_r >2). The most common abnormal finding related to hemodialysis access is stenosis at the anastomosis sites or within the vein itself.
- Evidence of wall defect with flow out into the surrounding tissue. These findings are consistent with a pseudoaneurysm.
- Low volume flow (<500 mL/min). Usually, the result of a severe stenosis; requires fistulagram.

Figure 4–47 shows examples of some of the abnormal findings described above.

INVASIVE TESTING AND TREATMENT OF PERIPHERAL ARTERIAL DISEASE

Peripheral Angiography

Peripheral angiography is performed very similar to cerebral angiography in which a catheter is used to cannulate an artery (most commonly the CFA). The catheter is then threaded through the arterial system with the use of a guidewire to the point of interest. In the case of lower extremity angiography, that point is typically the abdominal aorta, and for the upper extremities, it would be the aortic arch. Contrast is injected at the site, and fluoroscopy or cine film x-rays are used to obtain

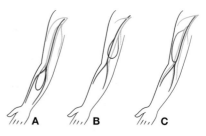

FIGURE 4–45. Dialysis grafts. **(A)** Forearm loop graft. **(B)** Upper arm loop graft. **(C)** Upper arm straight graft.

TABLE 4–3 • Common Duplex Scanning Protocols for Arteriovenous Fistulas and Grafts	
Arteriovenous Fistula Protocol (PSV, EDV, and Volume Flow)	**Arteriovenous Graft Protocol (PSV, EDV, and Volume Flow)**
Inflow artery	Inflow artery
Arterial anastomosis	Arterial anastomosis
Proximal fistula	Proximal graft
Mid fistula	Mid graft
Distal fistula	Distal graft Venous anastomosis Outflow vein
Central venous outflow	Central venous outflow
Formula for volume flow: Time average velocity × Area × 60	

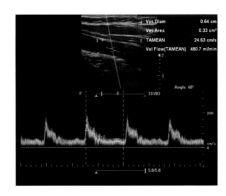

FIGURE 4–46. Correct measurement of volume flow with spectral Doppler. Note placement of calipers measuring vessel diameter and angle-corrected flow velocity.

images of the vascular anatomy. Once all the images are obtained, the catheter is removed from the artery and pressure is held to the site to prevent bleeding out into the surrounding tissue. The patient is typically instructed to lie supine for 3-6 hours following the procedure to further avoid any bleeding complications.

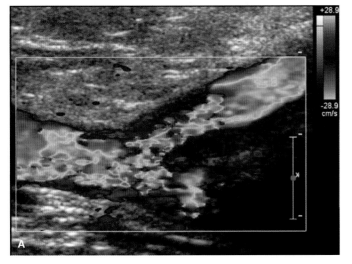

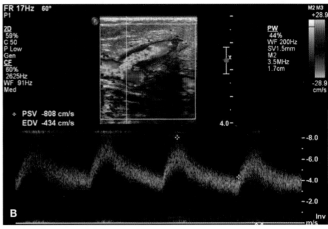

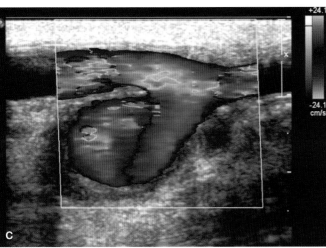

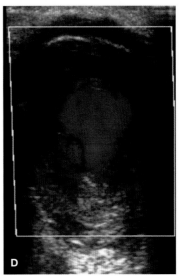

FIGURE 4–47. Duplex findings showing some of the complications associated with surgically created arteriovenous fistulas and grafts. **(A)** Color Doppler imaging showing a significant stenosis at the anastomosis site. **(B)** PW Doppler image of the same narrowed area showing elevated velocities. **(C)** Color Doppler image showing evidence of e pseudoaneurysm. **(D)** Color Doppler image showing evidence of a true aneurysm containing partial thrombus.

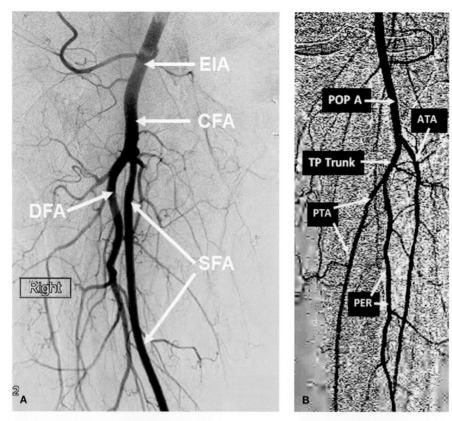

FIGURE 4–48. **(A)** Arteriogram demonstrating normal arterial anatomy in the thigh. **(B)** Arteriogram demonstrating a normal trifurcation of the tibial arteries below the knee.

Peripheral angiography is still considered the gold standard for lower extremity vascular disease unlike cerebrovascular angiography, in which other imaging modalities have replaced conventional angiography for diagnostic purposes.

The angiographic interpretation is the same regardless of the location of the arteries. Normal vessels should appear to fill with contrast entirely (Fig. 4–48). If disease is present in any arteries, there will be what is referred to as a "filling defect," where contrast cannot fill in areas where plaque is present (Fig. 4–49). A stenosis identified with angiography can be calculated as either percent diameter reduction or a percent area reduction and the calculations are the same as mentioned in Chapter 2. In order for a lesion to be considered hemodynamically significant, it must have at least a 50% diameter reduction, which is equal to a 75% area reduction.

Computed Tomography Angiography

Computed tomography angiography (CTA) uses ionizing radiation to produce angiographic type images of the peripheral arteries of the extremities and the aorta. IV contrast is injected systemically through an IV site generally in the antecubital fossa as the patient is passed through the CT scanner. With postprocessing, angiographic type images can be created very similar to conventional angiography and the interpretation is the same (Fig. 4–50).

Magnetic Resonance Angiography

Magnetic resonance angiography (MRA) is yet another way to evaluate the peripheral arteries with the use of radio waves and a strong magnetic field. Similar to CTA, MRA contrast such as gadolinium may be injected on occasion systemically into a peripheral vein as the patient is passed through the magnetic resonance imaging (MRI) scanner. Angiographic images are created that are very similar to conventional angiography and the interpretation is the same (Fig. 4–51).

Medical Therapy

Since ASO is a type of both cerebrovascular and peripheral vascular disease, the medical treatment is virtually the same as far as medications and life style modifications. The following is a list of these treatments:

- Controlling hypertension—Patients with hypertension will be placed on antihypertensive medications to control their blood pressure in an effort to reduce the strain to the blood vessel walls caused by hypertension.
- Life style modifications—Since smoking is one of the main causes of peripheral arterial disease, patients who use tobacco should be instructed to quit smoking. There are many smoking cessation classes and aides available to patients who wish to quit. Patients who are overweight

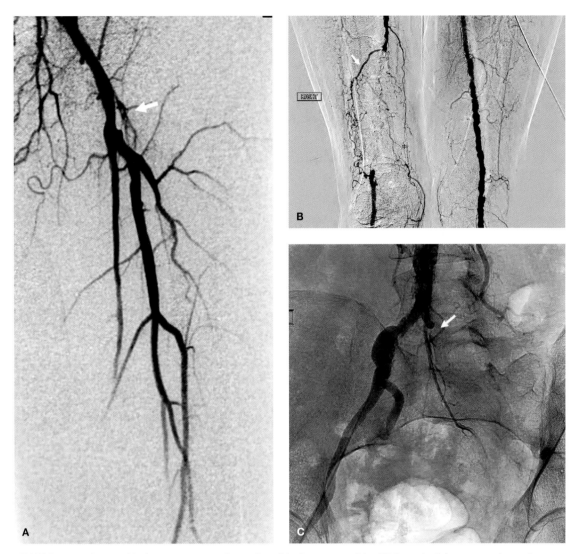

FIGURE 4–49. Abnormal findings on angiography studies of the lower extremities. **(A)** Stenosis of the common femoral artery identified by a filling defect (*arrow*). **(B)** The right side has a segmental occlusion of the superficial femoral artery with collateral flow reconstituting flow to the popliteal artery. The left side shows diffuse disease throughout the superficial femoral artery. **(C)** The right side shows a stenosis of the right common iliac artery with poststenotic dilatation. The left side shows an absent (occluded) common iliac artery (*arrow*).

should be instructed to modify their diets to a low calorie, low cholesterol diet.

- Anticoagulation therapy—Anticoagulation therapy can reduce the risk of peripheral arterial disease by decreasing the viscosity of the blood.
- Antiplatelet therapy—Patients can be placed on aspirin or another form of antiplatelet drug to slow down the progression of atherosclerotic disease.

Surgical Treatment

The decision to intervene with surgery or an interventional procedure is based on the patient's symptoms as well as the severity of the disease, which usually correlate. Typically, invasive therapies are not considered for just claudication-type symptoms unless they are severe and debilitating. Invasive therapies are usually reserved for more severe symptoms such as rest pain

or tissue loss and are often performed in an effort to preserve the limb and avoid amputation. There are two types of surgical approaches that are commonly performed for peripheral arterial disease: endarterectomy and surgical bypass graft.

Endarterectomy

Endarterectomy is a surgical procedure in which atherosclerotic plaque is removed from an artery with an open repair approach. This type of procedure is only effective when there is just an isolated focal lesion causing the reduction of blood flow and symptoms. For more diffuse disease, a surgical bypass graft is needed to restore normal blood flow.

Surgical Bypass

As discussed earlier in this chapter, surgical bypass grafts can either be synthetic or autogenous vein. The location of disease, extent of the disease, and availability of a vein conduit will all

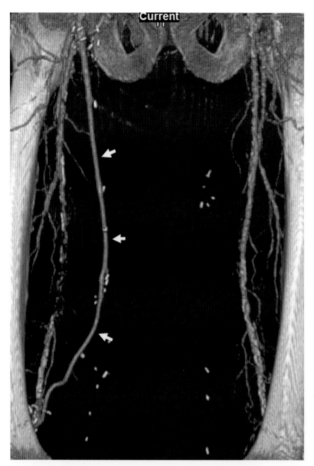

FIGURE 4–50. CT angiography study of the lower extremities demonstrating diffuse atherosclerosis bilaterally with a segmental occlusion of the right superficial femoral artery and a patent right femoral popliteal bypass graft (*arrows*).

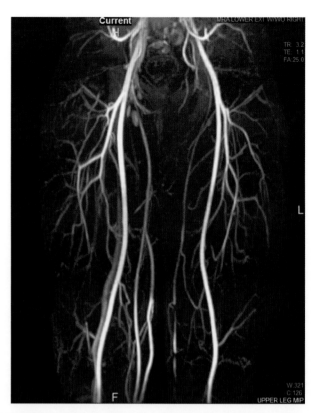

FIGURE 4–51. MR angiography study demonstrating normal arterial flow of the lower extremities.

help determine which type of bypass is performed. The most important point related to bypass grafts is that they must originate from an artery with good inflow and must connect distally enough to provide adequate outflow in order for them to be successful. Poor inflow and outflow are common reasons for graft failure.

Angioplasty and Stenting

Angioplasty and stenting is a minimally invasive technique used to dilate and restore normal flow to a focal stenotic lesion. Angioplasty is performed along with angiography as a guide to find the stenotic lesion. Once the lesion is located, a balloon-tipped catheter is advanced to the level of the stenosis under fluoroscopic guidance and a balloon is inflated to push the plaque up against the walls of the artery. This can be repeated a few times if necessary to restore normal flow through that segment of the artery (Fig. 4–52). A stent is often deployed following the angioplasty to keep that segment of the artery open. Stenting and angioplasty are typically reserved for the larger peripheral arteries (iliac arteries, femoral arteries, subclavian arteries) and not very useful for the smaller vessels (tibial arteries).

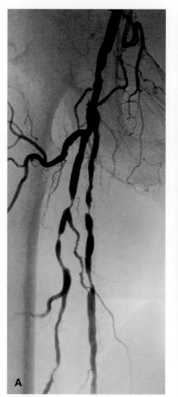
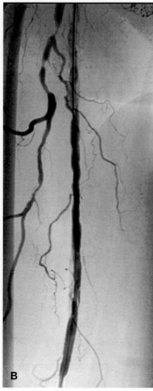

FIGURE 4–52. Angiography images showing the results of angioplasty. **(A)** Arteriogram image demonstrating multiple hemodynamically significant stenosis within the superficial and deep femoral arteries. **(B)** The same vessels status post balloon angioplasty showing resolution of the stenosis within the superficial femoral artery.

Questions

1. A normal spectral waveform of the brachial artery is

   (A) Multiphasic
   (B) Aphasic
   (C) Monophasic
   (D) Tardus parvus

2. Which of the following is a pathology specific to the upper extremity arteries?

   (A) TOS
   (B) Carotid body tumor
   (C) Raynaud's syndrome
   (D) Embolus

3. The type of flow pattern in which the velocities increase toward the center of the vessel and is found in most of the normal peripheral arteries is known as

   (A) Turbulent
   (B) Plug
   (C) Laminar
   (D) Occluded

4. What blood vessel at rest is most likely to have a high resistive waveform?

   (A) CFA
   (B) Common carotid artery
   (C) Renal artery
   (D) Hepatic artery

5. The DPA is a continuation of which artery?

   (A) ATA
   (B) PTA
   (C) Popliteal artery
   (D) CFA

6. All of the following are true regarding spectral broadening EXCEPT

   (A) Spectral broadening is commonly associated with stenosis
   (B) Spectral broadening refers to the filling of the spectral window with disturbed flow
   (C) Spectral broadening refers to a decrease in bandwidth with disturbed flow
   (D) Spectral broadening occurs with turbulent blood flow

7. What is the first branch originating from the aortic arch that is only present on the right side?

   (A) Subclavian artery
   (B) Brachiocephalic artery
   (C) Lateral thoracic artery
   (D) Internal mammary artery

8. Which artery is a continuation of the SFA as it passes through the adductor canal below the knee?

   (A) Popliteal artery
   (B) Tibioperoneal trunk
   (C) PFA
   (D) PTA

9. Which artery runs along the medial aspect of the lower leg and courses posterior to the medial malleolus?

   (A) Peroneal artery
   (B) Anterior tibial artery
   (C) DPA
   (D) PTA

10. The waveform shown in Figure 4–53 is

    (A) Monophasic
    (B) Aphasic
    (C) Triphasic
    (D) Preocclusive

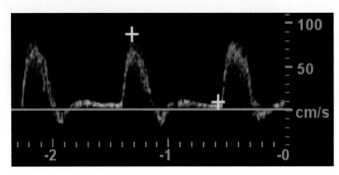

FIGURE 4–53.

11. The waveform shown in Figure 4–54 was obtained from the SFA and demonstrates

    (A) Increased PSV

    (B) A triphasic waveform

    (C) Laminar flow

    (D) Flow reversal

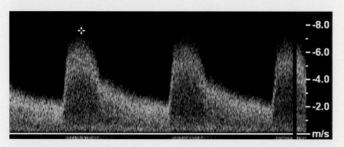

FIGURE 4–54.

12. The waveform shown in Figure 4–55 suggests

    (A) Normal laminar arterial flow

    (B) PST flow

    (C) Multiphasic flow

    (D) Distal occlusion

13. The waveform shown in Figure 4–56 suggest that

    (A) There is an occlusion just proximal to this area

    (B) There is an occlusion just distal to this area

    (C) There is a critical stenosis at this area

    (D) This is a normal waveform

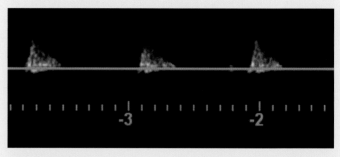

FIGURE 4–56.

14. A patient is sent to your laboratory to have his lower extremity bypass graft evaluated with duplex. While performing the examination, you notice that the velocity at the proximal anastomosis is 80 cm/s. You continue the examination and obtain a pulse wave Doppler signal about 1 cm distal to the proximal anastomosis and you get a velocity of 210 cm/s. What do these findings suggest?

    (A) Normal flow present within this bypass

    (B) 1% to 19% narrowing of this bypass

    (C) 20% to 49% narrowing of this bypass

    (D) 50% to 99% narrowing of this bypass

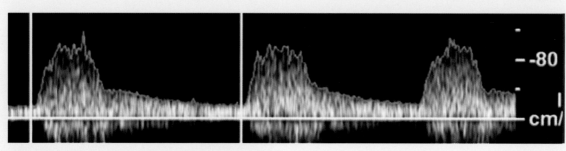

FIGURE 4–55.

15. **The following is a type of lower extremity bypass**

    (A) Brachial artery to cephalic vein

    (B) CFA to popliteal reversed saphenous vein

    (C) Cephalic vein to brachial vein

    (D) Femoral vein to internal iliac vein

16. **Which statement is true about the symptom of claudication?**

    (A) Exercise-induced pain caused by too much blood flow to the legs

    (B) Varies each time regarding distance the patient is able to walk

    (C) Always relieved by rest

    (D) Only occurs in the calves

17. **Rest pain can be relieved by**

    (A) Standing

    (B) Elevating legs

    (C) Exercise

    (D) Taking deep breaths

18. **The peak systolic blood pressure in an area of a limb distal to a significant obstruction or stenosis**

    (A) Will increase

    (B) Will decrease

    (C) Will remain the same

    (D) Will double

19. **Which is the most common cause of peripheral arterial disease of the lower extremities?**

    (A) Arteritis

    (B) Arterial spasm

    (C) ASO

    (D) Embolism

20. **The most common site of ASO in the lower extremities is**

    (A) The bifurcation of the common iliac arteries

    (B) The origin of the PFA

    (C) The trifurcation of the tibial arteries

    (D) The distal SFA through the adductor canal

Questions 21 through 34: Match the structures in Fig. 4–57 with the names of the arteries in Column B.

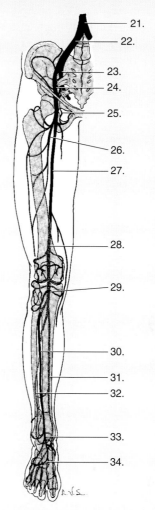

FIGURE 4–57. (Reproduced, with permission, from Lindner HH. *Clinical Anatomy*. East Norwalk, CT: Appleton & Lange; 1989:602. Copyright © McGraw Hill.)

COLUMN A	COLUMN B
21. _____	(A) CFA
22. _____	(B) Popliteal artery
23. _____	(C) Aorta
24. _____	(D) SFA
25. _____	(E) Internal iliac artery
26. _____	(F) PFA
27. _____	(G) External iliac artery
28. _____	(H) Common iliac artery
29. _____	(I) Tibioperoneal trunk
30. _____	(J) DPA
31. _____	(K) ATA
32. _____	(L) Peroneal artery
33. _____	(M) Plantar arch
34. _____	(N) PTA

35. An obese patient is sent to your laboratory to be evaluated for arterial disease of the lower extremities. When performing their PVR and segmental pressure study, you notice that their thigh PVR waveform indicates moderate disease but the pressure index at this level is 1.14. How could be a possible explanation for this?

    (A) The disease is not severe enough to lower the pressure

    (B) The technologist had to have made a mistake

    (C) It is most likely the result of cuff artifact

    (D) This is fine because a pressure of 1.14 is in the range of moderate disease

36. If a patient has a steal from an AVF graft with no underlying atherosclerotic disease, the pregraft compression digital PPG waveforms obtained during noninvasive arterial testing would show

    (A) Normal blood flow to the digits

    (B) Reduced blood flow to the digits

    (C) No difference in blood flow to the digits

    (D) Increased blood flow to the digits

37. The images in Figure 4–58 were obtained from a patient in order 1, 2, and 3 from proximal to distal in a lower extremity bypass graft. What do these findings suggest?

    (A) Normal

    (B) 1% to 19% stenosis

    (C) 20% to 49% stenosis

    (D) 50% to 99% stenosis

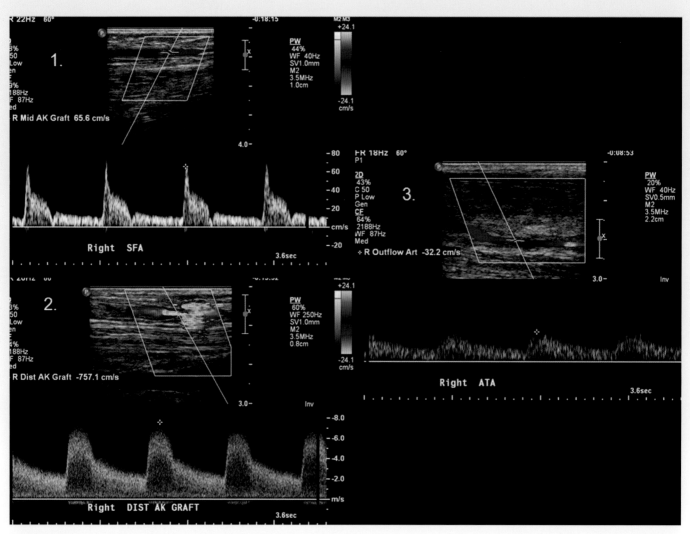

FIGURE 4–58.

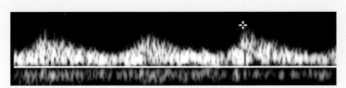

FIGURE 4–59.

38. **The waveform shown in Figure 4–59 was obtained in the lower extremity. How is this waveform best described?**

(A) Normal monophasic waveform of the lower extremity

(B) Abnormal monophasic waveform found distal to a stenosis

(C) Abnormal monophasic waveform found proximal to a stenosis

(D) Abnormal monophasic waveform found at a stenosis

39. **The images in Figure 4–60 were obtained from a patient in order 1, 2, and 3 from proximal to distal in an upper extremity arterial venous fistula. What is your diagnosis based on these findings?**

(A) Normal

(B) Less than 50% stenosis at the anastomosis

(C) More than 50% stenosis at the anastomosis

(D) Occlusion at the anastomosis

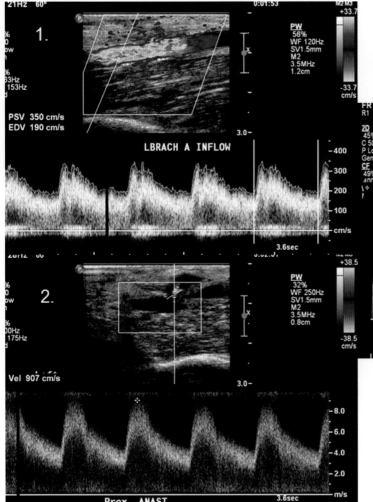

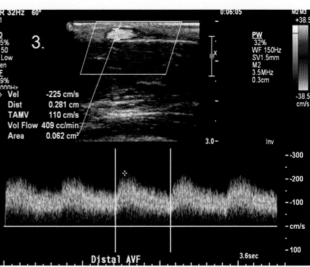

PSV Ratio = 2.6

FIGURE 4–60.

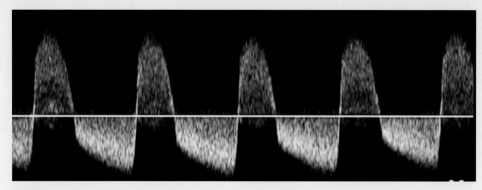

FIGURE 4–61.

40. The spectral Doppler waveform shown in Figure 4–61 is characteristic for which abnormality?

(A) AVF steal

(B) Stenosis

(C) Pseudoaneurysm

(D) Vasospasm

41. What is the procedure in which a balloon-tipped catheter is advanced to the level of a focal stenotic lesion under fluoroscopic guidance and a balloon is inflated to push the plaque up against the walls of the artery in an effort to restore normal blood flow to the limb?

(A) CT angiography

(B) Angioplasty

(C) Digital subtraction angiography

(D) MR angiography

42. The brachial artery bifurcates just below the antecubital fossa into which two arteries?

(A) Subclavian and axillary arteries

(B) Deep and superficial palmar arteries

(C) Brachiocephalic and subclavian arteries

(D) Radial and ulnar arteries

43. Noninvasive physiologic testing that involves placing a PPG on one of the digits of each hand recording waveforms and pressures while the arms are moved through a series of positions is used to evaluate for which syndrome?

(A) Subclavian steal syndrome

(B) TOS

(C) Raynaud's syndrome

(D) Fibromuscular dysplasia

44. In a blood vessel with a nonhemodynamically significant stenosis, if the diameter decreases, what happens to the flow volume?

(A) Flow volume increases

(B) Flow volume decreases

(C) Flow volume remains unchanged

(D) Volume increases but velocity decreases

45. Which statement is accurate related to a vessel that has a hemodynamically significant stenosis?

(A) There is no change in pressure distal to the segment

(B) There is an increase in the pressure gradient across the segment

(C) There is an increase in pressure at area of stenosis

(D) There is a decrease in velocity at area of stenosis

46. Which surgical procedure has the highest potential for problems such as AVF s and retained valves?

(A) Aorta-femoral bypass

(B) In-situ saphenous vein bypass

(C) Reversed saphenous vein bypass

(D) Synthetic bypass

47. The waveform shown in Figure 4–62 is a characteristic waveform for which condition?

    (A) Raynaud's syndrome

    (B) TOS

    (C) Takayasu's arteritis

    (D) Moyamoya disease

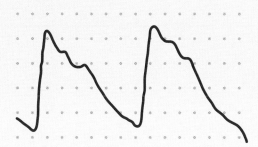

FIGURE 4–62.

48. An abnormal connection between an artery and a vein that can occur spontaneously or as a result of trauma is known as

    (A) Anastomosis

    (B) Pseudoaneurysm

    (C) AVF

    (D) Dissection

49. What is the name of the most widely utilized ratio used to evaluate overall perfusion to the lower extremity arteries?

    (A) Resistive index

    (B) Pulsatility index

    (C) ABI

    (D) Pressure gradient index

50. Which of the following may be used to diagnose the severity of a stenotic lesion with duplex?

    (A) PSV

    (B) Resistive index

    (C) Pulsatility index

    (D) ABI

51. All of the following are physical findings that can be associated with obstructive arterial disease of the lower extremities EXCEPT

    (A) Shiny tight appearance to the skin

    (B) Hair loss to the foot

    (C) Ulcer on the heel

    (D) Palpable pulse (grade 3)

52. Which of the following is NOT a common risk factor associated with arterial occlusive disease?

    (A) Tobacco use

    (B) Hypertension

    (C) Diabetes

    (D) Hypolipidemia

53. While reviewing the segmental pressures on a patient you notice that the patient has a right thigh pressure of 155 mm Hg and a right calf pressure of 90 mm Hg. The patient's brachial pressure is 120 mm Hg. Based on just these findings, what level of disease does this patient have?

    (A) Aortoiliac

    (B) Femoral-popliteal

    (C) Distal small vessel

    (D) Multilevel

54. What is the first component that is lost on a PVR waveform when arterial disease exists?

    (A) Anacrotic limb

    (B) Catacrotic limb

    (C) Dicrotic limb

    (D) Bicrotic limb

55. All are finding that suggest an arterial venous fistula is mature and ready for hemodialysis use EXCEPT?

    (A) Diameter of the draining vein 4 mm or more

    (B) PSV ratio less than 2

    (C) Flow volume 500 mL/min or more

    (D) Continuous flow in the venous side of the fistula

56. Figure 4–63 shows a resting noninvasive arterial examination of a 76-year-old patient with intermittent claudication bilaterally. Based on the examination data below, what is the extent of this patient's disease?

(A) Aorta and bilateral severe iliac occlusive disease

(B) Right mild femoral popliteal and mild tibial artery occlusive disease and left moderate iliac occlusive disease

(C) Right mild iliac and moderate femoral popliteal occlusive disease and left mild femoral popliteal occlusive disease

(D) Right severe iliac and femoral popliteal occlusive disease and left mild iliac occlusive disease

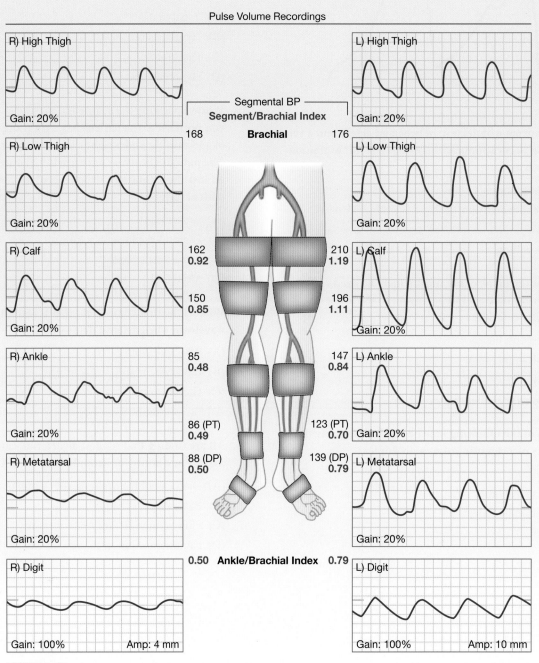

Pulse Volume Recordings

| R) High Thigh | | L) High Thigh |
| Gain: 20% | | Gain: 20% |

Segmental BP
Segment/Brachial Index
168 **Brachial** 176

| R) Low Thigh | | L) Low Thigh |
| Gain: 20% | | Gain: 20% |

| R) Calf | 162 **0.92** / 210 **1.19** | L) Calf |
| Gain: 20% | 150 **0.85** / 196 **1.11** | Gain: 20% |

| R) Ankle | 85 **0.48** / 147 **0.84** | L) Ankle |
| Gain: 20% | 86 (PT) **0.49** / 123 (PT) **0.70** | Gain: 20% |

| R) Metatarsal | 88 (DP) **0.50** / 139 (DP) **0.79** | L) Metatarsal |
| Gain: 20% | | Gain: 20% |

0.50 **Ankle/Brachial Index** 0.79

| R) Digit | | L) Digit |
| Gain: 100%   Amp: 4 mm | | Gain: 100%   Amp: 10 mm |

FIGURE 4–63.

Pulse Volume Recording

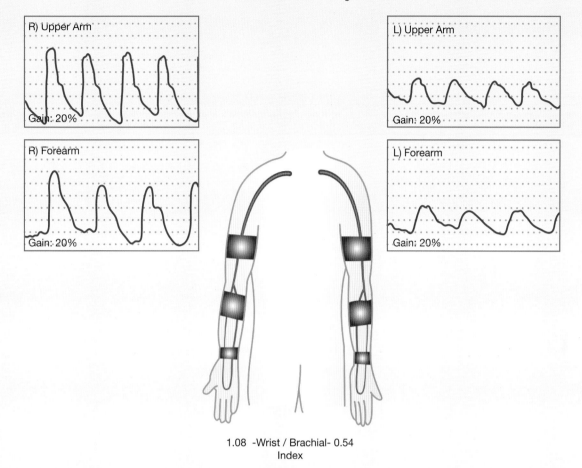

FIGURE 4–64.

57. **Figure 4–64 shows segmental pressures and PVR waveforms from a patient with ischemic type symptoms of the left hand. Based on this data, what is the location of the disease present?**

(A) Left subclavian and/or axillary arteries

(B) Left radial artery

(C) Left ulnar artery

(D) Left digits

58. **Figure 4–65 shows a segmental pressure and PVR examination. Based on these findings, what level of disease can be ruled out?**

(A) Left femoral popliteal disease

(B) Left iliac disease

(C) Left small vessel disease

(D) Aortoiliac disease

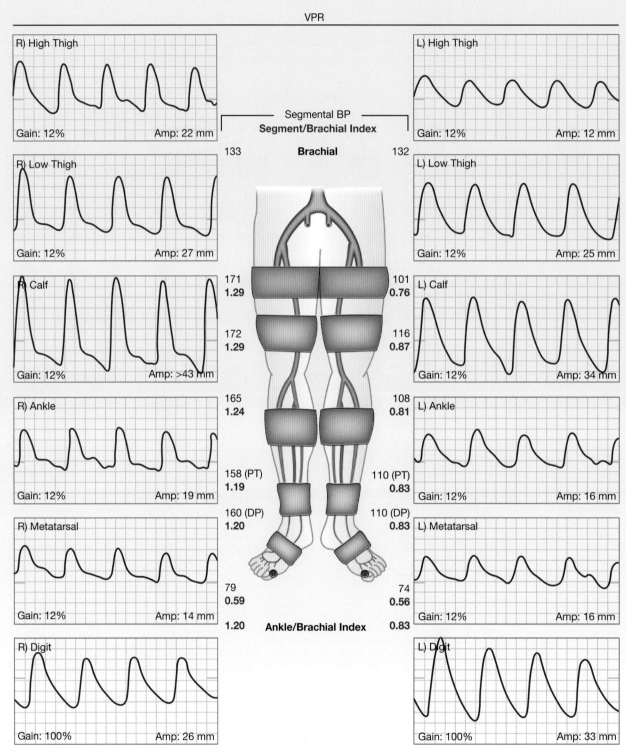

FIGURE 4–65.

59. Based on the analog Doppler waveform in Figure 4–66, what level of disease is present on the patient's right side?

(A) Right iliac disease

(B) Right femoral popliteal disease

(C) Right tibial disease

(D) There is no disease present on the right side

60. Blue toes are an indication of which type of acute arterial obstruction?

(A) Popliteal entrapment

(B) Raynaud's syndrome

(C) Compartment syndrome

(D) Embolus

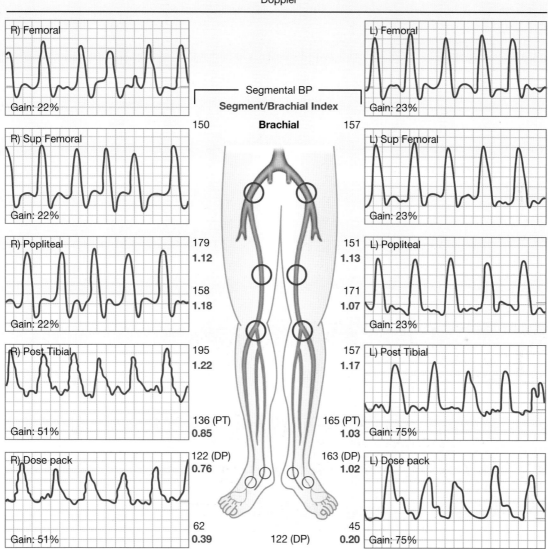

FIGURE 4–66.

61. **A reversed saphenous vein bypass graft involves**

    (A) Harvesting the saphenous vein, removing the valves, and connecting to the arteries in its normal anatomical orientation

    (B) Leaving the saphenous vein in its normal anatomical position, removing valves, ligating any branches, and connecting to the arteries

    (C) Harvesting the saphenous vein, reversing its normal anatomical orientation, and connecting to the arteries

    (D) Harvesting the saphenous vein, reversing its normal anatomical orientation, removing the valves, and connecting to the arteries

62. **The analog Doppler signal distal to an area of severe stenosis in the lower extremities will likely be**

    (A) Multiphasic

    (B) Monophasic

    (C) Quadphasic

    (D) Superphasic

63. **A normal toe pressure is _____ of the higher brachial pressure.**

    (A) 10% to 30%

    (B) 40% to 60%

    (C) 60% to 80%

    (D) Equal

Questions 64 through 70: Match the structures in Fig. 4–67 with the names of the arteries in Column B.

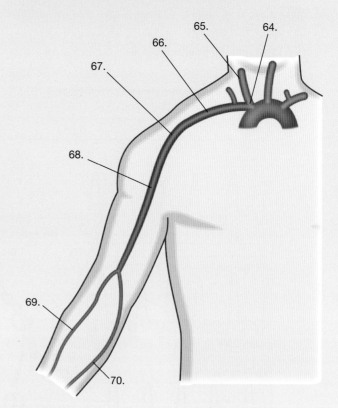

FIGURE 4–67.

COLUMN A	COLUMN B
64. _____	(A) Radial artery
65. _____	(B) Common carotid artery
66. _____	(C) Ulnar artery
67. _____	(D) Innominate artery
68. _____	(E) Brachial artery
69. _____	(F) Axillary artery
70. _____	(G) Subclavian artery

71. **When using the four-cuff technique during a segmental pressure examination, which of the following is consistent with a normal finding?**

    (A) The high thigh pressure is 30 mm Hg higher than the higher brachial pressure

    (B) The high thigh pressure is equal to the higher brachial pressure

    (C) The high thigh pressure is 30 mm Hg lower than the brachial pressure

    (D) The high thigh pressure is 30 mm Hg higher than the lower brachial pressure

72. **In relation to arteries and veins, which statement is true?**

    (A) Arteries have thinner walls than veins

    (B) Arteries have internal valves

    (C) Arteries have a much higher internal pressure

    (D) Arteries are more readily collapsible

73. **What type of pulse wave waveform is characteristic for the diagnosis of a pseudoaneurysm?**

    (A) Poststenotic waveform within neck of pseudoaneurysm

    (B) Triphasic waveform within the pseudoaneurysm

    (C) Monophasic waveform within the neck of the pseudoaneursym

    (D) To-and-fro waveform within the neck of the pseudoaneursym

74. **Which statement is accurate related to blood pressure cuff artifact?**

    (A) If the width of the blood pressure cuff is less than 20% the diameter of the limb, it can result in a falsely lowered peak systolic pressure

    (B) If the width of the blood pressure cuff is more than 20% the diameter of the limb, it can result in a falsely elevated peak systolic pressure

    (C) If the width of the blood pressure cuff is less than 20% the diameter of the limb, it can result in a falsely elevated peak systolic pressure

    (D) Blood pressure cuff size has no effect on peak systolic pressure

75. **Figure 4–68 shows PVR waveforms with various categories of disease. Identify the category of disease by matching them to the correct corresponding letters of each waveform.**

    _____ Normal

    _____ Mild

    _____ Moderate

    _____ Severe

76. **Which syndrome causes displacement and compression of the vessels due to the medial head of the gastrocnemius muscle?**

    (A) TOS

    (B) Popliteal entrapment syndrome

    (C) Adductor canal compression syndrome

    (D) Compartment syndrome

77. **A dampened waveform with a delay to peak systole is obtained in the CFA. The cause is most likely due to which of the following?**

    (A) Distal occlusion

    (B) Pseudoaneurysm

    (C) Aortoiliac disease

    (D) AVF

78. **A patient is sent to your laboratory for a lower extremity arterial study with and without exercise for thigh claudication symptoms. Her baseline ABIs at rest were 0.96 on the right and 0.97 on the left. Postexercise, her ABIs drop to 0.79 on the right and 0.75 on the left. They return to baseline values after 15 minutes. Based on these findings, what level of disease does this patient have?**

    (A) Single level

    (B) Multilevel

    (C) The patient has no significant disease

    (D) Femoral-popliteal

79. **Which penile-brachial index (PBI) is consistent with vasculogenic impotence?**

    (A) Less than 0.80

    (B) Less than 0.65

    (C) Less than 0.75

    (D) Less than 0.90

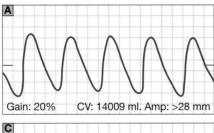

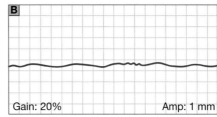

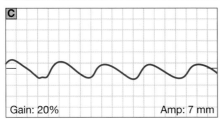

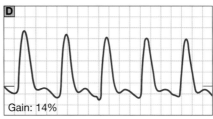

FIGURE 4–68.

80. During a penile duplex examination, what is the normal postinjection response of the cavernous arteries?

    (A) Decrease in diameter
    (B) Increase in PSV
    (C) Decrease in end-diastolic velocity
    (D) Change to multiphasic flow

81. All of the following parameters must be met during a noninvasive upper extremity arterial examination to confirm the diagnosis of TOS EXCEPT

    (A) Position dependent
    (B) Symptomatic
    (C) Complete loss of flow
    (D) Reduction of flow

82. Submerging a patient's hands in ice water resulting in a more than 16 mm Hg drop in peak systolic pressure is an examination performed for which syndrome?

    (A) TOS
    (B) May–Thurner syndrome
    (C) Superior vena cava syndrome
    (D) Raynaud's syndrome

83. What is the main advantage of an orthograde saphenous vein bypass graft over a reversed saphenous vein bypass?

    (A) The internal valves do not have to be removed
    (B) No size discrepancy at both anastomosis sites
    (C) No issue with missed accessory branches
    (D) They have a lower rate of failure

84. Retrograde flow in the native artery proximal to the distal anastomosis of a lower extremity bypass graft is consistent with what finding?

    (A) It is a normal finding
    (B) Distal resistance
    (C) Proximal disease
    (D) AVF

85. Which of the following is a type of AVF that can be used for hemodialysis?

    (A) Cephalic artery to radial artery
    (B) Basilic vein to cephalic vein
    (C) Cephalic vein to brachial artery
    (D) Basilic vein to brachial vein

86. What is the normal volume flow through a mature AVF used for hemodialysis?

    (A) More than 200 mL/min
    (B) More than 400 mL/min
    (C) More than 100 mL/min
    (D) More than 500 mL/min

87. Which imaging modality is considered the "gold standard" for peripheral artery imaging?

    (A) Conventional angiography
    (B) CT angiography
    (C) MR angiography
    (D) Arterial duplex

88. The effect of the absence of contrast around areas of disease during an angiography study is known as

    (A) Digital subtraction
    (B) Cine film
    (C) Filling defect
    (D) Run off

89. Figure 4–69 shows an angiogram of the distal thigh just above the knee. What pathology is identified in this image?

(A) Normal angiogram of the distal thigh

(B) Critical stenosis of the distal SFA

(C) Segmental occlusion of the distal SFA with collateral flow

(D) Fibromuscular dysplasia of the distal SFA

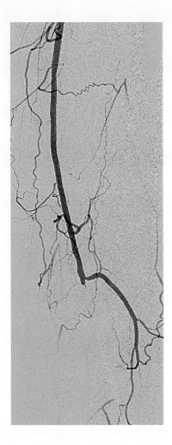

FIGURE 4–69.

90. The findings in Figure 4–70 are consistent with what diagnosis?

(A) Normal peripheral arterial flow

(B) Hemodynamically significant stenosis

(C) AVF

(D) Pseudoaneurysm

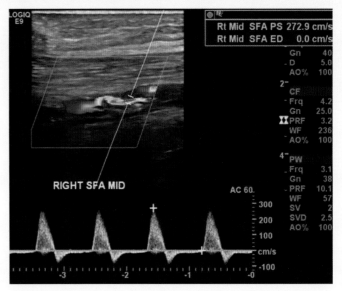

FIGURE 4–70.

91. A 76-year-old patient presented with a bruit in the right groin area status post cardiac catheterization. The images in Figure 4–71 were obtained for the patient's right groin. What do these findings most likely represent?

(A) Pseudoaneurysm

(B) Dissection

(C) Arteriovenous fistula

(D) Hemodynamically significant stenosis

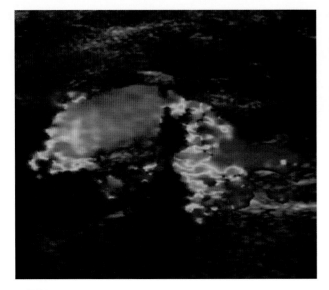

FIGURE 4–71.

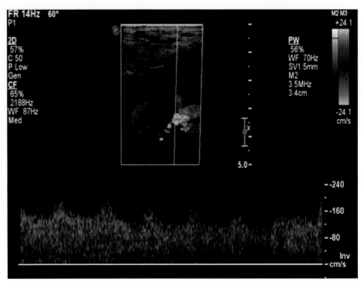

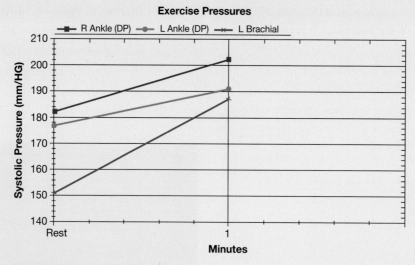

FIGURE 4–72.

92. **Figure 4–72 demonstrates the results of pre- and postsystolic pressures during an exercise examination. What do these findings suggest?**

(A) Normal response to exercise

(B) Single-level peripheral arterial disease

(C) Multilevel peripheral arterial disease

(D) Mild peripheral arterial disease

93. **The segmental pressures shown in Figure 4–73 indicate which level of disease?**

(A) Right iliac disease and left femoral popliteal disease

(B) Right femoral popliteal disease and left iliac disease

(C) Right tibial disease and left iliac disease

(D) Bilateral multilevel disease

Segmental BP					
Right	**mm Hg**	**Index**	**Left**	**mm Hg**	**Index**
Brachial	118		Brachial	122	
Thigh	151	1.24	Thigh	95	0.78
Calf	100	0.82	Calf	92	0.75
Ankle (PTA)	99	0.81	Ankle (PTA)	96	0.79
Ankle (DPA)	97	0.80	Ankle (DPA)	95	0.78

FIGURE 4–73.

Questions 94 through 96: Match the PVR components in Figure 4–74 in column A with the correct terms in column B.

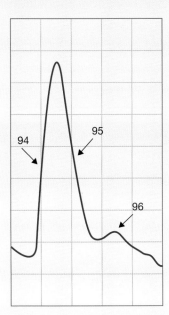

FIGURE 4–74.

COLUMN A

94. _____

95. _____

96. _____

COLUMN B

(A) Catacrotic limb

(B) Dicrotic limb

(C) Anacrotic limb

97. **What is the condition that involves a congenital narrowing of the thoracic aorta where it arches down toward the abdomen?**

(A) Takayasu's arteritis

(B) TOS

(C) TAO

(D) Coarctation of the aorta

98. **What is the second most common area for ASO to develop in the lower extremities?**

(A) Aorta and iliac arteries

(B) Distal femoral artery

(C) PTA

(D) PFA

99. **A 55-year-old male with severe uncontrolled hypertension is having symptoms of right lower extremity numbness and loss of sensation. While performing a lower extremity duplex examination, a linear echogenic structure is visualized in the external iliac artery that appears to be mobile with cardiac pulsations. What is most likely the diagnosis?**

(A) ASO

(B) Arteriovenous malformation

(C) Arterial dissection

(D) TAO

100. **What anatomical structure serves as the landmark for where the external iliac artery becomes the CFA in the lower extremities?**

(A) Adductor canal

(B) Profunda femoris

(C) Inguinal ligament

(D) Arcuate ligament

101. **What is the syndrome that produces a mass effect on the osteofascial compartments on an extremity resulting in a decrease in blood flow and is often caused by trauma?**

(A) TOS

(B) Compartment syndrome

(C) Raynaud's syndrome

(D) Subclavian steal syndrome

102. **The most clinically significant complication associated with a peripheral aneurysm is**

(A) Rupture

(B) Dissection

(C) Embolism

(D) Infection

103. **A patient with severe bilateral iliac artery disease is most likely to receive which type of lower extremity bypass?**

(A) Femoral popliteal bypass

(B) Femoral to femoral bypass

(C) Aorta-bifemoral bypass

(D) Axillary femoral bypass

104. **Which of the following can cause a spectral waveform in the lower extremity to change its shape to monophasic?**

(A) Normal resting flow

(B) Vasoconstriction

(C) Decreased cardiac output

(D) Postexercise

105. While performing a lower extremity arterial duplex examination on a patient, a velocity of 90 cm/s is obtained within the distal SFA. About 1 cm distal to that a velocity of 200 cm/s is obtained. What would be considered the percent stenosis using the velocity ratio criteria?

    (A) Normal
    (B) More than 50% stenosis
    (C) More than 75% stenosis
    (D) Less than 50% stenosis

106. What instrumentation uses infrared light that reflects off the red blood cells as they flow through the body to create a waveform?

    (A) PVRs
    (B) Power Doppler
    (C) PPG
    (D) Strain gauge plethysmography

107. A stenosis of the lower extremity arteries is most likely hemodynamically significant when the velocity ratio is

    (A) Less than 2.0
    (B) More than 2.0
    (C) More than 1.5
    (D) Less than 1.5

108. The hypogastric artery is also known as what artery?

    (A) PFA
    (B) Common iliac artery
    (C) External iliac artery
    (D) Internal iliac artery

109. The first branch originating from the most proximal portion of the subclavian artery is the

    (A) Thyrocervical trunk
    (B) Vertebral artery
    (C) Internal mammary artery
    (D) Lateral thoracic artery

110. An ABI of 0.60 correlates with which symptom?

    (A) Rest pain
    (B) Tissue loss
    (C) Claudication
    (D) Gangrene

111. Figure 4–75 is a color Doppler image of the left axillary artery in a patient who has decreased pulses distally. What does this finding indicate?

    (A) Arterial dissection
    (B) Critical stenosis
    (C) Arteriovenous malformation
    (D) Arterial occlusion

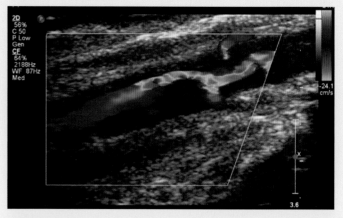

FIGURE 4–75.

112. Figure 4–76 was obtained during a duplex examination of a lower extremities bypass graft. Based on the findings in this image, what is most likely the diagnosis?

    (A) Normal
    (B) Occlusion
    (C) Stenosis
    (D) Pseudoaneurysm

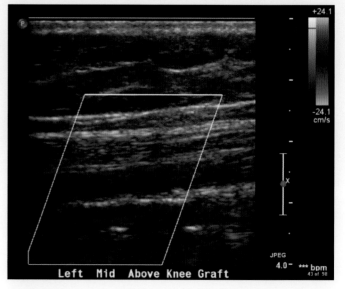

FIGURE 4–76.

113. **What pathology of the popliteal artery is identified in Figure 4–77?**

    (A) No pathology seen

    (B) Dissection with thrombosed false lumen

    (C) Aneurysm with partial thrombus

    (D) Complete occlusion

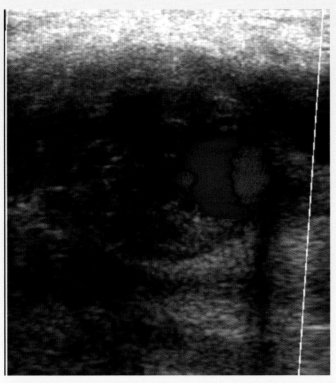

FIGURE 4–77.

114. **The signs known as the "six Ps" which indicate the presence of an acute arterial occlusion are**

    (A) Pain, Pallor, Paralysis, Pus, Pulselessness, Poikilothermia

    (B) Pain, Pallor, Paralysis, Paresthesia, Pulselessness, Palpable

    (C) Pain, Pallor, Paralysis, Paresthesia, Pulselessness, Poikilothermia

    (D) Painless, Pallor, Paralysis, Paresthesia, Pulselessness, Poikilothermia

115. **What is the most common reason for a stenosis to develop within a lower extremity bypass graft?**

    (A) ASO

    (B) Myointimal hyperplasia

    (C) Fibromuscular dysplasia

    (D) Arteritis

Answers and Explanations

1. **(A)** The normal spectral waveform of the brachial artery is high resistant and can either be triphasic or biphasic, described as multiphasic. The only difference between triphasic and biphasic is the third component of the waveform that can be lost with age due to decrease in the elasticity of the arteries. There is much disagreement about waveform terminology, so multiphasic is less specific.

2. **(A)** TOS is specific to the upper extremities. Carotid body tumors only occur at the carotid bifurcation, and the other two choices can occur in the upper or lower extremities.

3. **(C)** Laminar blood flow is the normal flow found in most of the peripheral arteries and consists of a parabolic velocity profile which means that flow increases toward the center of the vessel and decreases toward the vessel walls.

4. **(A)** The common femoral is a peripheral artery and at rest should have high resistant flow in normal patients.

5. **(A)** The DPA is a continuation of the ATA.

6. **(C)** Spectral broadening does not refer to a decrease in bandwidth with disturbed flow. It refers to an increase in bandwidth with disturbed flow.

7. **(B)** The brachiocephalic (aka innominate) artery is the first branch origination from the thoracic aortic arch and is only present on the right side.

8. **(A)** The popliteal is a continuation of the SFA as it passes through the adductor canal below the knee into the popliteal fossa.

9. **(D)** The PTA runs along the medial aspect of the lower leg and courses posterior to the medial malleolus.

10. **(C)** The waveform shown in Figure 4–53 is a typical triphasic (multiphasic) waveform.

11. **(A)** The PSV is increased in this monophasic waveform. Also, note the spectral broadening present. Not enough information is given to determine if there is reversal of flow or not; based on the spectral Doppler, the flow is all going in one direction.

12. **(B)** The waveform shown in Figure 4–55 is a classic post-stenotic waveform demonstrating an ill-defined border, spectral broadening and some reversal of flow.

13. **(B)** The waveform shown in Figure 4–56 is a monophasic waveform with no diastolic flow and diminished peak systolic flow suggesting a distal occlusion.

14. **(D)** A doubling in PSV between adjacent segments is consistent with a hemodynamically significant stenosis greater than 50%. The velocities obtained within these segments more than doubles going from 80 to 210 cm/s.

15. **(B)** Reversed vein grafts are common lower extremity bypasses. None of the other choices are lower extremity bypass grafts.

16. **(C)** Claudication is pain in the lower extremities as a result of hypoxia that is reproducible and induced by exercise. After a patient rests, they are then able to walk the same distance before the pain reoccurs.

17. **(A)** Ischemic rest pain can be relieved by lowering the legs dependently, such as standing or dropping the legs off the side of the bed. The arterial inflow is so poor that gravity is needed to get the blood to the feet.

18. **(B)** The peak systolic blood pressure in an area of a limb distal to a hemodynamically significant stenosis will decrease.

19. **(C)** ASO is the most common cause of peripheral arterial disease of the lower extremities.

20. **(D)** The most common site of ASO in the lower extremities is the distal SFA through the adductor canal.

21. **(C)** Aorta

22. **(H)** Common iliac artery

23. **(E)** Internal iliac artery

24. **(G)** External iliac artery

25. **(A)** CFA

26. **(F)** PFA

27. **(D)** SFA

28. **(B)** Popliteal artery

29. **(I)** Tibioperoneal trunk

30. **(K)** ATA

31. **(N)** PTA

32. **(L)** Peroneal artery

33. **(J)** DPA

34. **(M)** Plantar arch

35. **(C)** PVRs in general are more accurate than segmental pressures because they are not affected by the limitations of segmental pressures such as cuff artifact or calcified vessels. An obese patient will most likely have falsely elevated pressures due to the cuff size being too small for the limb. In an obese patient with underlying peripheral arterial disease, these elevated pressures may appear to be at a normal level. If the cuff size were appropriate for the limb in this same patient, it would result in a much lower pressure.

36. **(B)** The pregraft compression study in a patient with an AVF steal will have reduced blood flow to the arm and hand because the fistula is stealing that blood flow. When the graft is manually compressed during the post study, there should be an increase in blood flow in order to confirm the diagnosis of a steal.

37. **(D)** Spectral Doppler waveform number two shows a focal increase in velocity compared to number one resulting in a V_r more than 3 which is consistent with a more than 75% stenosis. Spectral Doppler waveform number three demonstrates tardus parvus flow supplying further evidence of a critical stenosis.

38. **(B)** The waveform shown in Figure 4–59 is a classic tardus parvus waveform that is found distal to a significant stenosis.

39. **(C)** There is an increase in velocity at the anastomosis site demonstrated in the spectral Doppler waveform number two resulting in a PSV ratio more than 2 which is consistent with a more than 50% stenosis at the anastomosis site. The spectral Doppler waveform number three demonstrates decreased volume flow (< 500 mL/min) as a result of the stenosis.

40. **(C)** The waveform shown in Figure 4–61 is a classic to-and-fro waveform that is found within the neck of a pseudoaneurysm.

41. **(B)** Angioplasty is the procedure in which a balloon-tipped catheter is inflated within a stenotic lesion in an attempt to restore normal blood flow to an area.

42. **(D)** The brachial artery bifurcates just below the antecubital fossa into the radial and ulnar arteries. The radial artery runs along the lateral side of the forearm while the ulnar artery runs along the medial side.

43. **(B)** Noninvasive testing for TOS involves performing physiologic testing with the use of PVRs or PPG while moving the patient's arms in several positions in an attempt to reduce the perfusion to the hand. The symptomatic position should be attempted; however, there are many common positions used during this examination such as the Adson maneuver with arms abducted out to sides, the costoclavicular maneuver with chest pushed forward and shoulders back, military position with elbow pointing to the rear and arms almost upright with palms facing forward, the hands straight up 180 degrees, and the arms straight out and abducted toward the rear.

44. **(C)** As the diameter of a blood vessel decreases, the flow remains a constant as long as the stenosis is not hemodynamically significant (see Chapter 1).

45. **(B)** In a normal vessel, the velocity of blood flow and the pressure do not change significantly. When a hemodynamically significant stenosis is present within an artery, there is an increase in the pressure gradient across the segment as well as an increase in the velocity of blood flow within the stenosis. The turbulent flow that exists past the stenosis caused the pressure distal to the stenosis to drop resulting in a pressure that is now lower than the pressure proximal to the stenosis. The difference between these two pressures is what is known as a pressure gradient and is what increases with a stenosis due to the change in pressures.

46. **(B)** An in-situ saphenous vein bypass is created by leaving the native vein in its normal anatomical position, removing the internal valves and ligating the accessory branches, and finally attaching each end to the proximal and distal native arteries. This type of surgical bypass has the highest potential for a missed branch and retained valves because the vein is not being completely removed and reversed, unlike the reversed saphenous vein bypass in which the vales do not have to be removed. There would be no concern for missed branches or retained valves with an artificial bypass graft.

47. **(A)** The waveform shown in Figure 4–62 is a classic peaked pulse waveform where the dicrotic notch is higher than normal and is commonly seen in patients with Raynaud's disease.

48. **(C)** An AVF occurs when there is an abnormal connection between a native artery and vein resulting in a high volume jet of flow passing between both systems. They can occur spontaneously or traumatically.

49. **(C)** The ABI is the most widely utilized ratio used to evaluate overall perfusion to the lower extremity arteries and is calculated by taking the ankle pressure and dividing it by the higher of the two brachial pressures.

50. **(A)** PSV, end-diastolic velocity, and PSV ratios are all used to determine the severity of a stenosis. RI and PI are indices used to quantify the distal bed. The ABI is not performed with duplex sonography.

51. **(D)** A palpable (grade 3) pulse indicates normal perfusion to a lower extremity, therefore is not an indication of an obstruction.

52. **(D)** Tobacco, hypertension, diabetes, and hyperlipidemia are all risk factors for cardiovascular disease. Hypolipidemia is a decrease in the amount of blood lipids.

53. **(B)** A pressure gradient more than 30 mm Hg indicates that there is disease present at or above the cuff with the lower pressure. A pressure gradient more than 30 mm Hg between the thigh and calf cuffs indicates femoral popliteal disease.

54. **(C)** The dicrotic limb is the first component that is lost in a PVR waveform when any arterial disease is present.

55. **(D)** In order for an AVF to be considered mature and ready for hemodialysis use by duplex, the draining vein should be at least 4 mm in size, there should be no narrowing at the anastomosis site that is confirmed by a

ratio of less than 2, and the volume flow should be at least 500 mL/min (ideally the volume flow should be >800 mL/min). Continuous flow on the venous side of the fistula would be an indication of an out flow venous obstruction not evidence of maturity.

56. **(C)** On the right, there is a decrease in the high thigh pressure (should be 30 mm Hg greater than the higher brachial with the four-cuff technique) with slight rounding and decrease in amplitude of the PVR waveform consistent with mild iliac disease. There is also a decrease in pressure of more than 30 mm Hg between the low thigh and calf cuffs with a dampened PVR waveform at the calf level consistent with moderate femoral popliteal disease. On the left, there is a decrease in pressure of more than 30 mm Hg between the low thigh and the calf cuff with an absent dicrotic notch on the PVR waveform consistent with mild femoral popliteal disease.

57. **(A)** Figure 4–67 demonstrates a 60 mm Hg pressure gradient between the two brachial cuffs as well as a dampened PVR waveform at the same level. A pressure gradient more than 15 mm Hg between arms or adjacent cuffs indicates that there is disease present at or above the cuff with the lower pressure. The 60 mm Hg pressure gradient between arms in this patient indicates that there is disease present within the left subclavian and/or axillary arteries.

58. **(D)** Aortoiliac disease can be ruled out in this patient because the right high thigh systolic pressure and PVR waveform are normal. If there were significant aorta disease, it would affect both the right and left inflow to the lower extremities.

59. **(C)** The analog Doppler waveforms are multiphasic and bidirectional down to the popliteal level. Below that level in the PTAs and DPAs, the waveforms are monophasic and unidirectional indicating tibial disease.

60. **(D)** Blue toes are a classic sign of an embolism that traveled through the blood steam to end up lodged within the smaller arteries of the digits.

61. **(C)** A reversed saphenous vein graft involves harvesting the saphenous vein, reversing its normal anatomical orientation, and connecting to the arteries. The anatomical reversing of the vein eliminates the need to remove the internal valves making them open in the correct direction of flow.

62. **(B)** A normal analog Doppler signal within a peripheral artery should be triphasic or biphasic with bidirectional flow because of the distal resistance that exists normally in a peripheral arterial system. When significant disease is present, the distal arterioles dilate resulting in a decrease in resistance changing the waveform to monophasic with flow continuous in one direction.

63. **(C)** A normal toe pressure is 60% to 80% of the higher brachial pressure.

64. **(D)** Innominate artery

65. **(B)** Common carotid artery

66. **(G)** Subclavian artery

67. **(F)** Axillary artery

68. **(E)** Brachial artery

69. **(A)** Radial artery

70. **(C)** Ulnar artery

71. **(A)** When using the four-cuff technique during a segmental pressure examination, the high thigh pressure is typically elevated due to the size of the limb. This higher pressure is reproducible and should be at least 30 mm Hg greater than the higher brachial pressure to be considered normal.

72. **(C)** Both arteries and veins have three distinct layers to their vessel walls. The innermost layer is known as the intima, the middle layer is the media, and the outer layer is the adventitia. Even though they have the same three layers, arterial walls are thicker than vein walls and have a much higher internal pressure than the veins as well. In addition to these differences, veins also have internal valves that help promote flow back to the heart that are not present in the arteries. Veins should be easily collapsible, while the rigid walls of the arteries make them much harder to compress.

73. **(D)** A to-and-fro waveform within the neck of the pseudoaneursym is a classic finding used for the diagnosis.

74. **(C)** Cuff artifact can occur when the width of the blood pressure cuff is either too large or too small for the limb. If the width of the cuff is less than 20% the diameter of the limb, it will result in a falsely elevated peak systolic pressure. If the width of the cuff is too large, it can also cause the peak systolic pressure to be falsely lower.

75. **(A)** Mild, **(B)** Severe, **(C)** Moderate, **(D)** Normal

76. **(B)** Popliteal entrapment syndrome occurs when the head of the gastrocnemius muscle compresses the popliteal artery resulting in a decrease in perfusion to the lower extremity when the calf muscle is contracted. The evaluation with noninvasive testing includes obtaining pressures and waveforms with the calf muscle relaxed and then repeated with the calf muscle contracted. If popliteal entrapment is present, there will be a reduction in blood flow during contraction.

77. **(C)** A dampened waveform with a delay to peak systole (tardus parvus) seen in the CFA indicates that significant proximal disease is present, most likely in the aortoiliac region.

78. **(B)** The normal response to exercise is an increase in the ABIs postexercise. A reduction in the ABIs indicates that disease is present. The greater the pressure drop, the more severe the disease. The recovery time also provides

information about the level of disease. If the recovery time exceeds 12 minutes that typically indicates that multiple levels of disease are present.

79. **(B)** A PBI of less than 0.65 is consistent with vasculogenic impotence.

80. **(B)** The normal response of the cavernous arteries during a penile duplex examination postinjection is that they will typically double in diameter size, have an increase in PSV of at least 30 cm/s, and will have increased diastolic flow.

81. **(C)** There are various degrees of TOS not all of which will result in a complete loss of blood flow to the hand; however in order to confirm the diagnosis, there must be a reduction in blood flow that is position dependent and it must be accompanied by symptoms.

82. **(D)** Raynaud's syndrome is commonly diagnosed using a cold immersion study which involves submerging a patient's hands in ice water that results in a more than 20% drop in peak systolic pressure.

83. **(B)** One of the main advantages of an orthograde saphenous vein bypass over a reversed saphenous vein bypass is that there is no size mismatch at the proximal and distal anastomosis sites. In general, the saphenous vein is larger in caliber at the proximal portion and small at the distal end. By leaving the vein in this anatomical position, it allows the larger end to be connected to the larger proximal arteries of the leg and the smaller end to the smaller tibial arteries. This does however now require the removal of the internal valves that does not have to occur with a reserved saphenous vein bypass.

84. **(A)** Retrograde flow in the native artery proximal to the distal anastomosis of a lower extremity bypass graft is a normal finding that can often be providing collateral flow to the proximal portion of the limb and beneficial to the patient.

85. **(C)** There are many types of AVFs that can be used for hemodialysis. Some of the more common are the cephalic vein to either the brachial or radial arteries and the basilic vein to either the brachial or radial arteries.

86. **(D)** The flow volume through an AVF needs to be high in order for the fistula to be used successfully during hemodialysis. The typical volume flow through a normal mature AVF is more than 500 mL/min and is often in the 1,000 mL/min range.

87. **(A)** There are many ways to image peripheral arteries; however, conventional angiography is still considered the "gold standard" when it comes to correlation of results.

88. **(C)** A "filling defect" is the effect that makes a vessel appear narrowed where plaque has replaced the lumen.

89. **(C)** This is an angiogram of the lower extremity demonstrating an occlusion of the distal SFA with a large collateral vessel.

90. **(B)** The duplex image shows an elevated PSV with aliasing on color Doppler and spectral broadening all findings that are consistent with a hemodynamically significant stenosis.

91. **(C)** The waveform seen in Figure 4–71 shows high peak systolic and high diastolic flow that is consistent with a traumatic AVF. These findings are also consistent with the patient's clinical presentation. A bruit heard in the area of a recent puncture site following a cardiac catheterization is a common presentation of these findings.

92. **(A)** Both the right and left ankle peak systolic pressures increased following exercise, which is the normal response in the absence of disease.

93. **(B)** The segmental pressures have a significant drop in systolic pressure (>30 mm Hg) between the right thigh and calf indicating femoral popliteal disease as well as a reduced systolic pressure and pressure index at the left thigh level indicating left iliac disease.

94. **(C)** Anacrotic limb

95. **(A)** Catacrotic limb

96. **(B)** Dicrotic limb

97. **(D)** Coarctation of the aorta is a congenital narrowing of the thoracic aorta where it arches down toward the abdomen.

98. **(A)** The aorta and iliac arteries are the second most common area of atherosclerotic disease in the lower extremities, with the distal SFA as the most common site.

99. **(C)** A finding of an echogenic linear structure that appears to move within the lumen of a blood vessel is consistent with an arterial dissection that can be caused by trauma or severe hypertension. Severe hypertension if untreated can cause an increased strain on the blood vessel walls causing them to separate resulting in a dissection.

100. **(C)** The inguinal ligament is the anatomical structure stretching from the anterior, superior border of the iliac crest to the pubic bone and serves as the landmark for where the external iliac artery becomes the CFA in the lower extremities.

101. **(B)** Compartment syndrome produces a mass effect on the osteofascial compartments on an extremity resulting in a decrease in blood flow and is often caused by trauma.

102. **(C)** Peripheral arterial aneurysms often contain a layer of thrombus as a result of the swirling pattern of blood flow found within the aneurysm. The thrombus within the lumen of the aneurysm can often be a source of emboli to the distal portions of the extremity. This type of embolism is the most clinically significant complication for peripheral aneurysms, unlike with abdominal aortic aneurysms where rupture is the most significant clinical complication.

103. (C) The intent of any lower extremity bypass graft is to get above the level of significant disease and below the level of the most significant disease. With bilateral iliac disease, the most logical type of bypass graft that would accomplish restoring normal blood flow to the lower extremities is an aorta-bifemoral bypass graft.

104. (D) Both proximal diseases as well as postexercise hemodynamics cause the distal arteriole beds to dilate, resulting in the peripheral artery waveform changing to a monophasic form.

105. (B) The formula for calculating a PSV ratio within the peripheral arteries is $PSV_{stenosis}/PSV_{proximal\ to\ stenosis}$. For this patient, the calculation would be 200/90 = 2.2. A PSV ratio more than 2 is consistent with a more than 50% stenosis.

106. (C) PPG uses infrared light that reflects off the red blood cells as they flow through the body to create a waveform and is typically used to obtain the digital waveforms and pressures during a noninvasive assessment of the lower extremities.

107. (B) Stenotic lesions within the lower extremity arteries are much more likely to be hemodynamically significant when the PSV is elevated and the velocity ratio is more than 2.

108. (D) Another name for the internal iliac artery is the hypogastric artery.

109. (B) The vertebral artery is the first branch originating from the most proximal portion of the subclavian artery followed by the costocervical artery, thyrocervical trunk artery, internal mammary artery, and the lateral thoracic artery.

110. (C) An ABI of 0.60 is most likely consistent with claudication symptoms.

111. (B) Figure 4–75 shows a color Doppler image of the axillary artery with a severely narrowed lumen with aliasing present. These findings are consistent with a critical stenosis of the axillary artery.

112. (B) The absence of color Doppler within the bypass graft suggests the presence of a total occlusion.

113. (C) Figure 4–77 demonstrates an enlarged popliteal artery with intraluminal thrombus consistent with a popliteal aneurysm.

114. (C) The symptoms associated with acute occlusive disease are known as the six Ps. They are: Pain, Pallor, Paralysis, Paresthesia, Pulselessness, Poikilothermia.

115. (B) Myointimal hyperplasia is the most common cause of stenosis within a lower extremity bypass graft.

Suggested Readings

1. Pellerito JS, Polak JF. *Introduction to Vascular Ultrasound*. 7th ed. Philadelphia, PA: Elsevier; 2020.

2. Kupinski AM. *Diagnostic Medical Sonography: The Vascular System*, 2nd ed. Baltimore, MD: Wolters Kluwer; 2018.

3. Hirsch AT, Haskal ZJ, Hertzer NR, et al. ACC/AHA 2005 Guidelines for the Management of Patients With Peripheral Arterial Disease (Lower Extremity, Renal, Mesenteric, and Abdominal Aortic): A Collaborative Report from the American Association for Vascular Surgery/Society for Vascular Surgery, Society for Cardiovascular Angiography and Interventions, Society for Vascular Medicine and Biology, Society of Interventional Radiology, and the ACC/AHA Task Force on Practice Guidelines (Writing Committee to Develop Guidelines for the Management of Patients With Peripheral Arterial Disease). *J Am Coll Cardiol*. 2006;47(6):1239–1312.

4. Rooke TW, Hirsch AT, Misra S, et al. 2011 ACCF/AHA Focused Update of the Guideline for the Management of Patients With Peripheral Artery Disease (Updating the 2005 Guideline): A Report of the American College of Cardiology Foundation/American Heart Association Task Force on Practice Guidelines. *J Am Coll Cardiol*. 2011;58(19):2020–2045.

5. Rumwell C, McPharlin M. *Vascular Technology: An Illustrated Review*. 5th ed. Pasadena, CA: Davies Publishing; 2017.

6. Raines JK, Almeida JI. *Noninvasive Vascular Diagnosis*. London: Springer; 2007.

7. Winsor TA. Influence of arterial disease on the systolic blood pressure gradients of the extremity. *Am J Med Sci*. 1950;220: 117–126.

8. Hirsch AT, Criqui MH, Treat-Jacobson D, et al. Peripheral arterial disease detection, awareness, and treatment in primary care. *J Am Med Assoc*. 2001;286(11):1317–1324.

9. Norgren L, Hiatt WR, Dormandy JA, et al. Inter-society consensus for the management of peripheral arterial disease (TASC II). *Eur J Vasc Endovasc Surg*. 2007;33(1):S1–S75.

10. Carter SA. Clinical measurements of systolic pressures in limbs with arterial occlusive disease. *J Am Med Assoc*. 1969;207:1869–1874.

11. Daigle RJ. *Techniques in Noninvasive Vascular Diagnosis*. 4th ed. Colorado: Summer Publishing; 2014.

12. Osmundson PJ, O'Fallon WM, Clements IP, et al. Reproducibility of noninvasive tests of peripheral occlusive arterial disease. *J Vasc Surg*. 1985;2(5):678–683.

13. Yao ST, Hobbs JT, Irvine WT. Ankle systolic pressure measurements in arterial disease affecting the lower extremities. *Br J Surg*. 1969;56:676–679.

14. Strandness DE, Sumner DS. *Hemodynamics for Surgeons*. New York, NY: Grune & Stratton; 1975.

15. Stein R, Hriljac I, Halperin JL, et al. Limitation of the resting ankle-brachial index in symptomatic patients with peripheral arterial disease. *Vasc Med*. 2006;11(1):29–33.

16. Hodgkiss-Harlow KD, Bandyk DF. Arterial duplex imaging of the lower extremity arteries and interventions. *J Vasc Ultrasound*. 2012;36(2):143–151.

17. Ligush J, Reavis SW, Preisser JS, et al. Duplex ultrasound scanning defines operative strategies for patients with limb-threatening ischemia. *J Vasc Surg*. 1998;28(3):482–490.

18. Mazzaariol F, Ascher E, Salles-Chunha SX, et al. Values and limitations of duplex ultrasonography as the sole imaging method of preoperative evaluation for popliteal and infrapopliteal bypasses. *Ann Vasc Surg*. 1999;13(1):1–10.

19. Moneta GL, Yeager RA, Antonovic R, et al. Accuracy of lower extremity arterial duplex mapping. *J Vasc Surg*. 1992;15(2):275–283.

20. Jager KA, Ricketts HJ, Strandness DE. Duplex scanning for the evaluation of lower extremity limb arterial disease. In: Bernstein EF, ed. *Noninvasive Diagnosis Techniques in Vascular Disease*. St. Louis, MO: Mosby; 1985:619–631.

21. Leng GC, Whyman MR, Donnan PT, et al. Accuracy and reproducibility of duplex ultrasonography in grading femoropopliteal stenosis. *J Vasc Surg*. 1993;17:510–517.

22. Sacks D, Robinson ML, Marinelli DL, et al. Peripheral arterial Doppler ultrasonography: diagnostic criteria. *J Ultrasound Med*. 1992;11(3):95–103.

23. Mueller SC, von Wallenberg-Pachaly H, Voges GE, et al. Comparison of selective internal iliac pharmaco-angiography, penile brachial index and duplex sonography with pulsed Doppler analysis for the evaluation of vasculogenic (arteriogenic) impotence. *J Urol*. 1990;143(5):928–932.

24. Cato R, Kupinski AM. Graft assessment by duplex ultrasound scanning. *J Vasc Technol*. 1994;18(5):307–310.

25. Singh P, Robbin ML, Lockhart ME, et al. Clinically immature arteriovenous hemodialysis fistulas: effect of US on salvage. *Radiology*. 2008;246:299–305.

26. Pietura R, Janczarek M, Zaluska W, et al. Colour Doppler ultrasound assessment of well-functioning mature arteriovenous fistulas for haemodialysis access. *Eur J Radiol*. 2005;55(1):113–119.

27. Robbin ML, Chamberlain MD, Lockhart ME, et al. Hemodialysis arteriovenous fistula maturity: US evaluation. *Radiology*. 2002;225:59–64.

28. Robbin ML, Oser RF, Clements MW, et al. Hemodialysis access graft stenosis: US detection. *Radiology*. 1998;208:655–661.

29. Shenoy S, Darcy M. Ultrasound as a tool for preoperative planning, monitoring, and interventions in dialysis arteriovenous access. *Am J Roentgenol*. 2013;201(4):W539–43.

30. Size G. *Inside Ultrasound: Vascular Reference Guide*. Pasadena, California: Davies Publishing, 2013.

31. Kim ES, Sharma AM, Scissons R, Dawson D, Eberhardt RT, Gerhard-Herman M, Hughes JP, Knight S, Marie Kupinski A, Mahe G, Neumyer M. Interpretation of peripheral arterial and venous Doppler waveforms: A Consensus Statement from the Society for Vascular Medicine and Society for Vascular Ultrasound. *Vascular Medicine*. 2020; Jul 15:1358863X20937665.

5

Peripheral Venous

PERIPHERAL VENOUS ANATOMY

Vessel Anatomy

Veins are thin-walled tubular structures that carry blood back to the heart. The venous system is a low-pressure system with a typical intraluminal pressure of 5-15 mm Hg, a pressure that is significantly lower than that of the arteries. Because of this lower internal pressure, veins are easily collapsible. The size and shape of veins can vary depending on the patient and certain conditions. The shape of the veins is determined by the transmural pressure. The transmural pressure is the difference between the internal pressure of the veins and the external pressure of the surrounding tissue. Veins, similar to arteries, have three distinct layers. These layers are composed of different materials than the arteries, and are typically much thinner. The three layers are:

- Tunica intima—Innermost layer of the veins composed of endothelial cells.
- Tunica media—Middle layer of the veins composed of smooth muscle and fiber.
- Tunica adventitia—Outermost layer of the veins composed of elastic tissue surrounded by a fibrous layer.

Veins also differ from arteries in that they contain internal valves that prevent blood from flowing in a retrograde fashion. There are more valves closer to the ankles due to increased hydrostatic pressure distally. These bicuspid valves are located in the intima layer of the majority of the upper and lower extremity veins with the exception of the brachiocephalic veins.

Lower Extremities

The venous anatomy of the lower extremities is composed of three components. Knowing the differences between these components and understanding their function is essential to all venous testing. The three components are:

- The deep system
- The superficial system
- Perforators

Deep System

The deep veins of the lower extremities and pelvis are paired with arteries and are deep below the muscle fascia. Their function is to provide the main source of blood return from the legs back to the heart.

The deep veins of the lower extremities start with the plantar veins in the foot. These veins join to form the posterior tibial veins (PTVs) that run along the medial aspect of the ankles and calves (Fig. 5–1). The calf veins are typically paired, and are adjacent to their corresponding artery; however, take note that anatomical variants can exist anywhere throughout the vascular system. Deeper in the calf just adjacent to the fibula are the paired peroneal veins that run parallel to the PTVs. The peroneal veins join the PTVs just below the knee to form the tibioperoneal trunk. The paired anterior tibial veins (ATVs) run along the lateral aspect of the calf between the tibia and fibula and join the tibioperoneal trunk to form the single popliteal vein. The popliteal vein courses behind the knee and then passes through the adductor canal. There are two sets of deep muscular veins that provide drainage for the calf muscles and connect to the deep system. The soleal sinuses drain blood from the lower calf muscle (soleus) and connect to the posterior tibial and peroneal veins. These veins serve as a reservoir for the "calf-muscle pump" before emptying. The gastrocnemius veins drain blood from the upper calf muscle (gastrocnemius) and connect to the popliteal vein (Fig. 5–2).

Once the popliteal vein passes through the adductor canal, it continues as the femoral vein (FV). The FV courses proximally

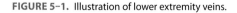

Common femoral vein

Great saphenous vein

Profunda femoris vein

Femoral vein

Tibioperoneal trunk

Popliteal vein

Gastrocnemius veins

Anterior tibial vein

Posterior tibial vein

Soleus sinus

Peroneal vein

FIGURE 5–1. Illustration of lower extremity veins.

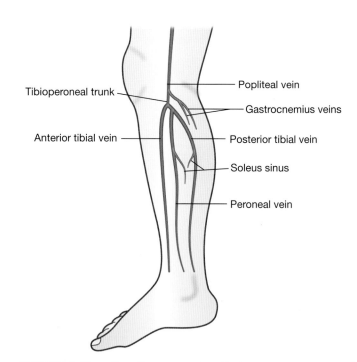

Tibioperoneal trunk

Popliteal vein

Gastrocnemius veins

Anterior tibial vein

Posterior tibial vein

Soleus sinus

Peroneal vein

FIGURE 5–2. Illustration of lower extremity calf veins.

about two-thirds of the way up the thigh to join the profunda femoris also known as the deep femoral vein (DFV). The confluence of these two veins gives rise to the common femoral vein (CFV). The CFV becomes the external iliac vein superior to the inguinal ligament. The external iliac vein continues into the pelvis where it is joined by the internal iliac vein to become the common iliac vein. The right and left common iliac veins eventually join in the lower abdomen to form the inferior vena cava (Fig. 5–3).

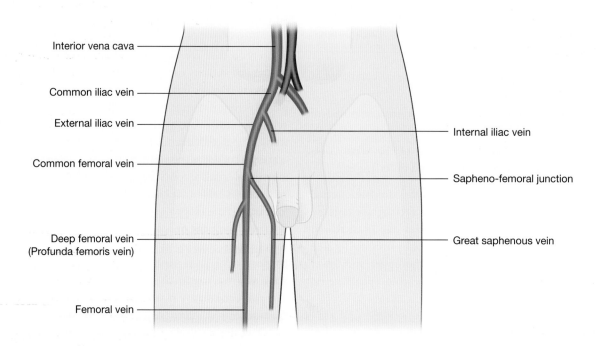

Interior vena cava

Common iliac vein

External iliac vein

Internal iliac vein

Common femoral vein

Sapheno-femoral junction

Deep femoral vein
(Profunda femoris vein)

Great saphenous vein

Femoral vein

FIGURE 5–3. Illustration of lower extremity veins showing the anatomy of the thigh and deep pelvic veins. The two common iliac veins join to form the IVC.

Superficial System

The superficial veins of the lower extremities are not paired with arteries and are located just under the surface of the skin anterior to the muscle fascia for the majority of their course. Their function is much different than that of the deep system. The main function of the superficial veins is to help regulate the body's temperature by releasing or conserving heat.

There are two main superficial veins of the lower extremities. They are the great saphenous veins (GSVs) and small saphenous veins (SSVs). The GSV is the longest vein in the body and originates anterior to the medial malleolus. It courses along the medial aspect of the leg all the way up to where it connects to the CFV at the saphenofemoral junction (SFJ). Along the course of the GSVs, there are many secondary branches that empty into the main branch (Fig. 5–4). One of the most mentionable of those branches is the posterior arch in the calf. This branch serves as a connection for several important perforators which will be discussed later in this chapter. The SSVs originate in the dorsum of the foot and course along the posterior aspect of the calf to eventually join the popliteal vein. There is an anatomical variant that is worth mentioning in regard to the SSV. Approximately two-thirds of people have a variant where the SSV continues above the knee and joins the great saphenous, called a thigh extension (TE) vein or the "vein of Giacomini." This tributary vein is not as prone to insufficiency as the main GSV and SSV trunks; however, its prevalence increases when one of the main trunks is incompetent.

> ### Venous nomenclature
>
> Over the years, there has been a change in some of the venous nomenclature. Specifically for the lower extremities, the FV was previously known as the superficial femoral vein. The GSVs and SSVs were previously known as the long or greater and lesser or short saphenous veins, respectively. In 2018, *Circulation* published a new consensus statement on venous ultrasound that changed "chronic DVT" or "chronic scarring" to "chronic postthrombotic change."

Perforators

Perforating veins are veins that provide a connection between the superficial and deep systems. All perforators contain a one-way valve that only allows blood to flow from the superficial system to the deep system. There are more than 100 perforators all along the course of the calf and thigh in most legs. They are typically very small in size and named in groups (Fig. 5–5). The posterior tibial perforators that connect to the posterior accessory GSV play a significant role in regard to venous stasis ulcers that will be discussed later in this chapter.

The perforators are grouped and named according to their location in the leg. In previous nomenclature, these vessels were named eponymously:

- Posterior tibial perforators (formerly Cockett's)
- Paratibial perforators (formerly Boyd's)
- Femoral canal (formerly Dodd's and Hunter's)

Upper Extremities

Deep System

The deep veins of the upper extremities start in the distal forearm and course proximally toward the antecubital fossa at the elbow joint. On the lateral side are the paired radial veins and on the medial side are the paired ulnar veins (Fig. 5–6). Similar to the lower extremities, the deep veins of the upper extremities are coupled with their corresponding arteries and deep below the muscle fascia. The radial and ulnar veins join at the antecubital fossa to form the brachial veins. There are typically two brachial veins surrounding one artery.

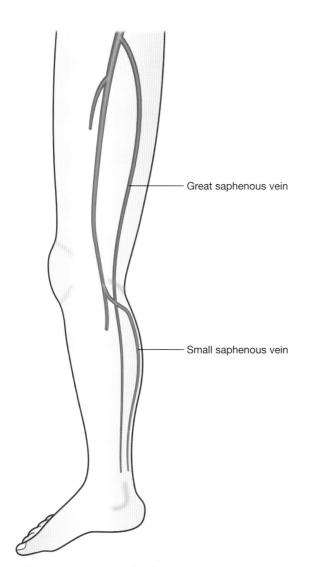

FIGURE 5–4. Illustration of superficial lower extremity veins.

Great saphenous vein

Small saphenous vein

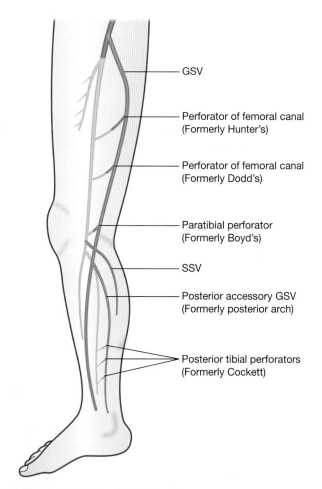

FIGURE 5–5. Illustration of perforator veins.

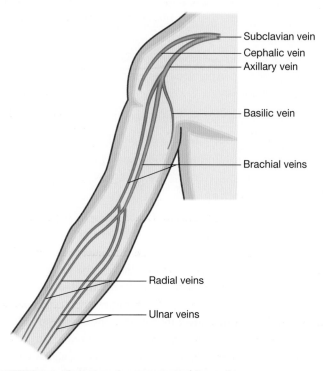

FIGURE 5–6. Illustration of upper extremity deep veins.

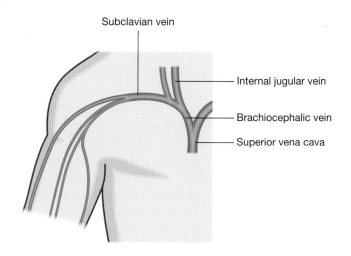

FIGURE 5–7. Illustration of upper extremity central veins.

The brachial veins course proximally and eventually become the axillary vein when joined by the basilic vein. The axillary vein courses centrally through the area of the axilla and becomes the subclavian vein after passing the border of the first rib. The subclavian vein courses more centrally inferior to the clavicle. At the base of the neck, the subclavian vein is joined by the internal jugular vein (IJV) and gives rise to the brachiocephalic vein bilaterally (Fig. 5–7). The left and right brachiocephalic veins join behind the sternum to form the superior vena cava (SVC).

Superficial System

Similar to the lower extremities, the superficial veins are not paired with arteries for the upper extremities. The two main superficial veins of the arm are the basilic and cephalic veins. The superficial veins of the arms begin at the metacarpal area and course proximally through the forearm and upper arm. The cephalic vein, which originates at an area called "the anatomic snuffbox," (Fig. 5–8) courses on the lateral aspect of the forearm and to join the axillary vein (Fig. 5–9). The basilic vein courses along the medial aspect of the forearm and upper arm joining the brachial vein to form the axillary vein. The median cubital vein connects the cephalic and basilic veins at the antecubital fossa.

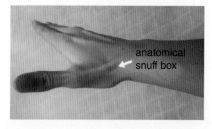

FIGURE 5–8. The "anatomic snuffbox." Arrow points to the location of the origin of the snuffbox. (Reproduced, with permission, from Parks EH. *Practical Office Orthopedics.* New York, NY; 2018; Figure 9–30. Copyright © McGraw Hill.)

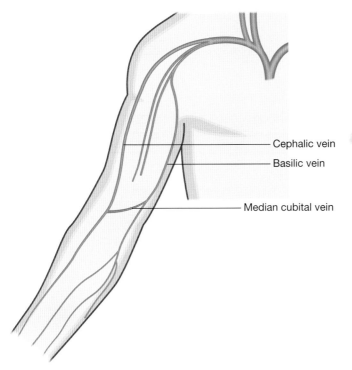

Cephalic vein

Basilic vein

Median cubital vein

FIGURE 5–9. Illustration of upper extremity superficial veins.

PATHOLOGY OF THE PERIPHERAL VENOUS SYSTEM

Thrombosis

Thrombus, sometimes referred to as a "clot," is a combination of red blood cells and fibrin that typically originates at the areas of valve cusps. Thrombus that develops in the deep venous system is known as deep vein thrombosis (DVT). In turn, thrombus that develops in the superficial system in known as superficial vein thrombosis. Most DVT becomes established in the calf due to stagnation and can propagate proximally. The clinical significance of DVT is that it can travel to the lung, causing a pulmonary embolism (PE) and death. The incidence of PE increases with DVT located above the knee. Treatment for DVT is typically blood thinners, first in the acute phase (up to 10 days) to prevent new clots from forming while the body breaks down the existing clot, and then longer term (10 days to 3 months) to prevent formation of new clot. Catheter-directed thrombolysis of occluded veins can be performed with newer thrombolysis catheters such as the Angiojet (Boston Scientific).

Pulmonary Embolism

PE is a blood clot that travels to the lung, causing death within 1 month in 10% to 30% of cases. The first symptom may be sudden death in about 25% of people who have a PE. The source for the majority of PEs is the deep veins of the lower extremities. Because of the urgent nature of an event such as a PE, it is critical that patients with DVT are treated immediately. PE can be a clinical diagnosis that is typically confirmed by a computed tomography (CT) angiography of the chest or nuclear medicine VQ lung scan. Thrombectomy can be performed using conventional angiography.

Pulmonary embolus most commonly originates from DVT, and DVT most commonly originates from the soleal vein in the calf. This clot propagates into the central venous system and travels superiorly. For this reason, calf veins (posterior tibial and peroneal veins) must be scanned with all lower extremity venous studies to rule out DVT.

Other Conditions

Phlegmasia Alba Dolens
Phlegmasia alba dolens is a condition that involves an obstructive iliofemoral DVT that causes extreme swelling with edema. This condition sometimes occurs during pregnancy.

Phlegmasia Cerulea Dolens
Phlegmasia cerulean dolens is also a condition that involves an obstructive iliofemoral DVT causing extreme swelling. This condition differs from phlegmasia alba dolens in that this condition is accompanied by cyanosis and reduces arterial inflow, which can be limb threatening. The cyanosis causes a blue or "cerulean" color, so this condition is sometimes called "painful blue leg."

Superior Vena Cava Syndrome
SVC syndrome is an obstruction of the SVC usually causing neck and facial swelling as well as difficulty breathing. SVC syndrome may be caused by indwelling catheters causing thrombus or stricture, or extrinsic compression from tumor or lymphadenopathy.

Venous Insufficiency

Venous valves promote blood flow return to the heart by not allowing blood to flow in a retrograde fashion back down to the ankles and the feet. When venous valves fail and become incompetent, they allow retrograde flow in the venous system. This is commonly known as venous reflux or chronic venous valvular insufficiency (CVVI). When insufficiency occurs, the blood in the distal veins starts to pool which increases the pressure within the venous system, causing venous hypertension. The increased pressure within the veins causes them to dilate and become varicose. As the pressure continues to increase, red blood cells and fluid may start to leak out into the surrounding tissue at the area just superior to the medial malleolus in an area known as the "gaiter zone." The breakdown of the red blood cells and fluid in this area can start to cause brawny pigment changes or even hardening of the skin, and over time can lead to venous stasis ulcerations. The most common cause of venous insufficiency is previous DVT that has scarred the lumen of the veins and has rendered the valves incompetent. This condition is known as postthrombotic change. Patients with CVVI sometimes present with "wet" venous ulcers in the gaiter zone.

PATIENT ASSESSMENT AND INTEGRATION OF DATA

Risk Factors

The three risk factors for the development of DVT are known as "Virchow's Triad." Virchow's Triad consists of:

- Trauma—This could include trauma to a vessel wall. For example, damage caused by an intravenous catheter. It could also be caused by trauma to an area of the body. For example, an injury to the calf during a motor vehicle accident.
- Stasis—Venous stasis refers to blood in the veins that is stagnant or not moving. Whenever blood flow slows down or stops completely, it is very likely to become thrombosed. Some examples of conditions that would cause venous stasis could be pregnancy due to extrinsic compression on the inferior vena cava by the fetus or immobility due to an inactive calf-muscle pump. With pregnancy, it is more common for stasis to occur in the later trimesters. Stasis caused by immobility is often the result of critical illness, postsurgery, or even extended airplane trips.
- Hypercoagulability—It is referred to as an abnormality of the molecular makeup of the blood that makes it much more prone to thrombosis. Hypercoagulability can be inherited as well as acquired. Example of an inherited blood disorder would be factor V Leiden. Oral contraceptives and patients with known or unknown cancer would be considered to have acquired hypercoagulability. Sometimes, the first sign of cancer in a patient is the presence of DVT in an otherwise healthy patient.

Signs and Symptoms

Acute Thrombosis

Many patients who have acute DVT are asymptomatic, although there are many patients who have symptoms that are suggestive of DVT without the presence of it. Clinical symptoms alone are insufficient for determining if DVT is present. There must be a confirmatory test to know for sure.

The main symptoms of acute DVT are:

- Pain
- Swelling
- Redness
- Superficial vein dilation

Chronic Postthrombotic Change

Chronic postthrombotic change is caused by chronic scarring to the lumen of the veins as a result of previous DVT.

The symptoms may vary depending on the venous systems involved.

The main symptoms of chronic venous disease are:

- Swelling
- Discoloration
- Ulcerations
- Varicose veins

Clinical Assessment

The clinical assessment of patients with suspected DVT typically starts with evaluating the probability of thrombosis based on risks and symptoms. Some centers utilize a clinical criteria method known as the Wells Criteria (Table 5–1). During this assessment, the physician will ask questions regarding risk factors, and a physical examination will be performed. The physical examination should include an inspection of the limb for specific symptoms suggesting DVT such as edema, redness, skin changes, ulcerations, and varicose veins. The edema and redness can be due to the accumulation of fluid and irritation of the interstitial tissue. Skin color changes can range from brawny discoloration at the gaiter zone to lipodermatosclerosis, which is thickening and hardening of the skin. Ulcerations

TABLE 5–1 • Wells Criteria—Clinical Scoring Method Used to Access the Probability of Deep Vein Thrombosis	
+1 Point	**– 2 Points**
Active cancer	
Paralysis, paresis, or recent plaster immobilization of leg	
Recent bedridden > 3 days or major trauma or surgery in past 4 weeks	
Localized tenderness along the distribution of the deep veins	Alterative diagnosis as likely or more likely than deep vein thrombosis
Entire lower limb swelling	
Calf swelling > 3 cm compared to the asymptomatic leg	
Pitting edema on symptomatic leg	
Collateral superficial veins on symptomatic leg	
Probability of DVT	
High probability ≥3 points Intermediate probability 1–2 points Low probability ≤0 point	

Primary Varicose Veins
= Confined ↑ pressure to the superficial system
w/ Absence to deep vein system obstruction.

Secondary Varicose vein
= Obstruction in the deep venous system
that led to an ↑ pressure in the Supf. System.

Protocols   **171**

are commonly seen directly above the medial malleolus due to incompetent perforators in that area, and are oftentimes very difficult to heal. Varicose veins are the result of increased pressure and dilation of the superficial veins of the limb. The increased pressure can be confined to just the superficial system in the absence of a deep system obstruction. In this case, the varicose veins are considered "primary varicose veins," which are often caused by an inherent weakness to the vein walls or by congenital defects to the internal valves themselves. Obstructions in the deep system that lead to increased pressure in the superficial system can also cause varicose veins known as "secondary varicose veins."

Clinical assessment for chronic venous insufficiency (CVI) and chronic valvular venous insufficiency (CVVI) has been created by the American Venous Forum and is called CEAP classification (Table 5–2).

PROTOCOLS

Venous Duplex

Venous duplex is a relatively inexpensive, noninvasive examination that is easily performed and has become the preferred method of assessment for DVT. Venous duplex can be used to evaluate the peripheral veins for the presence of acute thrombus as well as chronic changes to the vessels.

Lower Extremities

Patient Positioning
The patient is placed in the supine or reverse Trendelenburg position with the leg of interest slightly bent at the knee and externally rotated (Fig. 5–10).

Scanning Technique
Typically using a 5- to 7-MHz linear transducer, venous duplex examinations utilize both 2D grayscale imaging and Pulse Wave (PW) spectral Doppler to assess the lower extremity veins. Color Doppler can be used as a tool to help identify vessels and can also be helpful in demonstrating partial obstructions related to chronic scarring or nonocclusive thrombosis. The majority of the examination is performed in the transverse plane. Manual compression of the veins with the ultrasound transducer is performed at close intervals typically about 2 cm apart. Normal veins should completely compress (or "coapt") wall to wall if free of thrombus (Fig. 5–11). Anything other than complete compression is suspicious for thrombus or chronic postthrombotic change.

The scan should start at the groin crease which is at or slightly superior to the inguinal ligament. It is at this level where the GSV joins the CFV. This confluence is known as the SFJ and serves as the landmark for the starting point of the examination (Fig. 5–12). As the transducer is moved distally along the medial aspect of the upper thigh, there will be a separation of the two veins that join to form the CFV. They are the FV and the DFV, which is also known as the profunda femoris

TABLE 5–2 • CEAP Classification	
Clinical Classification	
C0	No venous insufficiency
C1	Telangiectasias and/or reticular veins < 3 mm diameter
C2	Varicose veins > 3 mm diameter
C3	Edema
C4	Skin changes (can be subdivided into minor and major)
C5	Healed skin ulcers
C6	Open skin ulcers
Etiologic Classification	
Ep	CVVI major cause of clinical symptoms
Es	CVI/CVVI secondary to DVT or other pathologic process
Ec	CVI/CVVI has congenital origin
En	Unknown etiology
Anatomic Classification	
Ad	CVI/CVVI affects the deep veins
As	CVI/CVVI affects the superficial veins
Ap	CVI/CVVI affects the perforator veins
Ads/p/sp	More than one combination
An	No venous anatomy ideintified
Pathophysiologic Classification	
Pr	Reflux or reverse venous flow
Po	Chronic venous obstruction
Pro	Pathologic combination
Pn	No venous pathology

vein (Fig. 5–13). Shortly after the separation of these two veins, the DFV dives deep into the thigh out of sight leaving only the FV visualized. Continuing down the thigh, the entire length of the FV should be evaluated from proximal to distal (Fig. 5–14). At the level of the adductor canal, the FV will start

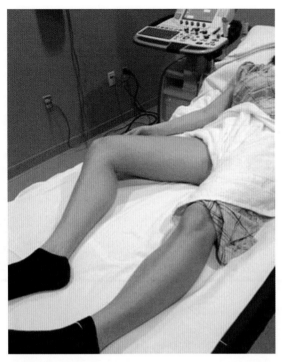

FIGURE 5–10. Proper positioning for a lower extremity venous duplex examination with the patient supine and the limb externally rotated with the knee slightly bent.

to dive deep below the muscle and eventually become the popliteal vein at the knee.

> **Controversies in Vascular:**
>
> When referencing proximal and distal in this chapter, it is important to point out that this is referring to the anatomical orientation in relationship to the heart. Some laboratories might reference these same locations as central and peripheral by referring to venous flow dynamics instead.

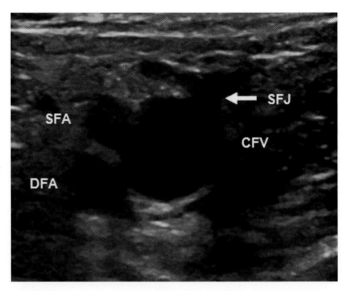

FIGURE 5–12. Common femoral vein (CFV) and saphenofemoral junction (SFJ) *arrow* with superficial femoral artery (SFA) and deep femoral artery (DFA).

A posterior approach with the ultrasound transducer is employed to visualize the popliteal vein behind the knee. In the majority of patients, this will make it appear as if the vein is anterior to its corresponding artery, but take note that it only appears this way because of the posterior approach (Fig. 5–15). The deep veins of the lower extremity are typically oriented posterior to their corresponding arteries throughout their course. While continuing distally, it is often possible to visualize the intramuscular veins that empty into the popliteal vein. These veins are known as the gastrocnemius veins. There are typically two sets of veins paired with an artery that run deep within the gastrocnemius muscle of the calf (Fig. 5–16). These veins are considered deep veins and are responsible for venous drainage of the calf muscles. The patient should not lie prone while

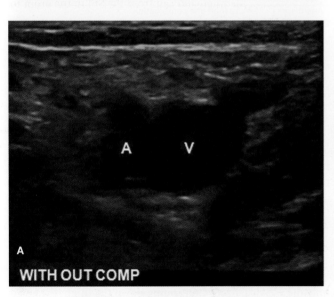

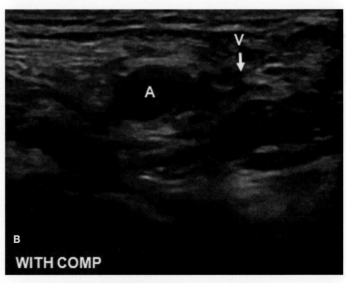

FIGURE 5–11. **(A)** Normal transverse image without compression of the common femoral vein and saphenofemoral junction adjacent to the common femoral artery. **(B)** Same transverse level with graded compression applied with the transducer showing the veins completely compressed wall to wall (*arrow*) with the artery remaining.

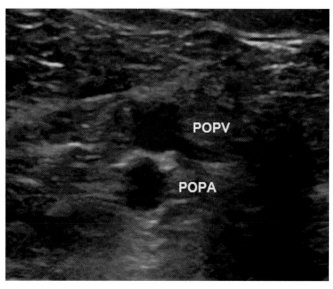

FIGURE 5–15. Popliteal vein (POPV) with popliteal artery (POPA).

FIGURE 5–13. Femoral vein (FV) with superficial femoral artery (SFA) and deep femoral vein (DFV) with deep femoral artery (DFA).

scanning the popliteal fossa as it collapses the more central veins and may lead to a false positive diagnosis.

The ATV joins the tibioperoneal trunk to form the popliteal vein. Continuing distally in the popliteal fossa, the ATV can be seen entering the popliteal vein superiorly, followed by the tibioperoneal trunk which eventually splits into the common tibial and common peroneal trunks. These common trunks are usually paired with one artery. These common trunks will eventually split in the upper calf into two sets of veins with

separate paired arteries known as the PTVs and peroneal veins (Fig. 5–17). The PTVs are located on the medial aspect of the calf just medial to the tibia and course from the medial malleolus to the upper calf. The peroneal veins are located deeper in the calf just anterior to the fibula. Both sets can typically be visualized in the same plane parallel to each other and their entire lengths should be evaluated (Fig. 5–18). It is also common to visualize the soleal sinus veins in the lower calf emptying into the PTVs and peroneal veins (Fig. 5–19). If ATVs are incorporated in the evaluation of the lower extremities, the transducer should be moved to the anterolateral aspect of the lower leg to visualize the paired veins with the artery (Fig. 5–20).

The GSVs and SSVs can both be visualized superficially anterior to the muscle fascia. The GSV can be followed on the medial aspect of the thigh and calf from the SFJ in the groin to just above the ankle. The SSV can be followed on the posterior

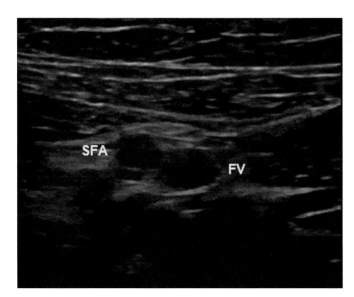

FIGURE 5–14. Femoral vein (FV) with superficial femoral artery (SFA).

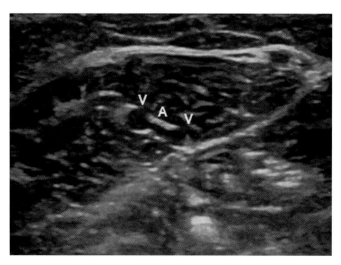

FIGURE 5–16. Paired gastrocnemius veins with corresponding artery.

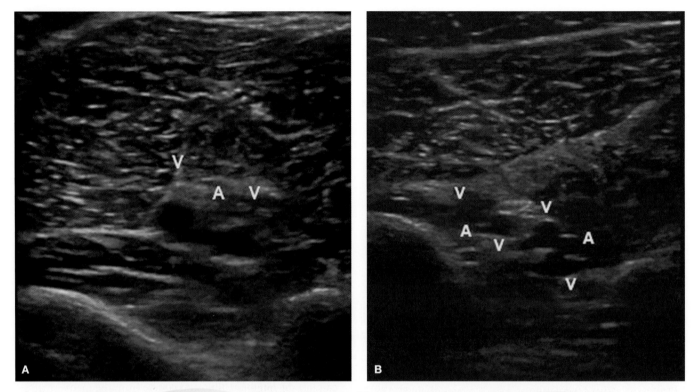

FIGURE 5–17. (A) Tibioperoneal trunk. **(B)** Peroneal (right side of the screen) and tibial veins at the level of the upper calf (left side of the screen).

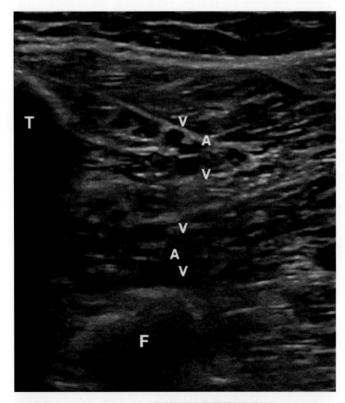

FIGURE 5–18. Paired posterior tibial veins medial to the tibia (T) and peroneal veins anterior to the fibula (F) with corresponding arteries at the level of the midcalf.

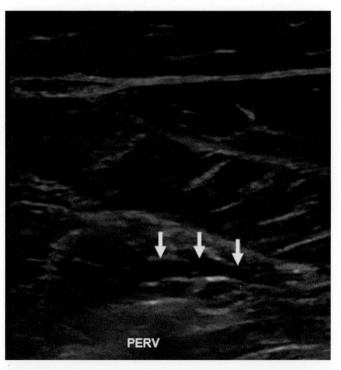

FIGURE 5–19. Soleal sinus emptying into the peroneal vein (*arrows*).

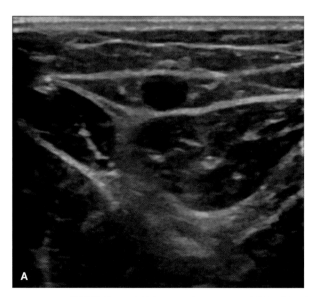

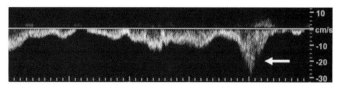

FIGURE 5-22. Normal lower extremity venous spectral Doppler waveform with distal augmentation (*arrow*).

FIGURE 5-20. Paired anterior tibial veins with corresponding artery.

aspect of the calf from its junction to the popliteal to just above the ankle (Fig. 5–21).

PW Doppler is performed in the longitudinal view typically at the areas of the common femoral, femoral, and popliteal veins. The waveforms in these areas should be spontaneous, phasic, and show an augmentation response to distal compression (Fig. 5–22). It is important to note that scanning protocol may vary site to site.

Limitations

The main limitation of lower extremity duplex examinations is the same that exists with any ultrasound examination and

that is lack of penetration due to body habitus and/or edema. Additional limitations would consist of incisions from recent surgery, dressings, and venous access lines located in the areas of interest. Subcutaneous emphysema, or air trapped in the subcutaneous tissues, may be another reason for limited visualization of the venous structures. In the technically difficult patient, the curvilinear transducer may be used to perform both the grayscale graded compressions as well as the color and spectral Doppler.

Upper Extremity

Patient Positioning

The patient is typically placed in the supine position with the arm of interest slightly externally rotated and abducted (Fig. 5–23).

Scanning Technique

Venous Duplex examinations utilize both 2D grayscale imaging and PW spectral Doppler to assess the upper extremity veins. Color Doppler plays a much larger role in the assessment of the upper extremity veins, specifically the central veins. The evaluation of the central veins with ultrasound can be limited due to the bony anatomy surrounding these vessels. The subclavian and brachiocephalic veins cannot easily be compressed and must rely on color and spectral Doppler for evaluation.

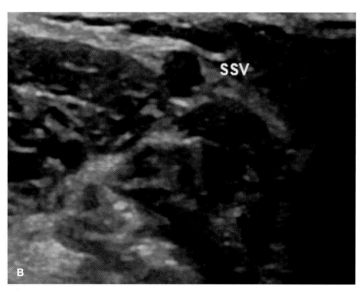

FIGURE 5-21. **(A)** Great saphenous vein. **(B)** Small saphenous vein.

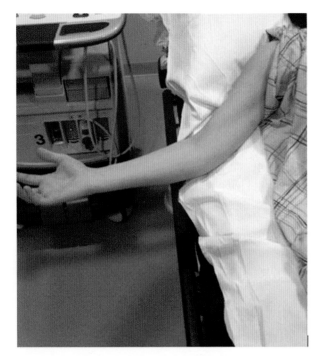

FIGURE 5-23. Proper positioning for an upper extremity venous duplex examination with the patient supine and the limb externally rotated and abducted.

The remainder of the examination is performed in the transverse plane. Similar to the lower extremity duplex examination, manual compression of the veins with the ultrasound transducer is performed at close intervals typically about a centimeter apart. Normal veins should completely compress (or "coapt") wall to wall, if free of thrombus.

The scan begins on the lateral portion of the neck just below the angle of the mandible where the IJV is located anterior to the common carotid artery (CCA) (Fig. 5–24). As the

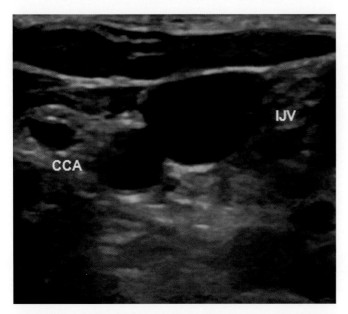

FIGURE 5-24. Internal jugular vein (IJV) with common carotid artery (CCA).

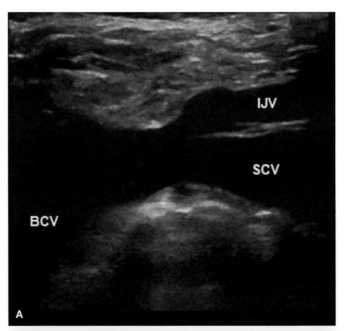

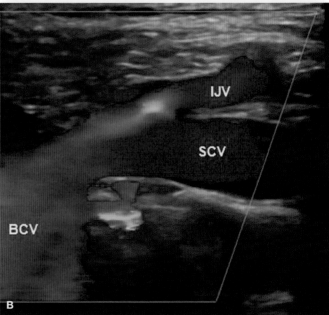

FIGURE 5-25. **(A)** 2D image of the left internal jugular vein (IJV) and subclavian vein (SCV) joining the brachiocephalic vein (BCV) centrally above the clavicle. **(B)** Color Doppler image of the same area.

transducer is moved down the lateral aspect of neck to its base just above the clavicle, the confluence of the IJV and the subclavian which together gives rise to the brachiocephalic vein will be identified (Fig. 5–25). Using a smaller footprint probe in this area is oftentimes very helpful to improve visualization. As the transducer continues to move above the clavicle laterally toward the axilla, the course of the subclavian vein can be followed (Fig. 5–26). At this level, it will not be possible to compress these veins due to the bony structures. As mentioned earlier, color and PW spectral Doppler should be used to evaluate patency. This should be done with the vessels in the longitudinal plane.

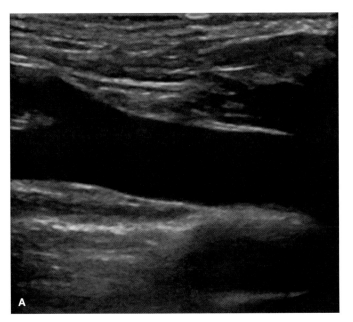

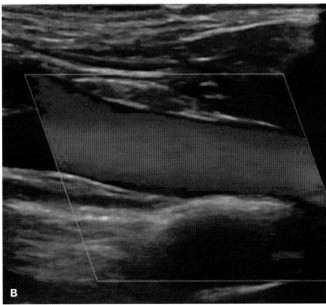

FIGURE 5–26. **(A)** Longitudinal view of the left subclavian vein (2D). **(B)** Left subclavian vein with color Doppler.

The spectral waveforms for the IJV, subclavian veins, and brachiocephalic veins should be phasic with a pulsatile component (Fig. 5–27). This is due to their close proximity to the heart. These waveforms should be very carefully analyzed for changes that could indicate a more proximal obstruction; such changes include loss of pulsatility or continuous flow. While following the entire course of the subclavian vein, the transducer will be moved below the clavicle continuing out toward the axilla. At the point where the cephalic vein joins the subclavian vein, the axillary vein will be visualized (Fig. 5–28). From this point forward, it will again be possible to use compression to evaluate the remainder of the upper extremity veins. A spectral Doppler waveform should also be obtained within the axillary vein at this level. The axillary vein waveform is more phasic and less pulsatile than the central veins (Fig. 5–29).

As the transducer is moved distally just below the axilla, the confluence of the basilic vein and the brachial veins is identified. The basilic vein courses medially, anterior to the muscle fascia, and parallel to the brachial veins. There is typically a paired set of brachial veins surrounding a single brachial artery (Fig. 5–30). Often times, it is possible to visualize the brachial nerve in this area as well. This is important to note because it can be mistaken for a noncompressible brachial vein. Continuing distally at the area just below the antecubital fossa, the radial and ulnar veins which join to form the brachial veins will be visualized. The paired radial veins will continue down to the hand along the lateral aspect of the forearm while the paired ulnar veins will run along the medial aspect (Fig. 5–31). To image the entire cephalic vein,

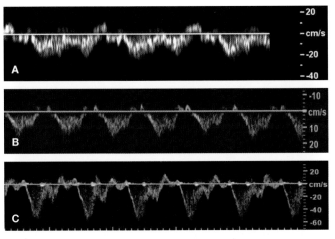

FIGURE 5–27. **(A)** Normal internal jugular vein spectral Doppler waveform. **(B)** Normal subclavian vein spectral Doppler waveform. **(C)** Normal brachiocephalic vein spectral Doppler waveform.

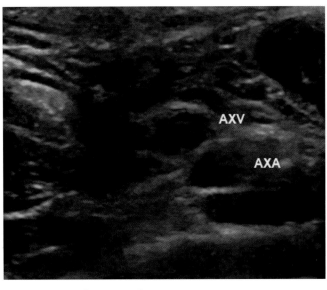

FIGURE 5–28. Axillary vein and artery.

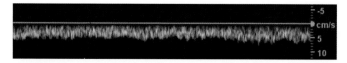

FIGURE 5-29. Normal axillary vein spectral Doppler waveform.

the transducer will be moved to the lateral side of the arm. The cephalic vein runs along the lateral aspect of the upper extremity from the wrist to where it terminates in the axillary vein. It is normally very superficial just underneath the skin anterior to the muscle fascia, so gentle pressure with a lot of gel is essential (Fig. 5-32).

Limitations

The limitations of upper extremity venous duplex studies are similar to those that exist with lower extremity examinations. The additional limitation of the upper extremity studies is related to the evaluation of the central veins. As mentioned earlier, in this section, the evaluation of the central veins can be limited by the bony anatomy of the chest. For this reason, it is critical to evaluate changes in PW Doppler waveforms in these areas.

Evaluation for Chronic Venous Insufficiency

Patient Positioning

It is important that the lower extremity being imaged is in a non–weight-bearing dependent position when evaluating a patient for venous insufficiency. This can be accomplished by simply standing the patient upright, placing the bed or stretcher in a reverse Trendelenburg position, or for certain portions of the examination having the patient sit on the edge of the bed with their lower leg hanging over (Fig. 5-33). Another method involves standing the patient on a stool with the leg dangling, but it is essential to be sure that the patient can balance and is not at risk for falling.

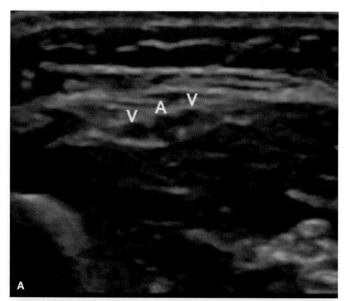

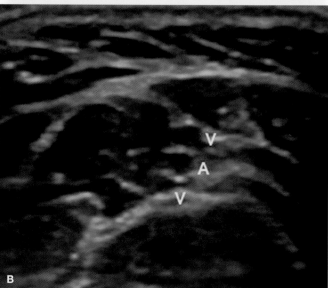

FIGURE 5-31. **(A)** Paired radial veins with corresponding artery. **(B)** Paired ulnar veins with corresponding artery.

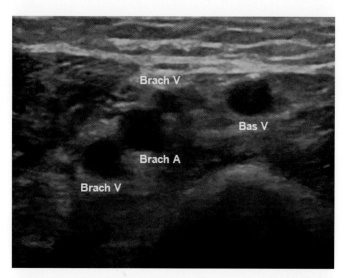

FIGURE 5-30. Paired brachial veins with corresponding artery along with the basilic vein.

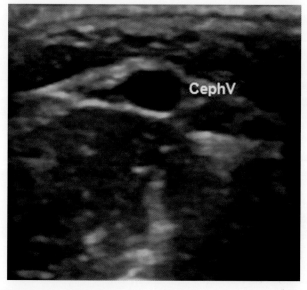

FIGURE 5-32. Cephalic vein.

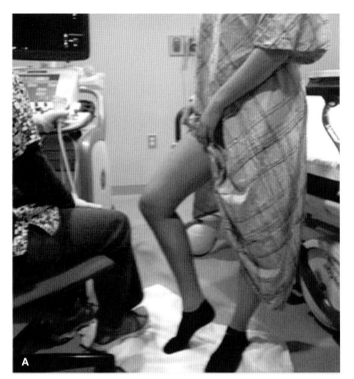

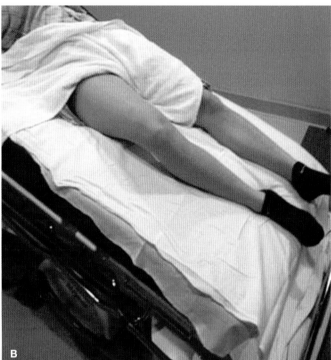

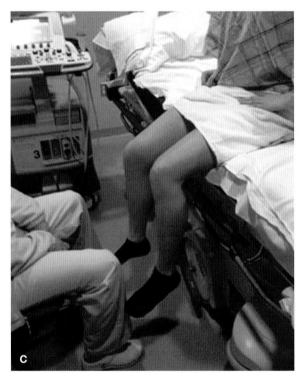

FIGURE 5–33. Proper positioning for the evaluation of venous insufficiency. **(A)** Standing and nonweight bearing. **(B)** Reverse Trendelenburg position. **(C)** Sitting on edge of bed with lower limbs in a non–weight-bearing position.

Scanning Technique

Venous Duplex examinations to evaluate for venous insufficiency utilize a 5- to 7-MHz linear transducer in both 2D grayscale imaging and PW spectral Doppler to assess the lower extremity veins for patency and flow direction. The protocol for evaluation of venous insufficiency usually involves the deep and superficial veins as well as the perforating veins of the calf at a minimum. Color Doppler can be used as a tool to help identify if venous reflux is present; however, spectral Doppler must be used to quantify it. Color Doppler is also very useful when evaluating perforator vein flow direction. The majority of the examination is performed in the longitudinal plane while obtaining spectral Doppler waveforms with distal calf compression to evaluate the venous flow response. Distal compression can be obtained manually or by the use of an automatic cuff inflator. An important technique to note here is that it is important to have the sample gate opened up to the size of the vessel being evaluated when obtaining the spectral waveform.

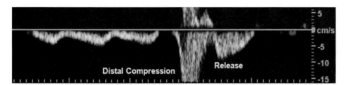

FIGURE 5–34. Normal venous flow response to distal augmentation showing no reversal (reflux) of flow. Note that the flow stays on the same side of the baseline as the augmentation.

This will allow you to capture any reversal of flow along the vessel walls as well as in the center of the vessel. In some cases, proximal compression and/or Valsalva maneuvers will also be used to evaluate flow response. The Valsalva maneuver is performed by having the patient take in a deep breath and bearing down as if they are having a bowel movement.

After performing graded compression to rule out DVT, the insufficiency scan typically begins at the level of the SFJ and ends with evaluation of the perforators. Protocols vary in relation to which vessels are examined and at which levels but the technique is always the same. In the longitudinal plane, a spectral Doppler waveform with distal compression is obtained and recorded from the vein being evaluated. The normal response should be very little or no reversal of blood flow following the release of distal compression (Fig. 5–34). Reversal of blood in the caudal direction should be less than 0.5 or 1.0 second depending on the literature source used. Depending on departmental protocol, the patient either performs a Valsalva maneuver or the technologist performs manual compression proximal to the vein being evaluated and the blood flow response is recorded. The normal response should be cessation of flow during the maneuver or compression followed by augmentation and resumption of flow in the correct direction upon release (Fig. 5–35).

Perforator veins, as mentioned earlier in this chapter, are connecting veins that connect the superficial veins to the deep veins. In a normal state, they only allow blood to flow from the superficial system to the deep system. When perforators are incompetent, the flow dynamic can be completely reversed. When assessing the perforators with duplex, an attempt should always be made to identify the direction of flow prior to any manipulation. This can be done by finding the perforator in transverse and using color Doppler (Fig. 5–36). The direction of flow should be recorded and documented. If reflux is present,

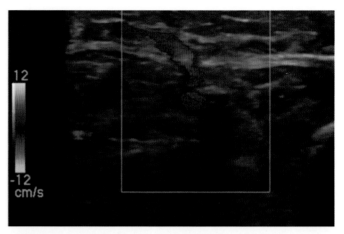

FIGURE 5–36. Normal perforator with flow going away from the transducer (superficial system to the deep system).

it should be measured in the same fashion as the other lower extremity veins. When normal, they should have very little to no reversal. For perforators, the reversal of blood flow should be less than 0.35 or 0.5 second depending on the literature source used. The other important characteristic to mention about perforators is that they are typically small in size when they are competent. Average size for a perforator is less than 3 mm. Perforators that are larger than 3 mm can be considered suspicious for incompetence. Whenever a perforator is identified, its diameter should be measured (Fig. 5–37).

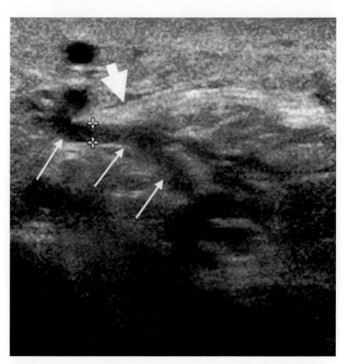

FIGURE 5–37. The *thin arrows* show the perforating vein connecting the posterior tibial vein (deep system) to a portion of the superficial system. Note that the perforator perforates the muscle fascia (indicated by the *wider arrow*) to join the deep system. All identified perforators should have their diameter measured to determine if an increase in size is present which might indicate incompetence.

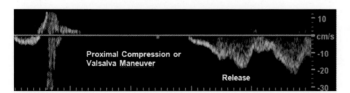

FIGURE 5–35. Normal venous flow response to proximal compression or Valsalva maneuver showing cessation of flow during with augmented flow following the release.

INTERPRETATION OF RESULTS

Normal Sonographic Findings

The most common purpose for evaluating the peripheral veins of the upper and lower extremities is to determine if there is any thrombus present. The normal appearance of veins should consist of no or very little internal echoes, free moving valves, and the veins should coapt with a small amount of pressure from the ultrasound transducer. Full compression of the veins is the single most reliable parameter used to rule out the presence of thrombosis. Additional normal findings observed are thin vein walls and normal size. The deep peripheral veins are typically slightly larger than their corresponding arteries.

Acute Thrombosis

The most common findings consistent with acute thrombosis are:

- Low-level echoes inside the vessel
- Venous distention
- Loss of compressibility

These common characteristics associated with acute thrombosis are often described as anechoic/hypoechoic, dilated, and noncompressible (Fig. 5–38). When discovered in one of the deep veins, it is referred to as acute DVT or "acute DVT." Conversely in the superficial system it is referred to as acute superficial vein thrombosis. Another indication that the thrombus is in its early acute stage is when motion is observed indicating that

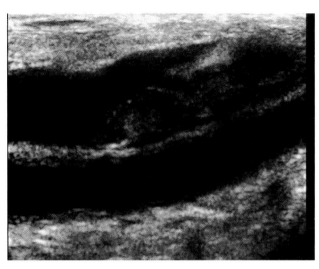

FIGURE 5–39. Sonographic image of an acute thrombus that is poorly attached to the vein wall. In real time, you would be able to appreciate the motion of the clot.

the clot is poorly attached to the vein wall. This is usually the tail end of a thrombus that extended from a more distal location (Fig. 5–39). Important to note that because the majority of acute clot becomes established in the calf first, it is important to always scan the calf area as part of the normal venous protocol. Clot in the soleal or gastrocnemius veins may also be discovered as a result of scanning the calf muscle. Although it is commonly said that acute DVT is hypoechoic, echogenicity is a relative term and does not predict acute DVT versus chronic postthrombotic change (Fig. 5–40).

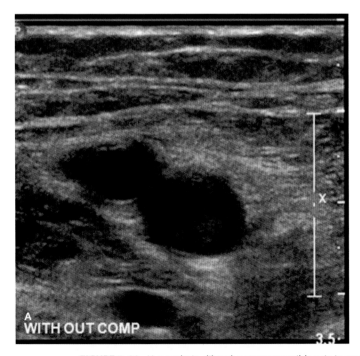
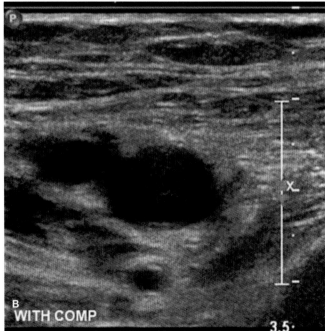

FIGURE 5–38. Hypoechoic, dilated, noncompressible vein is consistent with acute deep vein thrombosis. **(A)** Shows transverse view of the femoral vein with no compression applied. **(B)** Shows the same transverse view of the femoral vein with compression applied and the vein remaining noncompressible.

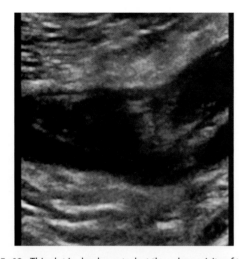

FIGURE 5–40. This clot is clearly acute, but the echogenicity of this clot would best be described as heterogeneous. Clot echogenicity alone should not be used to predict acute versus chronic.

Chronic Postthrombotic Change

The most common findings consistent with chronic changes are:

- Presence of synechiae
- Clot is firmly adherent to vein wall
- Larger developed collateral veins
- Contracted vein or recanalization of vein

As a thrombus ages, the vessel gets smaller in size and the thrombus becomes more rigid and permanent. Over time, the thrombus continues to break down and is absorbed by the body. Oftentimes, fibrous bands known as "synechiae" are left behind scarring the lumen of the vein (Fig. 5–41). Although the vascular literature describes the thrombus as becoming more echogenic, remember that echogenicity is the worst predictor of acute versus chronic.

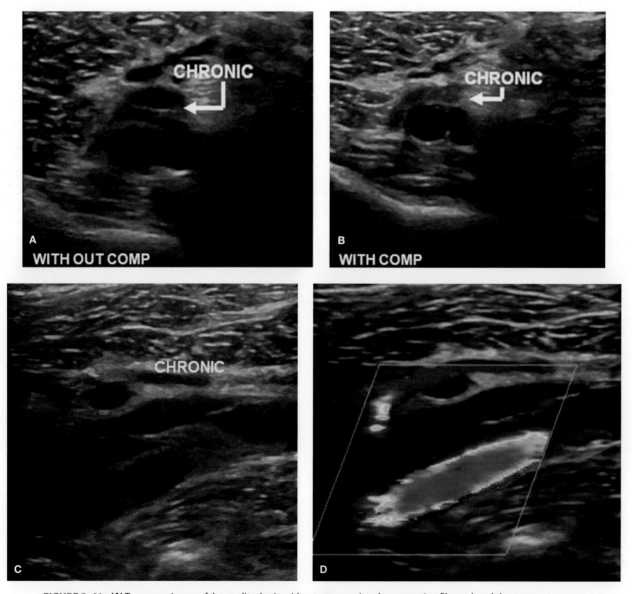

FIGURE 5–41. (A) Transverse image of the popliteal vein without compression demonstrating fibrous bands known as "synechiae" through the vessel lumen indicating chronic changes following the breakdown of a previous DVT. **(B)** Same popliteal vein showing partial compression around the residual fibrous material. **(C)** A sagittal view of the popliteal vein showing even a clearer view of the fibrous bands. **(D)** A sagittal view utilizing color Doppler to demonstrate the recanalization of the vessel lumen.

May–Thurner Syndrome

A less common cause of DVT is iliac vein compression syndrome, also called May–Thurner syndrome. With this syndrome, the left external iliac artery compresses the left external iliac vein, causing left iliofemoral DVT. Evaluation of the left CFV in a patient with May–Thurner will reveal continuous flow.

Pelvic Congestion Syndrome

An often-overlooked pathology is pelvic congestion syndrome. This most commonly affects premenopausal and multiparous women and presents as pelvic pain with no discernible cause. The syndrome occurs from varicose ovarian veins, most commonly on the left due to the left ovarian vein insertion into the left renal vein. The diagnosis is made by ruling out other causes of pelvic pain, and the treatment involves coils or glue to decrease the size of the ovarian vein. Ultrasound reveals dilated, tortuous veins more than 10 mm in size adjacent to the uterus. Although CT is more sensitive to pelvic congestion syndrome, ultrasound requires no ionizing radiation.

Analysis of Venous Waveforms

In addition to evaluating the grayscale images of the peripheral veins, a great deal of diagnostic information can be obtained by analyzing the spectral venous waveforms. Changes in venous flow can occur when thrombus is present. In certain instances, changes in the venous waveform can also suggest the presence of an obstruction more proximal that would not otherwise be discovered with ultrasound. For this reason, it is important to evaluate these waveforms during your examination.

Lower Extremities

A normal spectral waveform for the lower extremity peripheral veins should:

- Have augmentation in response to distal compression
- Be phasic with respiration
- Not have flow that is continuous or pulsatile

Any change from this normal flow pattern can indicate an obstruction. An increase of venous flow should occur past the transducer, when distal augmentation is applied (Fig. 5–42). In a more recent change, augmentation is not performed in all laboratories. Current literature suggests that distal augmentation provides very little diagnostic information and can

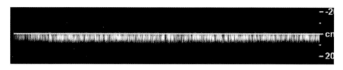

FIGURE 5–43. Represents a continuous spectral venous waveform that suggests the possibility of a proximal obstruction.

be eliminated from standard DVT protocols. It is important to note though that augmentation is still needed for venous insufficiency studies. An absent or reduced augmentation suggests the presence of an obstruction between the two points. It was stated in Chapter 1 that flow increases and decreases as a person inhales and exhales due to changes in pressure in the abdomen and chest. Those changes are represented on the spectral waveform with normal venous flow, termed phasicity (Fig. 5–42). When there is a loss of respiratory phasicity on a spectral venous waveform, the waveform is considered continuous. Continuous venous waveforms can indicate the possibility of a more proximal obstruction (Fig. 5–43). For example, if a normal phasic waveform was obtained in the right CFV and on the left more of a continuous type flow pattern was obtained, it might suggest that there is an obstruction of the left external or common iliac vein. One important thing to point out about changes in waveforms and the suggestion of proximal and distal obstructions is that it does not always mean that the obstruction is being caused by a thrombus. Oftentimes, the obstruction can be caused by extrinsic compression to the vein. For example, a large uterine fibroid can cause obstruction of one of the common iliac veins. In this case, the changes in the venous waveform of the CFV on that same side would be very similar to those of a patient with a thrombus of the common iliac vein.

Upper Extremities

A normal spectral waveform for the upper extremity peripheral veins varies depending on which vein is being interrogated. The veins that are furthest away from the heart will have spectral waveforms that are identical to the lower extremity veins with the characteristic of demonstrating augmentation in response to distal compression and having phasic flow. These types of waveforms will be found in the axillary and brachial veins. The veins closer to the heart such as the internal jugular, brachiocephalic, and subclavian veins will show cardiac pulsations combined with respiratory patterns.

Any change from each vessel's normal waveform can indicate that an obstruction is present. So, in essence each vessel is its own baseline when evaluating waveforms of the upper extremity veins. Lack of phasicity indicates more central proximal obstruction same as the lower extremity veins. One nuance to upper extremity veins is in relationship to the central veins closer to the heart. Not only does a continuous waveform indicate a proximal obstruction but a loss of pulsatility does, as well. For this reason, it is imperative that upper extremity veins are

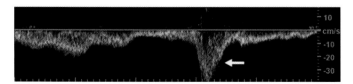

FIGURE 5–42. Normal lower extremity venous spectral Doppler waveform with distal augmentation (*arrow*).

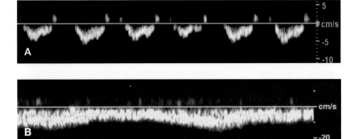

FIGURE 5–44. (A) Normal pulsatile venous flow in the subclavian vein. **(B)** Phasic venous flow with loss of pulsatility in the subclavian vein suggestive of a proximal obstruction.

always evaluated bilaterally. This will allow for comparison of the waveform to the contralateral side to identify subtle changes. For example, if a normal pulsatile waveform was obtained in a patient's right subclavian vein and on the left there was a phasic waveform with very little pulsatility, it might suggest that there was an obstruction more proximal (Fig. 5–44).

Findings Associated with Venous Insufficiency

Deep and Superficial Systems

When evaluating lower extremity veins for venous insufficiency, PW spectral Doppler should be used to identify and quantify any reversal of blood flow in the caudal direction following distal compression. The normal response of blood flow in the deep and superficial veins following distal compression is very little or no reversal of blood flow. When the reversal of blood flow exceeds 1.0 second (1,000 ms) for the deep system and 0.5 seconds (500 ms) for the superficial system in the standing position, it is considered significant venous reflux (Fig. 5–45). Another way to evaluate for venous reflux with PW spectral Doppler is to perform proximal compression or have the patient perform the Valsalva maneuver. As mentioned earlier in this chapter, the normal response to both should be cessation of flow followed by augmentation and resumption of flow in the correct direction upon release. When venous reflux is present, during the maneuver there will be reversal of blood flow (e.g., in the caudal direction) that will resume its normal direction when released (Fig. 5–46).

Augmentation can be performed manually, but the amount of compression varies from sonographer to sonographer and study to study. Equipment can be purchased that automates

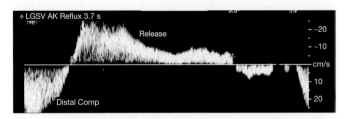

FIGURE 5–45. Doppler spectral waveform represents augmentation caused by distal compression followed by prolonged reversal of flow upon release. The reversal of flow is sustained for 3.7 seconds which is consistent with significant venous reflux.

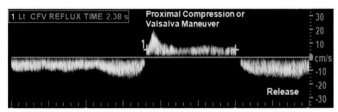

FIGURE 5–46. Doppler spectral waveform represents prolonged reversal of flow (reflux) during proximal compression or Valsalva maneuver followed by resumption of normal flow direction upon release.

the augmentation process which allows for better reproducibility (Fig. 5–47).

Perforating Veins

Blood flows from the superficial system to the deep system through the perforating veins in a normal patient. There should be very little or no flow in the opposite direction during or following distal compression. PW spectral Doppler should also be used on perforators when reflux is present in order to quantify it. In certain instances, the perforators can have completely reversed blood flow, from the deep system to the superficial, during distal compression (Fig. 5–48). For this reason, color Doppler should always be used first to establish the direction of blood flow. When the reversal of blood flow exceeds 0.35 seconds (350 ms), it is considered significant venous reflux. The other important thing to note about perforators is that normal competent perforators are typically small in size. Most competent perforators are less than 3 mm in diameter. When perforators become incompetent, they tend to dilate and increase in size. Perforators with a diameter that exceeds 3 mm

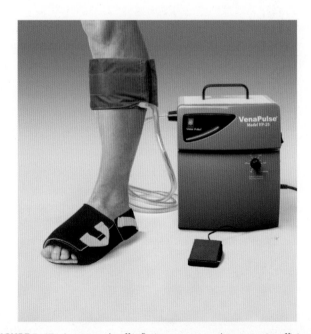

FIGURE 5–47. Automated cuff inflation systems make venous insufficiency studies more consistent and more ergonomic. (Image provided by ACI Medical, LLC, San Marcos, CA, manufacturer of the VenaPulse® Hands-Free Augmentation Device.)

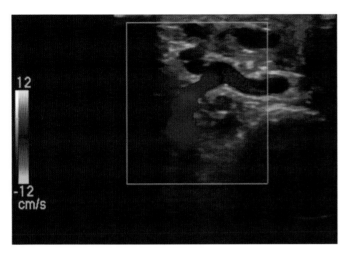

FIGURE 5–48. Reversed color flow in perforating vein. Flow is moving toward the probe from deep to superficial consistent with an incompetent perforator.

are highly suspicious for incompetence (Fig. 5–49). Table 5–3 provides a handy chart for CVI.

Miscellaneous Findings and Differential Diagnosis

Some patients present to the vascular lab with pain and say "it hurts right here" while pointing to a specific spot on the leg. Although in some cases the pain is vascular related, it may also be related to a nonvascular cause, such as hematoma, torn muscle, or tendon, or some other cause. A good clinical history can

Vein	Normal reflux time as measured by spectral Doppler
Deep veins	≤ 1 second (1,000 ms)
Superficial veins	≤ 0.5 seconds (≤ 500 ms)
Perforating veins	≤ 0.35 seconds (≤ 350 ms)

TABLE 5–3 • Criteria for Chronic Venous Insufficiency (CVI) and Chronic Venous Valvular Insufficiency (CVVI)

aid in the diagnosis. It is important to always scan the area of pain in addition to the normal venous protocol.

Below is a list of some of the more common nonvascular findings and their descriptions:

- Baker's cyst—A cystic structure usually located medially in the popliteal fossa. They are typically anechoic but may contain hyperechoic material that can indicate rupture (Fig. 5–50).
- Edema—Fluid in the interstitial tissue. Will appear sonographically as anechoic spaces throughout the surrounding tissue (Fig. 5–51).
- Lymph nodes—Can typically be identified when they are enlarged. They are most commonly seen in the groin area and will appear sonographically as a hypoechoic border with a hyperechoic center (Fig. 5–52).

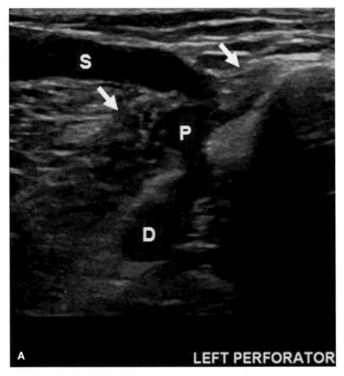

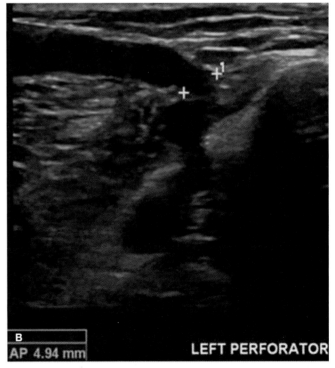

FIGURE 5–49. (A) A large perforating vein (P) crossing the muscle fascia (*arrows*) that is connecting the superficial system (S) to the deep system (D). **(B)** Same perforating vein showing a diameter measurement (+ calipers).

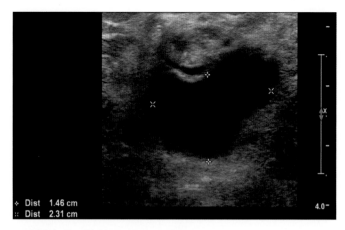

FIGURE 5–50. Baker's cyst in popliteal fossa.

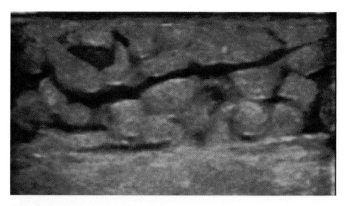

FIGURE 5–51. Interstitial tissue edema.

- Hematoma—A localized collection of blood. It can appear anechoic, complex, or hyperechoic depending on its age. Blood typically appears anechoic at first, but over time the echogenicity tends to increase (Fig. 5–53).
- Abscess—A localized collection of pus typically caused by infection. It most commonly appears as a complex mass that is very heterogeneous, and may contain foci of air (Fig. 5–54).

It is important to note that all the findings above can only be inferred by the ultrasound findings. They must be correlated with the patient's clinical presentation and history in order to make a diagnosis.

OTHER VENOUS TESTING

Photoplethysmography Testing

Photoplethysmography (PPG) testing can be used to evaluate the venous system for venous insufficiency. The PPG sensor uses infrared light that is reflected off the blood cells in the cutaneous vessels and is used to detect the return of blood flow following flexion maneuvers to evaluate for venous insufficiency. The changes in the amount of blood refilling the veins are recorded on a display or paper strip.

Patient Positioning

The patient is in the seated position with the leg of interest hanging down in a dependent non–weight-bearing position. The PPG sensor is placed on the medial aspect of the lower limb about 5-15 cm above the medial malleolus.

Examination Technique

With the leg in a dependent position, the patient is asked to perform 5-10 plantar flexion and dorsiflexion maneuvers which activates the calf-muscle pump and empties the blood from the lower limb. On the display or paper strip, the tracing should fall considerably as the lower leg empties during the flexion maneuvers and then gradually returns to baseline during the recovery period with the leg relaxed. If reflux is revealed during the examination, a tourniquet can be employed at different levels to compress the GSVs and SSVs in an effort to identify superficial versus deep venous insufficiency. When evaluating the GSV,

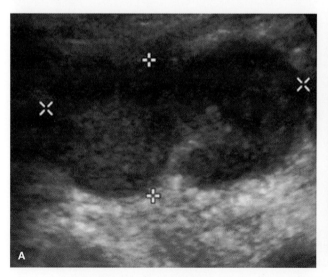

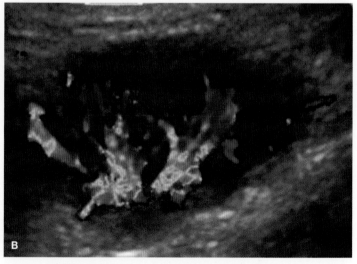

FIGURE 5–52. (A) Prominent lymph node seen on ultrasound. Calipers indicate the anterior–posterior and medial–lateral borders. **(B)** Same lymph node with color Doppler shows increased vascularity in this patient with lymphoma.

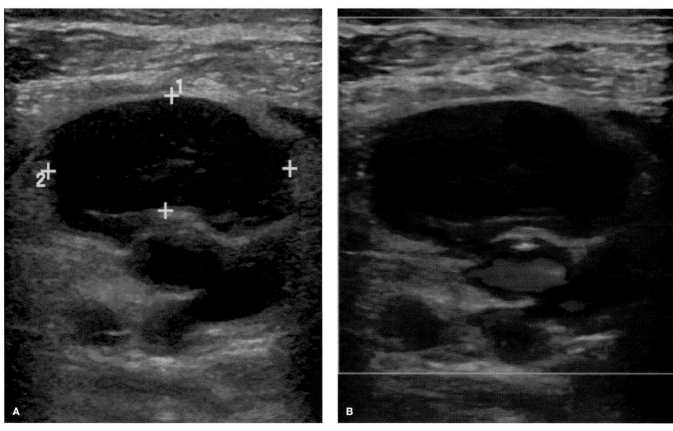

FIGURE 5–53. **(A)** Transverse image of the right groin status post cardiac catheterization shows an avascular structure consistent with a hematoma. Calipers indicate the anterior–posterior and medial–lateral borders. **(B)** Color Doppler image of the same area showing the absence of color flow in the structure as well as normal color flow in the native CFA.

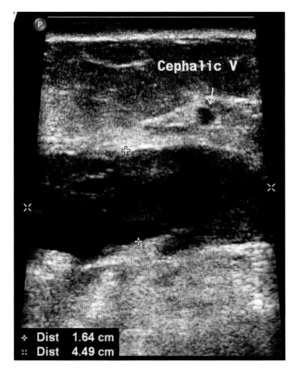

FIGURE 5–54. Sonographic image of the upper arm shows a complex mass posterior to the cephalic vein. These findings when compared to the patients' clinical presentation were consistent with an abscess.

the tourniquet is placed in the upper thigh just above the knee. When evaluating the SSV, the tourniquet would be lowered to the upper calf area just below the knee.

Interpretation of Results

The amount of time it takes for the venous blood to return back to baseline during the recovery period is known as the venous refill time (VRT). The VRT is measured to determine if venous reflux is present. Normally, it takes more than 20 seconds for a full recovery period (Fig. 5–55). The following are the diagnostic criteria used:

- More than or equal to ≥ 20 seconds (VRT) = Normal response
- Less than 20 seconds (VRT) = Venous reflux suspected
- Less than 10 seconds (VRT) = Severe venous reflux suspected

If the results are normal, the test is complete. When an abnormal VRT is achieved, a tourniquet is often applied to differentiate between superficial and deep venous reflux. With the tourniquet placed on the thigh, the GSV is eliminated as a contributing factor. If the results are abnormal without the tourniquet and change to normal with the tourniquet, then it is most likely the GSV that

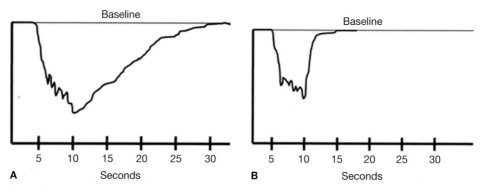

FIGURE 5–55. **(A)** PPG examination demonstrating a normal venous refill time (VRT) of greater than 20 seconds. **(B)** PPG examination demonstrating an abnormal VRT of less than 20 seconds.

is causing the reflux. If the results do not change, then it is most likely the deep system that is causing the reflux. The same would apply to the SSV with the tourniquet below the knee.

Vein Mapping

Vein mapping consists of ultrasound evaluation of the superficial veins of the upper and lower extremities to identify a surgical conduit for procedures such as a lower extremity bypass, coronary artery bypass, or arteriovenous fistula formation. The examination typically involves the evaluation of the size, patency, depth, and length in an effort to determine the feasibility of its use in one of the above-mentioned surgical procedures. The entire examination is performed in the transverse plane with diameter measurements performed at various levels throughout the course of the veins (Fig. 5–56). The veins that

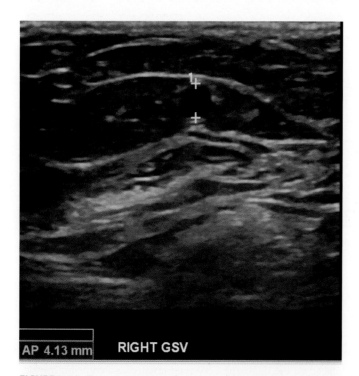

AP 4.13 mm   **RIGHT GSV**

FIGURE 5–56. Transverse sonographic image of the right great saphenous vein with an anterior–posterior diameter measurement (+ calipers) during a vein mapping examination.

are commonly evaluated are the GSVs, SSVs, cephalic veins, and basilic veins. Which veins are evaluated will depend on the surgical procedure that is being planned.

Venography

Venography is in little use today and has been mostly replaced by venous duplex. It can at times be used as a confirmatory test in difficult-to-scan patients. It is also often used when thrombolysis is being considered. Venography is an invasive test that requires the injection of radiographic contrast directly into the veins through a catheter placed in either the foot or the groin while a series of fluoroscopic x-rays are obtained. It can be used to evaluate for the presence of thrombus as well as to determine if venous reflux is present. The approach of each is slightly different. For the evaluation of thrombus, an ascending venogram is performed. In this case, the venous access is in the dorsum of the foot where the contrast is injected. With a positive finding, a filling defect with the contrast will be seen indicating that thrombus is present in that area (Fig. 5–57). For the evaluation of venous reflux, a descending venogram is performed. The difference is that the venous access is moved to the patient's groin area. If reflux is present, contrast filling in a retrograde fashion will be witnessed.

TREATMENT OF PERIPHERAL VENOUS DISEASE

Acute Deep Vein Thrombosis

The initial and primary treatment of acute DVT is anticoagulation with heparin, or low–molecular-weight heparin (LMWH) such as Lovenox, or whatever the current recommended medication is. The type of treatment usually depends on several factors such as location of the acute DVT, patient compliance, and even physician preference. Intravenous heparin requires a hospital stay that starts with a bolus followed by 4-5 days of therapy until a stable international normalized ratio (INR) is achieved. After the initial therapy, the patient is often treated with oral anticoagulation, such as warfarin, Eliquis, Xarelto, etc., for

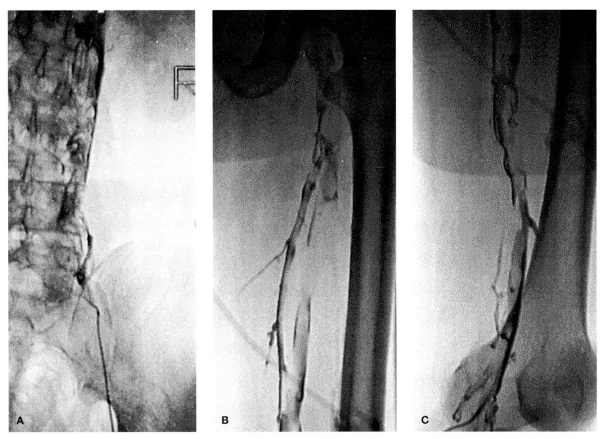

FIGURE 5–57. Venogram images of the right lower extremity. **(A)** Pelvic veins. **(B)** Groin and upper thigh veins. **(C)** Lower thigh and upper knee veins. Filling defect in all areas is consistent with thrombosis.

several months to prevent reoccurrence. The typical duration is 3-6 months and sometimes up to a year. The duration is determined by the patient's situation. Higher-risk patients tend to be on oral anticoagulation longer, sometimes even for the duration of their lives. Blood thinners do not destroy existing clot; they simply work to prevent new clot from forming. More aggressive treatments for acute DVT include thrombolysis and thrombectomies. Thrombolysis is a catheter-based procedure where thrombolytic agents are introduced to the area of the clot in an effort to dissolve it (Fig. 5–58). A thrombectomy is surgical removal of

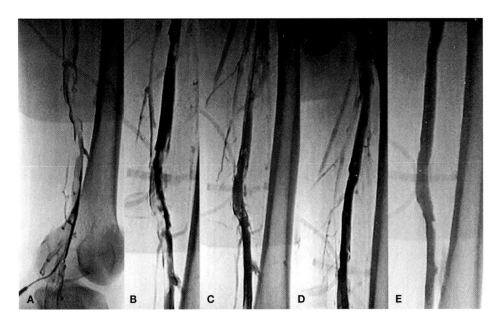

FIGURE 5–58. Venogram images of the right thigh. **(A)** Shows the femoral vein with a filling defect indicating thrombosis. **(B–D)** Shows the same femoral vein with improved flow over a progressive period of time while thrombolytic agents are infused through a catheter. **(E)** Shows the femoral vein post thrombolysis procedure.

the clot. These more aggressive type treatments are performed to reduce the chances of chronic postthrombotic change.

Venous Insufficiency

The treatment of venous insufficiency differs depending on the location of the incompetent valves. The majority of the treatments related to venous insufficiency are for the superficial and perforating veins. There are some treatment options for the deep vein incompetence such as valve replacements and venoplasty with stenting; however, their benefits have varied greatly. The treatments for venous insufficiency within the superficial veins are vein stripping, endovenous laser treatment (EVLT), radiofrequency ablation (RFA), phlebectomy, and sclerotherapy. Vein stripping is the surgical removal of the varicose incompetent veins. EVLT and RFA are very similar procedures with the main difference being the source from which the vein is thermally ablated. EVLT uses a laser whereas RFA uses high radio frequencies. These procedures start with venous access through a distal vein under ultrasound guidance. Once access is obtained, the catheter with the thermal element is advanced to a comfortable level near the junction with the deep system. Anesthesia is injected around the vein throughout its course. This provides some protection from the heat to the surrounding tissue and also ensures that the vein has good contact with the thermal element. As the element is activated, it is slowly pulled back until it is completely removed from the vein at the original access point. The extreme heat causes thermal injury inside the vein which will result in complete ablation of the vein. A phlebectomy is a procedure that involves a mini incision over the area of a varicose vein where a vein retractor can be inserted to remove the varicose vein. Sclerotherapy is a chemical ablation of small surface veins through a series of injections. Incompetent perforating veins can be treated with EVLT or RFA. Another procedure that is commonly performed for incompetent perforating veins is subfascial endoscopic perforator vein ligation also known as a SEPS procedure. This involves an endoscopic approach to locate the problematic perforator and ligate it. This is often done in an area of a venous stasis ulcer in an effort to promote healing.

Questions

1. The following vein is a component of the superficial venous system

   (A) CFV

   (B) PTV

   (C) Popliteal vein

   (D) GSV

2. In relation to arteries and veins, which statement is true?

   (A) Arteries and veins have internal valves

   (B) Veins have a tunica media and adventitia but lack a tunica intima

   (C) Arteries have a much higher internal pressure

   (D) Arterial walls collapse with gentle probe pressure

3. The CFV becomes the external iliac vein above the level of what structure?

   (A) Adductor canal

   (B) Inguinal ligament

   (C) Profunda hiatus

   (D) Popliteal fossa

4. A normal venous spectral waveform of the lower extremities is

   (A) Phasic

   (B) Continuous

   (C) Pulsatile

   (D) Bidirectional

5. The deep vein that runs along the anterolateral portion of the lower leg between the tibia and fibula and joins the tibioperoneal trunk is the

   (A) PTV

   (B) ATV

   (C) Peroneal vein

   (D) Gastrocnemius vein

6. The paired PTVs in the lower leg join in the upper portion of the calf to form the

   (A) Tibioperoneal trunk

   (B) Common peroneal trunk

   (C) Common tibial trunk

   (D) Soleal sinuses

7. The innermost layer of the vein wall is known as the tunica

   (A) Media

   (B) Adventitia

   (C) Superficial

   (D) Intima

8. Which of the following best describes a normal waveform of the brachiocephalic veins?

   (A) Phasic

   (B) Pulsatile

   (C) Continuous

   (D) Oscillating

9. The vein that runs along the lateral aspect of the upper extremity and joins the axillary vein just before becoming the subclavian vein is known as the

   (A) Cephalic vein

   (B) Brachial vein

   (C) Basilic vein

   (D) Innominate vein

10. All of the following veins contain internal valves EXCEPT the

    (A) IJV

    (B) Brachial vein

    (C) Brachiocephalic vein

    (D) Cephalic vein

11. Which perforators connect to the posterior accessory GSV and typically play a significant role in regard to venous stasis ulcers?

    (A) Paratibial perforator

    (B) Perforator of femoral canal

    (C) Superficial epigastric vein

    (D) Posterior tibial perforator

12. During expiration, as abdominal pressure decreases and thoracic pressure increases

    (A) There is no significant change in venous blood flow return

    (B) Venous blood flow return in the lower extremities increases while decreasing in the upper extremities

    (C) Venous blood flow return in the lower extremities decreases while increasing in the upper extremities

    (D) Flow is suspended in both the upper and lower extremities

13. Most deep venous thrombi become established in the

    (A) Groin
    (B) Thigh
    (C) Calf
    (D) Foot

14. The condition involving an outflow obstruction of the venous system that presents with extreme swelling, cyanosis, and reduced arterial inflow is known as

    (A) Dependent rubor
    (B) Phlegmasia alba dolens
    (C) Phlegmasia cerulea dolens
    (D) Venous insufficiency

15. Which location of DVT is more likely to travel to the lung as a pulmonary embolus?

    (A) Peroneal vein DVT
    (B) CFV DVT
    (C) PTV DVT
    (D) Gastrocnemius vein DVT

16. The three predisposing conditions known as "Virchow's Triad" are

    (A) Trauma, hypertension, and hypercoagulability
    (B) Trauma, sclerosis, and hypercoagulability
    (C) Thrombosis, stasis, and hypertension
    (D) Trauma, stasis, and hypercoagulability

17. All of the following are classic symptoms of DVT EXCEPT

    (A) Pain
    (B) Edema
    (C) Paralysis
    (D) Redness

18. When the calf-muscle pump and venous valves become inadequate at returning blood back to the heart, it leads to the pooling of blood in the lower extremities. A condition known as

    (A) DVT
    (B) Phlegmasia alba dolens
    (C) Phlegmasia cerulea dolens
    (D) Venous insufficiency

19. An ascending venogram is used to evaluate for

    (A) Thrombosis
    (B) Venous insufficiency
    (C) Baker's cyst
    (D) Varicose veins

20. After initial treatment of DVT, patients are often treated with oral anticoagulation in an effort to

    (A) Serve as a thrombolytic
    (B) Prevent chronic scarring of the vein lumen
    (C) Prevent reoccurrence
    (D) Prevent post thrombotic syndrome

Questions 21 through 28: Match the structures in Figure 5–59 with the names of the veins in Column B.

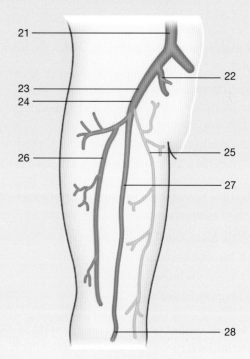

FIGURE 5–59.

COLUMN A	COLUMN B
21. _____	(A) CFV
22. _____	(B) External iliac vein
23. _____	(C) GSV
24. _____	(D) DFV
25. _____	(E) FV
26. _____	(F) Internal iliac vein
27. _____	(G) Inferior vena cava
28. _____	(H) Popliteal vein

29. All of the following are sonographic findings associated with chronic postthrombotic change EXCEPT

    (A) Partially compressible

    (B) Synechiae

    (C) Recanalization lumen

    (D) Dilated vein

30. While scanning a patient's upper extremity veins, you obtain a phasic spectral Doppler waveform within the right subclavian vein and a pulsatile spectral Doppler waveform within the left subclavian vein. What does this suggest?

    (A) An obstruction proximal to the left subclavian vein

    (B) An obstruction proximal to the right subclavian vein

    (C) An obstruction distal to the left subclavian vein

    (D) An obstruction distal to the right subclavian vein

31. Which veins of the upper extremity should have cardiac pulsations coupled with respiratory patterns normally?

    (A) Basilic vein

    (B) IJV

    (C) Cephalic vein

    (D) Radial vein

32. Tailed thrombus with motion seen on duplex is a finding consistent with

    (A) Acute vein thrombosis

    (B) Chronic post thrombotic change

    (C) Venous insufficiency

    (D) PE

Questions 33 through 40: Match the structures in Figure 5–60 with the names of the veins in Column B

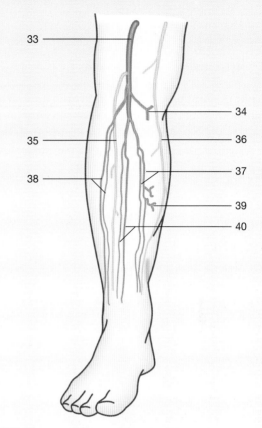

FIGURE 5–60.

COLUMN A	COLUMN B
33. _____	(A) Gastrocnemius veins
34. _____	(B) PTVs
35. _____	(C) Popliteal vein
36. _____	(D) SSV
37. _____	(E) Soleal veins
38. _____	(F) Peroneal veins
39. _____	(G) Inferior vena cava
40. _____	(H) ATVs

41. **The distention of the distal veins that occurs when a patient has venous insufficiency is a result of**

    (A) Decreased hydrostatic pressure

    (B) Abnormal vein walls

    (C) Pooling and stasis of blood

    (D) Decreased transmural pressure

42. **While performing a PPG venous examination on a patient without a tourniquet, you obtain an abnormal VRT. In order to determine where the insufficiency is occurring, you proceed to apply a tourniquet just above the knee and get a normal VRT. Where is the patient's insufficiency occurring?**

    (A) Deep system

    (B) GSV

    (C) SSV

    (D) There is no insufficiency

43. **The venous valves are attached to which layer of the vessel walls?**

    (A) Tunica intima

    (B) Tunica media

    (C) Tunica adventitia

    (D) Tunica interstitial

44. **The radial and ulnar veins join at about the level of the antecubital fossa to form which vessel?**

    (A) Basilic vein

    (B) Axillary vein

    (C) Brachial vein

    (D) Brachiocephalic vein

Questions 45 through 55: Match the structures in Figure 5–61 with the names of the veins in Column B.

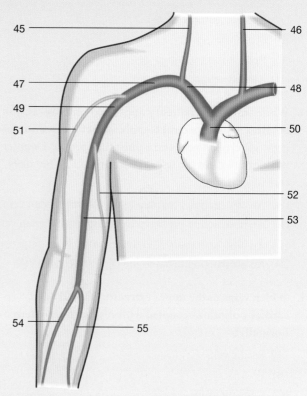

FIGURE 5–61.

COLUMN A	COLUMN B
45. _____	(A) SVC
46. _____	(B) Right internal jugular vein
47. _____	(C) Cephalic vein
48. _____	(D) Ulnar vein
49. _____	(E) Right brachiocephalic vein
50. _____	(F) Radial vein
51. _____	(G) Brachial vein
52. _____	(H) Basilic vein
53. _____	(I) Subclavian vein
54. _____	(J) Left IJV
55. _____	(K) Axillary vein

56. A study that is positive for superficial venous reflux will demonstrate a flow reversal time of

    (A) Less than 5 seconds
    (B) More than 0.05 second
    (C) More than 0.5 second
    (D) More than 0.005 seconds

57. Varicosities that are a result of insufficiency that started in the deep system and extended into the superficial system by way of the perforator veins are known as

    (A) Primary varicose veins
    (B) Secondary varicose veins
    (C) Spontaneous varicose veins
    (D) First varicose veins

58. All of the following are symptoms associated with chronic venous insufficiency EXCEPT

    (A) Varicose veins
    (B) Discoloration at the gaiter zone
    (C) Swelling
    (D) Heel ulceration

59. What is the treatment known as sclerotherapy?

    (A) Surgical removal of superficial veins
    (B) Ablation of superficial veins by the use of radiofrequency-induced heating
    (C) Ablation of superficial veins through a series of injections with a chemical agent
    (D) Removal of superficial veins through mini surgical incisions

60. Sonographic findings consistent with acute thrombosis are

    (A) Hypoechoic, dilated, and noncompressible
    (B) Hyperechoic, dilated, and noncompressible
    (C) Hypoechoic, nondilated, and compressible
    (D) Hyperechoic, nondilated, and noncompressible

61. The image in Figure 5–62 of the midcalf represents which of the following?

    (A) Normal response to compression
    (B) Acute DVT PTV
    (C) Acute DVT peroneal vein
    (D) Acute DVT posterior tibial and peroneal veins

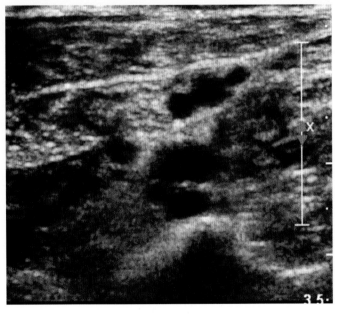 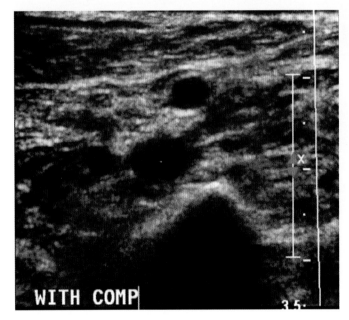

FIGURE 5–62.

62. **The waveform in Figure 5–63 is a normal waveform for which vessel?**

    (A) CFV

    (B) Brachial vein

    (C) Popliteal vein

    (D) Brachiocephalic vein

64. **The arrow in Figure 5–65 of the lower extremity is pointing to what anatomical landmark?**

    (A) Gastrocnemius junction

    (B) Saphenopopliteal junction

    (C) SFJ

    (D) Inguinal ligament

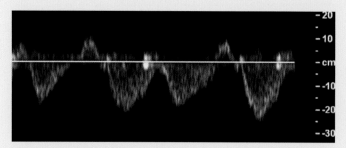

FIGURE 5–63.

63. **The image in Figure 5–64 of the midthigh represents which of the following?**

    (A) Normal response to compression

    (B) Acute DVT

    (C) Chronic postthrombotic change

    (D) Baker's cyst

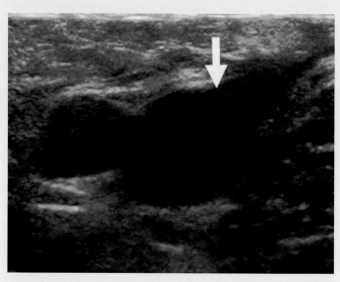

FIGURE 5–65.

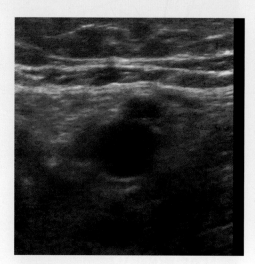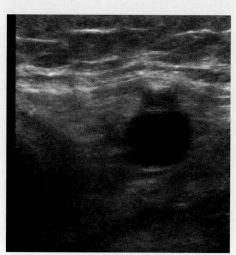

FIGURE 5–64.

65. Which of the following is the longest vein in the body?

    (A) SSV

    (B) GSV

    (C) Inferior vena cava

    (D) FV

66. Varicose veins that occur when there is no DVT are called

    (A) Primary varicose veins

    (B) Secondary varicose veins

    (C) Cardinal varicose veins

    (D) Hydrostatic varicose veins

67. Which of the following veins act as a reservoir for the "calf-muscle pump"?

    (A) Popliteal vein

    (B) Gastrocnemius vein

    (C) SSV

    (D) Soleal vein

68. What is the most significant clinical concern for a patient with acute DVT?

    (A) Venous insufficiency

    (B) PE

    (C) Chronic postthrombotic change

    (D) Superficial thrombophlebitis

69. All of the following veins are paired EXCEPT the

    (A) Posterior tibial

    (B) Anterior tibial

    (C) Peroneal

    (D) Small saphenous

70. Which of the following statements about lower extremity venous duplex is always true?

    (A) If a vein fills with color flow, then there is no presence of DVT

    (B) Graded compression should always be performed in the transverse plane

    (C) A continuous flow, steady waveform is indicative of a normal lower extremity venous waveform

    (D) Respiratory phasicity in the lower extremity veins is always abnormal

71. Which of the following is not a predisposing risk factor for DVT?

    (A) Trauma

    (B) Cancer

    (C) Pregnancy

    (D) Headache

72. Which of the following is TRUE regarding lower extremity venous anatomy?

    (A) The SSV typically terminates at the peroneal vein

    (B) The GSV typically terminates at the DFV

    (C) The GSV typically terminates at the CFV

    (D) The GSV is part of the deep venous system

73. Figure 5–66 of the subclavian vein most likely represents

    (A) Attenuation artifact

    (B) Inactive valve

    (C) Venous dissection

    (D) Nonocclusive thrombosis

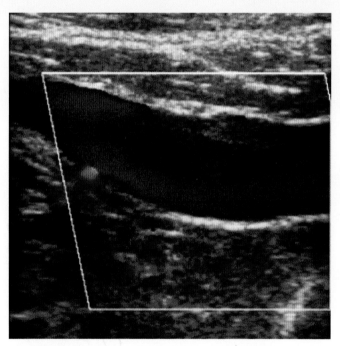

FIGURE 5–66.

74. The image in Figure 5–67 of the mid neck represents which of the following?

    (A) Acute DVT IJV
    (B) Chronic postthrombotic change IJV
    (C) Mirror artifact
    (D) Normal response to compression

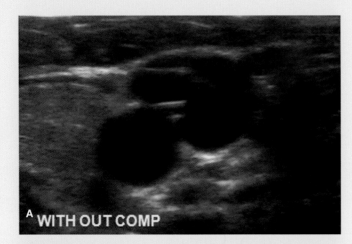

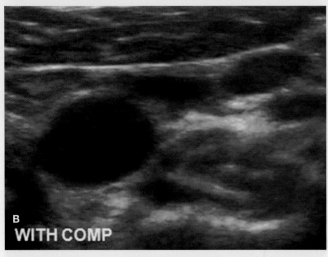

FIGURE 5–67.

75. The spectral Doppler venous waveform of the lower extremity in Figure 5–68 shows

    (A) Distal augmentation of flow
    (B) Pulsatile flow
    (C) Continuous flow
    (D) Normal respiratory phasic flow

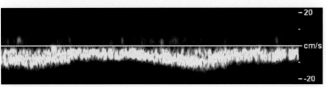

FIGURE 5–68.

76. The inferior vena cava is formed by the union of the

    (A) Superior vena cava and right heart
    (B) Left and right common iliac veins
    (C) External iliac vein and internal iliac vein
    (D) Portal venous system and systemic veins

77. Which of the following is an advantage of venous duplex over venography?

    (A) Venous duplex uses ionizing radiation
    (B) Venous duplex is noninvasive
    (C) Venous duplex uses an iodinated contrast agent
    (D) Venous angiography is painless

78. Venous stasis ulcers are most commonly located

    (A) In the proximal thigh
    (B) In the adductor canal
    (C) By the medial malleolus
    (D) In the popliteal fossa

79. A patient presents with large varicose veins that have enlarged over the past few years and are becoming increasingly painful. What is the LEAST likely examination to be done to determine the cause of his disease?

    (A) Venous duplex
    (B) PPG testing
    (C) Ascending venogram
    (D) Descending venogram

80. The normal response to venous flow during the Valsalva maneuver is

    (A) Cessation of flow
    (B) Augmentation of flow
    (C) Reversal of flow
    (D) Increase in flow

81. The flow in Figure 5–69 of a perforating vein identified just above the medial malleolus shows

    (A) Normal flow from the deep to the superficial system
    (B) Abnormal flow from the superficial to the deep system
    (C) Normal flow from the superficial to the deep system
    (D) Abnormal flow from the deep to the superficial system

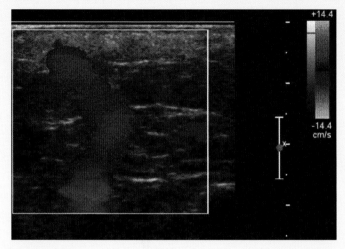

FIGURE 5–69.

Questions 82 through 84: Match the letters on the image in Figure 5–70 with the structures in column A.

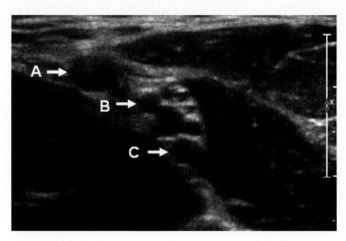

FIGURE 5–70.

COLUMN A

82. Brachial vein _____

83. Basilic vein _____

84. Brachial nerve _____

85. The image in Figure 5–71 of the posterior aspect of the proximal calf represents which of the following?

    (A) Normal response to compression
    (B) Acute DVT popliteal vein
    (C) Acute DVT gastrocnemius veins
    (D) Baker cyst

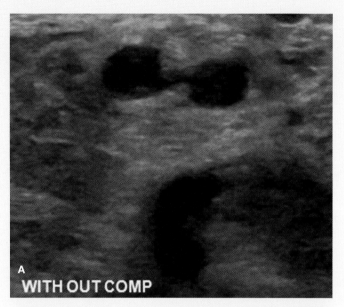

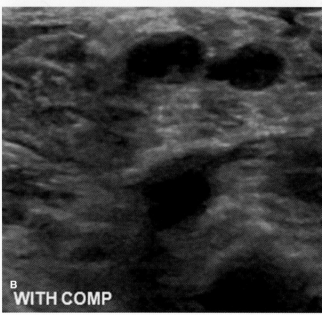

FIGURE 5–71.

86. Continuous flow in both the right and left CFVs would be highly suspicious of?

   (A) Thrombosis of the inferior vena cava
   (B) Congestive heart failure
   (C) Venous insufficiency
   (D) Thrombosis of the bilateral CFVs

87. Which of the following is not included in Virchow's Triad?

   (A) Hypercoagulability
   (B) Trauma
   (C) Stasis
   (D) Edema

88. Which of the following is the most accurate method to rule out DVT?

   (A) Graded compression
   (B) Spectral Doppler
   (C) Color Doppler
   (D) Continuous wave (CW) Doppler

89. Wet ulcers in the gaiter zone are indicative of

   (A) Deep venous thrombosis
   (B) High blood pressure
   (C) Pulmonary embolus
   (D) Venous insufficiency

90. During a venous duplex examination for venous insufficiency, a spectral Doppler waveform is obtained from the GSV above the knee. Following distal augmentation using an automatic cuff inflator, you demonstrate 1.5 seconds of retrograde flow. How would you best describe these findings?

   (A) Normal response to distal augmentation
   (B) Acute superficial thrombosis of the GSV
   (C) Equipment malfunction
   (D) Significant reflux within the GSV

91. A catheter-based procedure where thrombolytic agents are introduced to the vein at the area of a clot in an effort to dissolve it and reduce the chances of postthrombotic syndrome is known as

   (A) Thrombectomy
   (B) Thrombolysis
   (C) Anticoagulation
   (D) Phlebectomy

92. Which of the following is NOT a potential limitation of a lower extremity venous duplex examination?

   (A) Patient body habitus
   (B) Venous access lines
   (C) Bony anatomy
   (D) Recent incision

93. During a PPG examination for the evaluation of venous reflux, a normal VRT is

   (A) 20 seconds
   (B) 10 seconds
   (C) 15 seconds
   (D) 5 seconds

94. The majority of patients have how many perforating veins in each leg?

   (A) 20
   (B) 30
   (C) 50
   (D) More than 100

95. Proper positioning of a patient for a lower extremity duplex examination is

   (A) Supine with leg slightly bent at the knee and internally rotated
   (B) Prone with leg slightly bent at the knee and externally rotated
   (C) Prone with leg slightly bent at the knee and internally rotated
   (D) Supine with leg slightly bent at the knee and externally rotated

96. This spectral Doppler venous waveform of the lower extremities in Figure 5–72 indicates

   (A) Central obstruction
   (B) Peripheral obstruction
   (C) Normal venous flow
   (D) Phasic flow

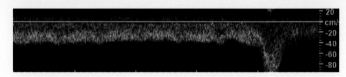

FIGURE 5–72.

97. This spectral Doppler venous waveform of the lower extremities in Figure 5–73 indicates

(A) Normal venous flow with augmentation

(B) Continuous flow

(C) Proximal obstruction

(D) Venous reflux

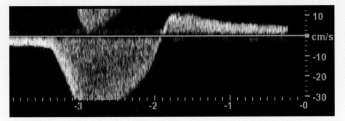

FIGURE 5–73.

98. The finding in Figure 5–74 indicates

(A) Normal GSV

(B) Thrombosed varicose vein

(C) Baker's cyst

(D) Acute DVT

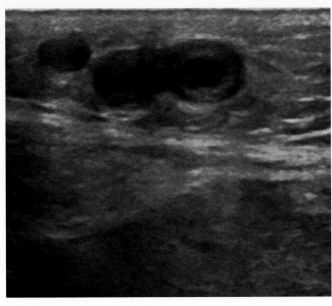

FIGURE 5–74.

99. This spectral Doppler venous waveform in Figure 5–75 of the lower extremity during a Valsalva maneuver indicates

(A) Normal venous flow

(B) Venous reflux

(C) Distal obstruction

(D) Partial obstruction

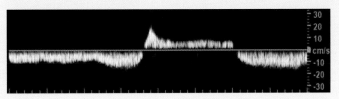

FIGURE 5–75.

100. The vein in Figure 5–76 most likely represents

(A) Popliteal vein

(B) Brachial vein

(C) Cephalic vein

(D) DFV

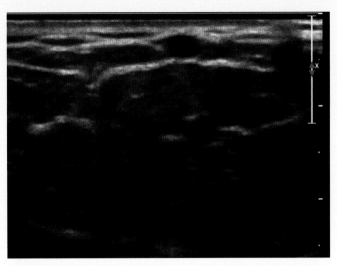

FIGURE 5–76.

Answers and Explanations

1. **(D)** The GSV is part of the superficial system in the lower extremities. The common femoral, posterior tibial, and popliteal veins are all part of the deep system of the lower extremities.

2. **(C)** Arteries have a much higher internal pressure than veins, and the thicker tunica media of their walls makes compression difficult. Only veins have valves.

3. **(B)** Above the inguinal ligament is the anatomical landmark where the CFV becomes the external iliac vein.

4. **(A)** A normal spectral waveform for the lower extremity veins should be phasic with changes in respiration and in one direction. Pulsatile waveforms suggest increased pressure in the venous system while continuous waveforms suggest the presence of a more proximal obstruction.

5. **(B)** The deep vein that runs along the anterolateral aspect of the lower leg between the tibia and fibula is the ATV. The PTV runs along the medial aspect of the lower leg.

6. **(C)** The common tibial trunk is formed in the upper calf by the paired PTVs. The common peroneal trunk is formed by the paired peroneal veins. These two common trunks eventually join to form the tibioperoneal trunk higher in the calf.

7. **(D)** The innermost layer of the vein wall is the tunica intima. The middle layer is the tunica media and the outermost layer is the tunica adventitia.

8. **(B)** The normal spectral waveform for the brachiocephalic (innominate) veins is pulsatile because of its close proximity to the heart. Upper extremity veins that are further from the heart such as the axillary vein will be more phasic.

9. **(A)** The cephalic vein runs along the lateral aspect of the arm until terminating in the axillary vein just before it becomes the subclavian. The basilic vein runs along the medial aspect of the arm and terminates at the axillary vein. The brachial vein is located in the upper arm and eventually becomes the axillary vein at the level of the axilla.

10. **(C)** There are no internal valves located in the brachiocephalic veins. The internal jugular, brachial, and cephalic veins all contain internal valves.

11. **(D)** Posterior tibial perforators connect to the posterior accessory GSV near the gaiter zone just above the medial malleolus. They commonly play a significant role in venous stasis ulcerations.

12. **(B)** Flow always goes from an area of higher pressure to an area of lower pressure. The pressure in the abdomen decreases as a person exhales. This causes venous flow to increase in the lower extremities. At the same time, the pressure in the chest increases causing venous flow in the upper extremities to decrease. The opposite is true when a person inhales.

13. **(C)** The majority of DVTs become established in the calf veins, specifically in the soleal sinuses. However, DVT can develop in any deep vein.

14. **(C)** Phlegmasia cerulea dolens is an outflow obstruction with extreme swelling accompanied by cyanosis and reduced arterial inflow. Phlegmasia alba dolens is an outflow obstruction with extreme swelling without cyanosis and reduced arterial inflow.

15. **(B)** The CFV DVT is more likely to travel to the lung as a PE because it is located above the knee. DVT located above the knee is more likely to become a PE.

16. **(D)** The three conditions that make up Virchow's Triad are trauma, stasis, and hypercoagulability.

17. **(C)** Paralysis is a symptom more related to arterial disease or stroke like symptoms. Pain, edema, and redness are all symptoms related to DVT.

18. **(D)** Venous insufficiency is the condition in which blood return back to the heart is inadequate. It leads to the pooling of blood in the distal veins which leads to increased pressure in the venous system.

19. **(A)** Ascending venograms are used to evaluate an obstruction caused by thrombosis. Descending venograms are used to evaluate incompetent venous valves.

20. **(C)** Oral anticoagulation is initiated after the initial treatment with a blood thinner like heparin or LMWH for a DVT in an effort to prevent reoccurrence. The duration of treatment will vary depending on the patient's condition and circumstances. It cannot prevent chronic postthrombotic change nor can it serve as a thrombolytic.

21. **(G)** Inferior vena cava

22. **(F)** Internal iliac vein

23. **(B)** External iliac vein

24. **(A)** CFV

25. **(C)** GSV

26. **(D)** DFV

27. **(E)** FV

28. **(H)** Popliteal vein

29. **(D)** Dilated vein is not a finding associated with chronic postthrombotic change. The findings that are associated with chronic changes are synechiae (webs), collateral veins, contraction of vein, and recanalization of vein.

30. **(B)** Normally subclavian veins have pulsatile flow with some respiratory patterns. Lack of pulsatility in a subclavian vein indicates a central obstruction on the side with the phasic waveform.

31. **(B)** Veins that are in close proximity to the heart will have cardiac pulsations coupled with respiratory patterns. For the upper extremities, this includes the internal jugular, brachiocephalic, and subclavian veins.

32. **(A)** When a clot appears to be poorly attached to a vessel wall, it is always considered to be an acute thrombus. It is typically the most distal portion of the clot that has propagated upward in the leg. The other findings associated with acute thrombosis are low-level echogenicity (although this is not reliable), dilated veins, and noncompressible vein.

33. **(C)** Popliteal vein

34. **(A)** Gastrocnemius veins

35. **(D)** SSV

36. **(G)** GSV

37. **(B)** PTVs

38. **(H)** ATVs

39. **(E)** Soleal veins

40. **(F)** Peroneal veins

41. **(C)** When a patient has venous insufficiency, the distal veins start to dilate because of pooling and stasis of blood in the distal veins of the calf. The hydrostatic pressure is increased distally. Vein walls are normally very elastic and will stretch when under these types of pressures, causing an increase in the transmural pressure.

42. **(B)** When an abnormal VRT (< 20 seconds) is achieved, it indicates that venous insufficiency is present. Tourniquets are often used to distinguish between deep venous reflux and superficial venous reflux. If an abnormal VRT is achieved without the tourniquet and a normal VRT is achieved with the tourniquet applied above the knee, it must be the GSV that is the problem because its contributory flow has been eliminated by the tourniquet.

43. **(A)** The venous valves are attached to the innermost layer known as the tunica intima. They are bicuspid valves that assist in promoting blood flow in one direction toward the heart.

44. **(C)** The radial and ulnar veins join to form the brachial vein at the level of the antecubital fossa (at the elbow joint). The basilic vein is a portion of the superficial system and the axillary and brachiocephalic veins are portions of the deep system up in the axilla and chest areas.

45. **(B)** Right IJV

46. **(J)** Left IJV

47. **(I)** Subclavian vein

48. **(E)** Right brachiocephalic vein

49. **(K)** Axillary vein

50. **(A)** SVC

51. **(C)** Cephalic vein

52. **(H)** Basilic vein

53. **(G)** Brachial vein

54. **(F)** Radial vein

55. **(D)** Ulnar vein

56. **(C)** A flow reversal time that exceeds 0.5 second (500 ms) in the superficial venous system is considered significant for reflux. A flow reversal time that exceeds 1 second in the deep system would be considered significant for reflux.

57. **(B)** Secondary varicose veins are the result of an obstruction in the deep venous system. In some cases, the pressure in the deep system gets so great that it backs up into the superficial system by way of the perforating veins. Primary varicose veins are isolated to the superficial system in the absence of a deep venous obstruction. Primary varicose veins are often due to congenital defects of the venous valves.

58. **(D)** Heel ulcerations are typically an indication of peripheral arterial disease not peripheral venous disease. Varicose veins, discoloration, and swelling are all symptoms associated with venous insufficiency.

59. **(C)** Sclerotherapy is a treatment for small superficial spider veins which involves the injection of chemical agents in an effort to ablate the vessel. Ablation and surgical removal of superficial veins are typically preformed on the larger superficial veins such as the GSV and its branches. The ablation of veins with the use of radiofrequency is known as RFA. This can also be accomplished with lasers through EVLT.

60. **(A)** The findings consistent with acute thrombosis are hypoechoic/anechoic, dilated, and noncompressible. Keep in mind that echogenicity is the least reliable factor.

61. **(C)** Figure 5–62 shows the paired PTVs surrounding the posterior tibial artery (more anterior) completely compressible with manual compression which is the normal response. The paired peroneal veins surrounding the peroneal artery (more posterior) show one vein compressing completely and the other anechoic, dilated, and noncompressible, which is consistent with acute DVT.

62. **(D)** The brachiocephalic vein should have cardiac pulsations with phasic flow patterns like the waveform in Figure 5–63

due to its close proximity to the heart. The common femoral, brachial, and popliteal will have more a phasic flow pattern similar to other veins further away from the heart.

63. **(B)** The FV in Figure 5–64 is anechoic, dilated, and noncompressible consistent with acute DVT.

64. **(C)** The arrow in Figure 5–65 is pointing to the area where the GSV joins the common FV known as the SFJ. This area is typically just below the inguinal ligament in the crease of the groin.

65. **(B)** The GSV is the longest vein in the body. It runs from the SFJ at the crease of the groin all the way down to the dorsum of the foot along the medial aspect of the leg.

66. **(A)** Primary varicose veins are isolated to the superficial system in the absence of a deep venous obstruction. Primary varicose veins are often due to congenital defects of the venous valves.

67. **(D)** Soleal veins are venous sinuses that serve as reservoirs for the calf-muscle pump just before it contracts to propel blood back toward the heart.

68. **(B)** The single biggest clinical implication of acute DVT is the patient risk for a blood clot that travels to the lung known as a PE. PE is potentially fatal.

69. **(D)** The SSV is a portion of the superficial system and is not paired. It is also not paired with a corresponding artery. The posterior tibial, anterior tibial, and peroneal veins are all part of the deep venous system in the calf. They are all paired and have a corresponding artery associated with them.

70. **(B)** Graded manual compression is the single most reliable diagnostic factor in determining DVT and should always be performed in the transverse plane to prevent the rolling of the vessel outside the field of view. Absence or presence of color Doppler can be somewhat unreliable in terms of a definitive diagnosis with lower extremity venous duplex studies. Normal venous waveforms should have respiratory phasicity. Continuous venous flow indicates that there is a possible proximal obstruction.

71. **(D)** Headache is not a predisposing risk factor for DVT. Trauma, cancer, and pregnancy all fall into one of the categories of "Virchow's Triad." "Virchow's Triad" identifies trauma, stasis, and hypercoagulability as the three predisposing risk factors to the development of thrombosis. Patients with cancer are oftentimes considered to have an acquired hypercoagulability. Pregnant patients can often experience stasis in the lower extremity veins due to the weight of the fetus on the inferior vena cava.

72. **(C)** The GSV is a superficial vein that typically terminates at the CFV in the groin at the SFJ. The SSV is also a superficial vein that typically terminates at the popliteal vein behind the knee.

73. **(D)** Figure 5–66 shows a filling defect with color Doppler in the subclavian veins with the presence of hypoechoic

material on the anterior wall. These findings are most consistent with partial nonocclusive thrombus of the subclavian vein.

74. **(B)** Figure 5–67 shows hyperechoic septations (synechiae) through the lumen of the IJV that are partially compressible with manual compression. These findings are consistent with chronic postthrombotic change of the IJV.

75. **(D)** Figure 5–68 shows a normal lower extremity venous waveform with normal respiratory phasic flow.

76. **(B)** The right and left common iliac veins join to form the inferior vena cava at the level of the umbilicus. The external and internal iliac veins join lower in the pelvis to form the common iliac veins on each side.

77. **(B)** Lower extremity venous duplex is a noninvasive, painless examination that utilizes only sound waves (ultrasound) to produce an image. There is no contrast needed, as with venography. For these reasons, ultrasound has become the preferred method of assessment for the lower extremity veins over venography and other modalities. Compression of the veins may cause patient discomfort, but for most patients it is not painful.

78. **(C)** Venous stasis ulcerations are most commonly located just above the medial malleolus in an area known as the gaiter zone. They are typically caused by an incompetent perforator in this area and can be very resistant to treatment.

79. **(C)** Varicose veins are a sign of venous insufficiency. Venous duplex, PPG, and descending venography can all be used to assess a patient for venous insufficiency. Ascending venography cannot be used to assess for venous insufficiency. Ascending venography is typically employed to evaluate for thrombosis.

80. **(A)** The normal response of venous flow during the Valsalva maneuver is cessation of flow followed by augmentation upon release. Reversal of flow during the maneuver would indicate venous reflux.

81. **(D)** Figure 5–69 shows a perforator with flow going from the deep system to the superficial system (toward the transducer), which is consistent with reversed and abnormal flow dynamics for perforating veins.

82. **(B)** Brachial vein

83. **(A)** Basilic vein

84. **(C)** Brachial nerve

85. **(C)** Figure 5–71 shows a pair of hypoechoic, dilated, noncompressible calf veins located within the upper calf muscle which is most consistent with acute DVT of the gastrocnemius veins.

86. **(A)** Continuous flow is present in the venous system when there is a proximal obstruction to flow. Because the continuous flow was bilateral, the mostly likely cause would be the result of a thrombus in the inferior vena cava which is proximal to both CFVs.

87. **(D)** Virchow's Triad identifies the three most common predisposing risk factors for thrombosis and they are trauma, stasis, and hypercoagulability. While edema is not a predisposing risk factor for thrombosis, it can be a symptom of it.

88. **(A)** Graded compression is the single most reliable method used when evaluating for DVT. Spectral and color Doppler can be used to further confirm the diagnosis.

89. **(D)** Wet ulcers that are commonly found in the gaiter zone are often referred to as venous stasis ulcers and are an indication that the patient has venous insufficiency.

90. **(D)** Retrograde flow following distal augmentation of greater than 0.5 seconds is an indication of significant venous reflux.

91. **(B)** Thrombolysis is a catheter-based procedure where thrombolytic agents are introduced into the vein to dissolve a clot and prevent further damage to the vessel lumen and internal valves. A thrombectomy is the surgical removal of a clot.

92. **(C)** Patient body habitus, a venous access line in the area of interest, and a recent incision from surgery are all potential limitations of a venous duplex examination. Bony anatomy is not a limiting factor for a lower extremity venous duplex examination; however, it can be for the central veins during an upper extremity duplex examination.

93. **(A)** During a PPG examination, the VRT should be 20 seconds or more to rule out venous reflux. Anything less than 20 seconds would be considered positive for reflux. A VRT less than 10 seconds indicates severe venous reflux.

94. **(D)** There are typically more than 100 perforating veins connecting the superficial system to the deep system. They are typically small in size (<3 mm) and not always visualized during a routine ultrasound.

95. **(D)** The proper position during a lower extremity venous duplex examination is with the patient supine with the leg of interest externally rotated. This allows for access to all the lower extremity veins.

96. **(A)** The venous waveform in Figure 5–72 shows continuous flow which indicates a central obstruction to venous flow.

97. **(D)** The venous waveform in Figure 5–73 shows reversal of flow following augmentation caused by distal compression consistent with venous reflux.

98. **(B)** Figure 5–74 shows a dilated superficial varicose vein with thrombus.

99. **(B)** Figure 5–75 shows reversal of flow during the Valsalva maneuver indicating reflux.

100. **(C)** Figure 5–76 represents the cephalic vein in the upper extremity.

Suggested Readings

1. Pellerito JS, Polak JF. *Introduction to Vascular Ultrasound.* 7th ed. Philadelphia, PA: Elsevier; 2020.

2. Kupinski AM. *Diagnostic Medical Sonography: The Vascular-System.* 2nd ed. Baltimore, MD: Wolters Kluwer; 2017.

3. Berdejo GL, Cruz J, Lipsitz EC. Sonography of the peripheral veins. In: Odwin CS, Fleischer AC, Krebs CA, eds. *Ultrasonography Examination.* China: The McGraw-Hill Companies, Inc; 2012:627–665.

4. Rumwell C, McPharlin M. *Vascular Technology: An Illustrated Review.* 5th ed. Pasadena, CA: Davies Publishing; 2017.

5. Oliver MA. Incidental findings during lower extremity venous duplex examination. *Vasc Ultrasound Today.* 2008;13:77–96.

6. Caggiati A, Bergan JJ, Gloviczki P, et al. Nomenclature of the veins of the lower limbs: an international interdisciplinary consensus statement. *J Vasc Surg.* 2002;36(2):416–422.

7. Delis KT, Knaggs AL, Khocabakhsh P. Prevalence, anatomic patterns, valvular competence and clinical significance of the Giacomini vein. *J Vasc Surg.* 2004;40(6):1174–1183.

8. Wells PS, Anderson DR, Bormanis J, et al. Value of assessment of pretest probability of deep-vein thrombosis of the lower limbs: an epidemiological study. *J Thromb Haemost.* 2005;3:1362–1367.

9. Dawson DL, Beals H. Acute lower extremity deep vein thrombosis. In: Zierler RE, ed. *Strandness's Duplex Scanning in Vascular Disorders.* Philadelphia, PA: Lippincott Williams & Wilkins; 2010:179–198.

10. Oliver MA. Medical management of acute deep vein thrombosis. *J Vas Tech.* 2002;26:227–229.

11. Dickson BC. Venous thrombosis: on the history of Virchow's triad. *Univ Toronto Med J.* 2004;81:166–171.

12. Kabnick LS. New horizons in the treatment of saphenous vein reflux. *J Vasc Tech.* 2002;239–246.

13. Lapropoulos N, Tiongson J, Pryor L, et al. Definition of venous reflux in the lower-extremity veins. *J Vasc Surg.* 2003;38(4):793–798.

14. Beraldo S, Satpathy A, Dodds SR. A study of the routine use of venous photoplethysmography in a one-stop vascular surgery clinic. *Ann R Coll Surg Engl.* 2007;89(4):379–383.

15. Bernardi E, Pesavento R, Prandoni P. Upper extremity deep venous thrombosis. *Semin Thromb Hemost.* 2006;32(7):729–736.

16. Carty CA, Steele JL, Clemens J. Standing versus supine evaluation for superficial venous reflux. *J Vasc Ultrasound.* 2013;37(3):119–124.

17. Deep Vein Thrombosis (DVT)/Pulmonary Embolism (PE)—Blood Clot Forming in a Vein. (n.d.) Available online at http://www.cdc.gov/ncbddd/dvt/data.html. Accessed August 22, 2013.

18. Meissner MH, Moneta G, Burnand K, et al. The hemodynamics and diagnosis of venous disease. *J Vasc Surg.* 2007;46 suppl S: 4S–24S.

19. Kearon C, Kahn SR, Agnelli G, et al. Antithrombotic therapy for venous thromboembolic disease: American College of Chest Physicians Evidence-Based Clinical Practice Guidelines. *Chest.* 2008;133(6 suppl):454S–545S.

20. Baldwin ZK, Comerota AJ, Schwartz LB. Catheter-directed thrombolysis for deep venous thrombosis. *Vasc Endovasc Surg.* 2004;38(1):1–9.

21. Agnelli G, Becattini C. Treatment of DVT: how long is enough and how do you predict recurrence. *J Thromb Thrombolysis.* 2008;25(1):37–44.

22. Lip GYH, Hull RD. Overview of the treatment of lower extremity deep vein thrombosis (DVT). Available online at UptoDate.com. Accessed September 25, 2018.

23. Needleman L, Cronan JJ, Lilly MP, et al. Ultrasound for lower extremity deep venous thrombosis. *Circulation.* 2018;137: 1505–1515.

24. Sharma K, Bora MK, Varghese J, et al. Role of transvaginal ultrasound and Doppler in diagnosis of pelvic congestion syndrome. *JCDR.* 2014;8(7):OD05–OD07.

25. Kim ES, Sharma AM, Scissons R, et al. Interpretation of peripheral arterial and venous Doppler waveforms: A Consensus Statement from the Society for Vascular Medicine and Society for Vascular Ultrasound. *Vasc Med.* 2020;1358863X20937665.

6

Abdominal Vascular Studies

INTRODUCTION

This chapter will review the anatomy and pathology of the abdominal vasculature. The liver and its blood vessels, aorta and its tributaries, and the vasculature of the kidneys will be discussed in detail. The abdomen contains two different circulatory system components: the systemic vasculature and the portal venous system. These two systems have a very important interconnected relationship in the presence of liver disease.

Some concepts apply to all of the studies contained within this chapter. For example, for each study type, a complete and thorough patient history must be taken, including reviewing previous studies, obtaining the medical and surgical history, and performing a clinical examination where indicated (e.g., listening for bruits, palpating pulsating masses). Angle correction should be used with spectral Doppler any time velocity information is desired. If angle correction is needed, the angle correction should not exceed 60 degrees.

ABDOMINAL AORTA

Anatomy

The aorta originates from the left ventricle of the heart and passes through the diaphragm to become the abdominal aorta (Fig. 6–1). The aorta is the largest artery in the body, with the normal adult abdominal aorta averaging 2 cm in diameter, decreasing in size until it terminates at the aortic bifurcation. Men tend to have slightly larger aortas than women, by about 3 mm.

The mesenteric vessels, which include the celiac artery (CA), superior mesenteric artery (SMA), and inferior mesenteric artery (IMA), originate from the aorta. The renal arteries, which supply blood to the kidneys, originate from the aorta just

inferior to the SMA origin. The gonadal arteries (testicular or ovarian) arise from the aorta anterolaterally and travel inferiorly to either the testicles or the ovaries, as appropriate.

At the level of the umbilicus, the aorta bifurcates into left and right common iliac arteries (CIA), which supply the legs and pelvic organs with blood (Fig. 6–2). The CIA typically measure less than 1.5 cm in diameter.

Pathology

Atherosclerotic Disease

The abdominal aorta is prone to atherosclerotic disease and plaque formation, with men at higher risk at an earlier age than women. Plaque and thrombus formation can lead to stenosis or occlusion, as well as the formation of emboli that can cause problems in the lower extremities (Fig. 6–3).

Abdominal Aortic Aneurysm

Approximately 30% of abdominal aortic aneurysms (AAAs) are discovered incidentally on clinical examination. Risk factors for AAA are the same as other vascular disorders, including hypertension, diabetes, and smoking. Smoking increases the likelihood a patient will develop an AAA, as well as the likelihood of AAA rupture. Rupture of AAA kills approximately 4,500 people in the United States annually. Ultrasound is the preferred imaging test for AAA screening because of its high sensitivity and specificity, low cost, and lack of ionizing radiation. Although it is generally accepted that a measurement of the abdominal aorta over 3 cm is an AAA, a better definition of AAA is a focal increase in size that is 1.5 times larger than the nearest unaffected part of the aorta. This distinction is important because females naturally have slightly smaller aortas than men. Therefore, it is possible to have an AAA even though the aorta measures less than 3 cm, as long as a contiguous segment is 1.5 times larger in diameter. In some cases, the patient may

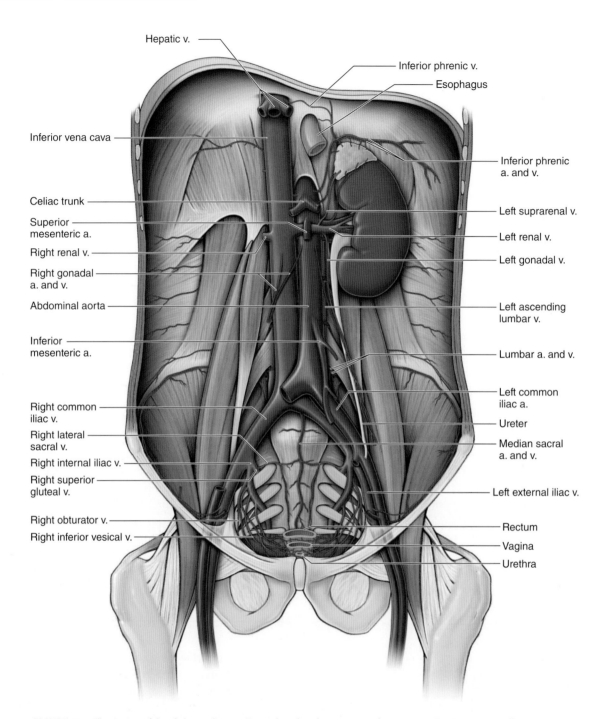

FIGURE 6–1. Illustration of the abdominal aorta. (Reproduced, with permission, from Morton DA, Foreman K, Albertine KH. *The Big Picture: Gross Anatomy*, 2nd ed. New York, NY; 2019; Figure 11–2. Copyright © McGraw Hill.)

have widened areas of the aorta that are less than 3 cm. This is called ectasia, and the patient is said to have an ectatic aorta (Fig. 6–4).

The most common presentation of AAA is fusiform dilatation, in which a focal portion of the aorta is dilated beyond 3 cm, outer wall to outer wall (Fig. 6–5). Another type of aneurysmal dilatation is called a saccular aneurysm, which is like a bubble coming off the aorta. Saccular aneurysms more commonly occur in the thoracic aorta, and are less common

in the abdominal aorta. The saccular aneurysm (Fig. 6–6) is a true aneurysm because it involves all three layers of the aorta, unlike a pseudoaneurysm, which does not involve all three layers. Pseudoaneurysms of the aorta are very rare (Fig. 6–7). The fusiform and saccular aneurysms are prone to thrombus formation, which may cause embolic showers to the distal lower extremities. An even more rare type of AAA is the mycotic aneurysm, which occurs as a result of an infectious process (Fig. 6–8).

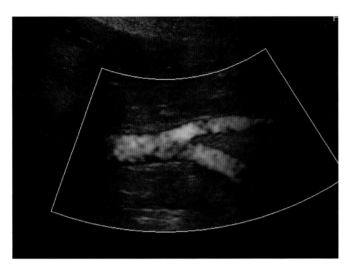

FIGURE 6–2. Coronal power Doppler of common iliac artery bifurcation.

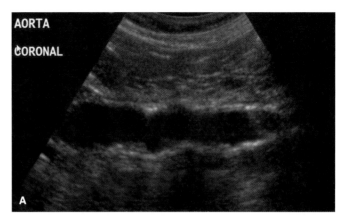

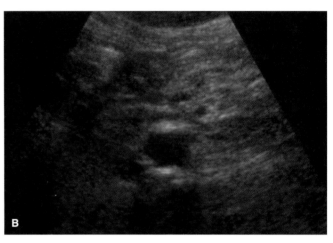

FIGURE 6–3. Calcified material in an atherosclerotic aorta without aneurysm. **(A)** Grayscale sagittal aorta with calcifications. **(B)** Transverse view of same aorta.

Patients with an AAA less than 5.5 cm require continued observation. Once the AAA reaches a size of 5.5 cm, intervention should be considered. Aneurysms over 6 cm have a 10% to 20% risk of rupture, and 7-cm aneurysms have a 20% to 40% risk. AAAs are slow growing, so the typical follow-up is between once every 6 months and once every 2 to 3 years, depending on the size of the aneurysm. Figure 6–9 is from a patient with a thrombosed fusiform AAA. Note the aneurysmal dilatation measuring approximately 5 cm in maximal diameter.

While open surgical repair used to be standard, endovascular aneurysm repair (EVAR) is now the preferred method of treatment due its less invasive nature. EVAR has lower short-term complications compared to open surgery, especially in patients who are at high risk for surgery. With EVAR, a synthetic graft is placed into the aneurysm via a groin catheter, eliminating the large incisions used for open repair (Figs. 6–10 and 6–11). EVARs are not infallible, and a leak from the stent

contained within the aneurysmal sac can occur, called an endoleak. Ultrasound with color Doppler can be used to monitor the EVAR and evaluate for an endoleak, without the radiation and need for contrast agents associated with computed tomography (CT). Some studies have touted ultrasonography

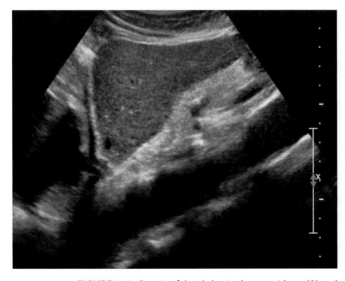

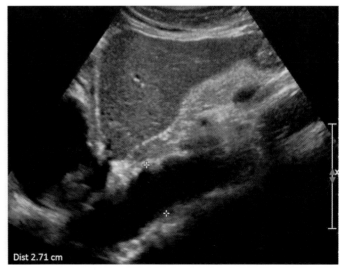

FIGURE 6–4. Ectasia of the abdominal aorta without **(A)** and with **(B)** calipers. Aorta is widened in parts but less than 3.0 cm in diameter.

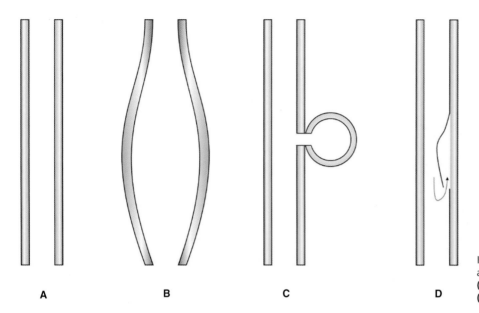

FIGURE 6–5. The most common types of abdominal aortic pathology. **(A)** Normal aorta. **(B)** Fusiform dilatation. **(C)** Saccular aneurysm. **(D)** Dissection.

(US) as comparable to CT in diagnosing endoleaks, and US has the additional advantage of being able to provide direction of flow information. Contrast-enhanced US (CEUS) may offer even greater real-time diagnostic capabilities for endoleaks.

There are different categories of endoleaks, Types I, II, III, and IV (Fig. 6–12). Types I and II are the most common types. With Type I, flow is leaking proximally or distally at the attachment point due to a poor seal at one end. With Type II, retrograde flow is leaking into the aneurysmal sack via a branch vessel. The lumbar arteries and IMA should be occluded as a result of placement of the graft; therefore, flow in these vessels is symptomatic of endoleak (Fig. 6–13). Types III and IV endoleaks are from a problem with the graft material itself. If the cause of the endoleak cannot be identified, it may be termed a "Type V."

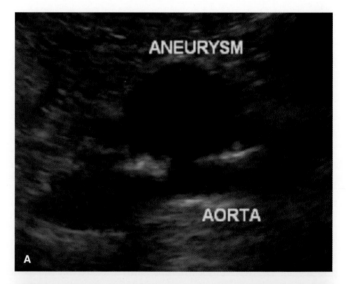

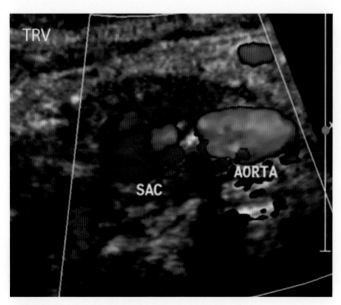

FIGURE 6–6. Color Doppler image of saccular aneurysm.

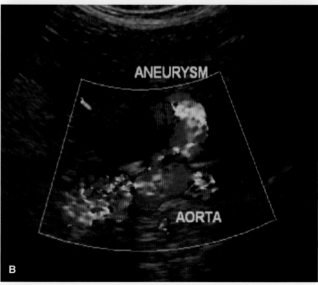

FIGURE 6–7. (A) Grayscale of pseduoaneurysm of aorta. **(B)** Color Doppler of same patient.

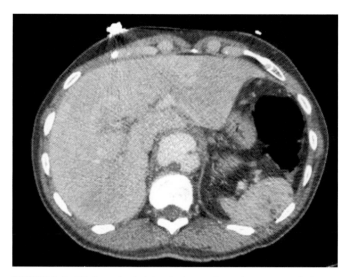

FIGURE 6–8. CT of proximal abdominal mycotic aortic aneurysm. Patient had clinical symptoms consistent with infectious process.

Dissection of the Aorta

Aortic dissection is a separation of the intima from the wall of the aorta, creating a flap that causes blood flow on both sides (Fig. 6–14). Most commonly, dissections of the abdominal aorta are an extension of a thoracic aortic dissection. Diseases such as

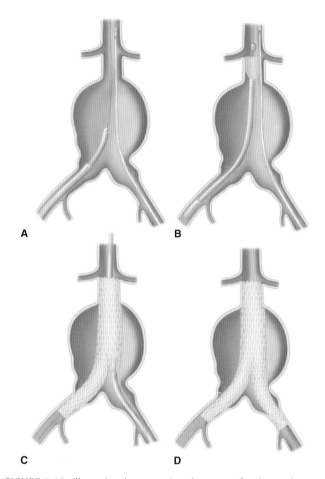

FIGURE 6–10. Illustration demonstrating placement of endovascular aneurysm repair (EVAR) graft. **(A)** Insertion of sheath into right iliac. **(B)** Deployment of aortoiliac limb of graft. **(C)** Deployment of other iliac limb of graft. **(D)** Complete EVAR. (Reproduced, with permission, from Brunicardi F, Andersen DK, Billiar TR, et al. *Schwartz's Principles of Surgery,* 11th ed. New York, NY; 2019; Figure 23–33. Copyright © McGraw Hill.)

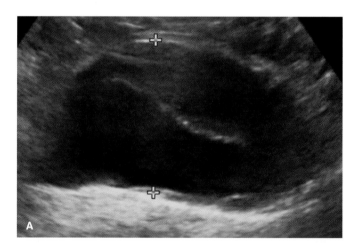

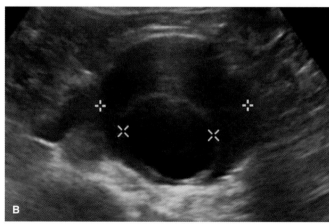

FIGURE 6–9. **(A)** Sagittal and **(B)** transverse ultrasound images of 5-cm abdominal aortic aneurysm (AAA) with thrombus.

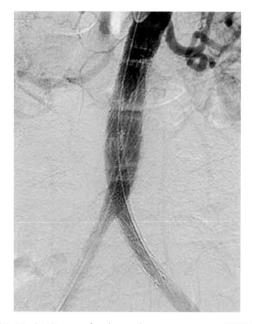

FIGURE 6–11. Angiogram of endovascular aneurysm repair (EVAR). (Reproduced, with permission, from Brunicardi F, Andersen DK, Billiar TR, et al. *Schwartz's Principles of Surgery,* 11th ed. New York, NY; 2019; Figure 23–32B. Copyright © McGraw Hill.)

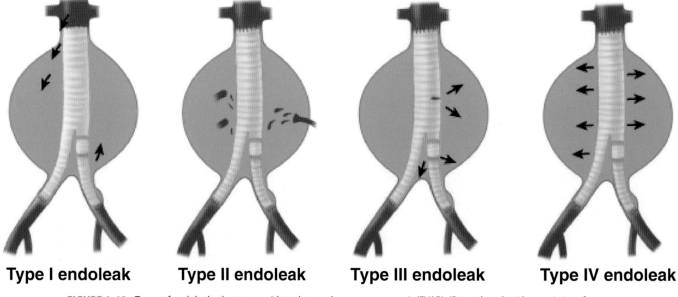

Type I endoleak   Type II endoleak   Type III endoleak   Type IV endoleak

FIGURE 6–12. Types of endoleaks that occur with endovascular aneurysm repair (EVAR). (Reproduced, with permission, from Brunicardi F, Andersen DK, Billiar TR, et al. *Schwartz's Principles of Surgery,* 11th ed. New York, NY; 2019; Figure 23–34. Copyright © McGraw Hill.)

Marfan's may make a patient prone to thoracic aortic dissection. Although the false lumen is often bigger than the true lumen, or original aortic lumen, the false lumen is prone to thrombose and may or may not have flow within it.

Scanning Protocol, Patient Assessment, and Integration of Data

Aorta studies should be performed on a fasting patient to minimize intestinal gas. Even with fasting, the aorta can be a difficult vessel to examine because of the depth of the vessel. Even in a relatively thin patient, the proximal aorta is deep and courses more superficially at the distal end. Therefore, depth and focal zone will need to constantly be adjusted as the probe is moved

distally. On a large patient, or in the presence of excessive bowel gas, a lot of probe pressure may be needed. It might not be possible to visualize parts of the aorta due to bowel gas or large body habitus; it is important to document any suboptimal areas. A curvilinear transducer that is 2 to 4 MHz will likely be needed, although in thin patients a 5 MHz may be used.

Evaluation of the abdominal aorta typically begins in a sagittal plane at the proximal aorta, and continues to mid and distal aorta. In the sagittal plane, the aorta is measured in its anteroposterior (AP) dimension, orthogonal to the long axis of the aorta, proximally, mid, and distally. All measurements of the aorta should be outer wall to outer wall. Depending on protocol, color and/or spectral Doppler may be obtained at one or

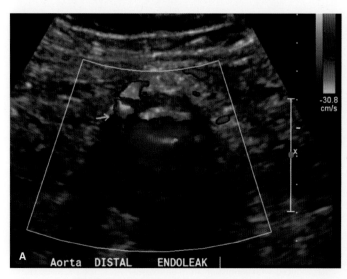

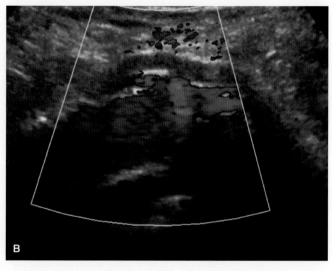

FIGURE 6–13. (A) Transverse color Doppler of Type II endoleak with reversal of flow from IMA. **(B)** Sagittal color Doppler image demonstrating endoleak.

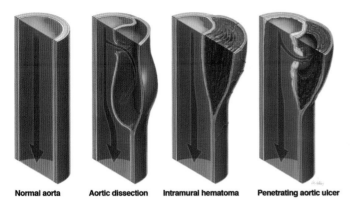

FIGURE 6-14. Illustration of aortic dissection. (Reproduced, with permission, from Brunicardi F, Andersen DK, Billiar TR, et al. *Schwartz's Principles of Surgery,* 11th ed. New York, NY; 2019; Figure 22–18. Copyright © McGraw Hill.)

Normal aorta   Aortic dissection   Intramural hematoma   Penetrating aortic ulcer

more levels. The proximal, mid, and distal aorta are also documented in the transverse plane. The measurement that should be obtained in the transverse plane is the maximal diameter. This measurement may not be true transverse, but is the widest measurement obtained. This is attributed to the fact that aneurysmal aortas may not be perfect circles in cross section. It is not necessary to measure the length of the aneurysm, and in fact it may cause confusion if a report is read incorrectly and the length assumed to be the maximum cross-sectional dimension. Length of an aneurysm should only be documented if the vascular surgeon or interventional radiologist requests it, such as for EVAR placement. Finally, the CIA should be measured in two planes, and color and spectral Doppler images obtained. The aorta should be evaluated for thrombus and calcific plaque, as well as dissection of the intima, all of which may be responsible for showering emboli to the lower extremities. If there is

a true lumen and a false lumen, both should be measured. See Figure 6–9 for an example of how the measurement should be performed. If dissection is suspected, a higher-frequency linear or curvilinear transducer should be used, perpendicular to the aorta wall, to optimize visualization of an intimal flap.

The spectral waveform of the aorta is dependent upon where the waveform is obtained. The proximal aorta has a lower-resistance waveform due to its low-resistance terminal bed, the liver, spleen, and kidneys, but the distal aorta and CIA have a high-resistance waveform because they supply the normally high-resistance lower extremities. The aorta velocities are typically 60 to 100-cm/s peak systolic velocity (PSV). While there have not been many studies done of grading the severity within the abdominal aorta, most laboratories utilize the same velocity criteria used with the evaluation of the lower extremity arteries. As with the lower extremities, a velocity ratio of 2 or more would indicate a 50% or more diameter stenosis. Although rare, total occlusion of the abdominal aorta can occur, and usually begins distally and progresses in a cephalad direction. Blood flow to the lower extremities is via collaterals with associated abnormal waveforms (Fig. 6–15).

MESENTERIC VESSELS

Anatomy

The CA, or celiac axis, is the first branch to originate from the abdominal aorta. It is usually seen at the 12:00–1:00 position in the transverse plane and is typically 1-2 cm in length (Fig. 6–16). As with all vascular anatomy, there is patient-to-patient variability. For example, the celiac axis sometimes originates closer to 1:00 than 12:00, or it may curve and be difficult to see in the transverse plane. The celiac axis gives off three vessels, only two

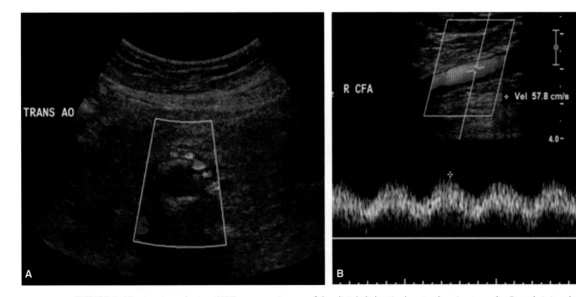

FIGURE 6-15. Aortic occlusion. **(A)** Transverse image of the distal abdominal aorta showing no color Doppler signal. CT, not shown here, confirmed aortic occlusion. **(B)** Tardus parvus waveform in the common femoral arteries is consistent with proximal occlusion.

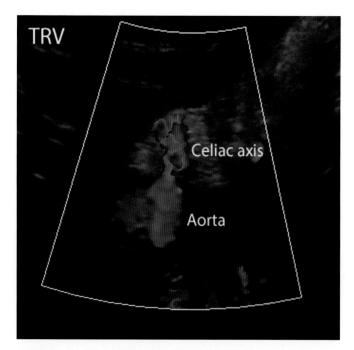

FIGURE 6–16. Color Doppler image of transverse celiac axis.

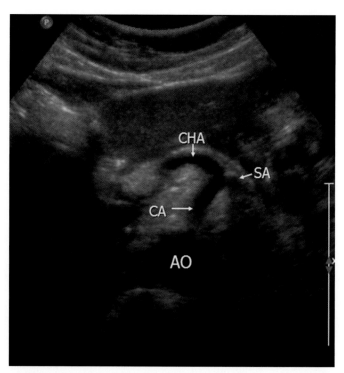

FIGURE 6–17. "Seagull sign" formed by celiac axis, common hepatic artery, and splenic artery.

of which are routinely seen by ultrasound. The two vessels that are routinely visualized are the splenic artery and the common hepatic artery (CHA). These vessels form the so-called "seagull sign" because the V-shape made by the common hepatic and splenic arteries resembles a bird drawn by a child (Fig. 6–17). The left gastric artery is the third, rarely visualized branch of the celiac axis. The splenic artery is a serpentine vessel that supplies blood to the spleen. The splenic artery travels along the posterior, superior border of the pancreas into the splenic hilum. Due to its serpiginous nature, the splenic artery is sometimes seen as circles on ultrasound, rather than a long vessel (Fig. 6–18). The CHA, which supplies oxygenated blood to the liver, originates from the CA and travels to the right, toward the liver. Distal to the CA, the CHA gives off the GDA. The GDA travels inferiorly and has anastomoses with the SMA. Distal to the GDA origin,

the CHA is now called the proper hepatic artery (PHA). Some laboratories call the PHA the main hepatic artery (MHA). The PHA gives off the right gastric artery, and then bifurcates into left hepatic artery (LHA) and right hepatic artery (RHA). The intrahepatic arterial branches travel within the liver along with a segment of bile duct and portal vein, forming the so-called portal triad (Fig. 6–19).

The next vessel to originate from the aorta, just inferior to the CA, is the SMA (Fig. 6–20). The SMA is typically visualized at the 12:00 position in transverse plane. The SMA supplies blood to part of the large and small intestines. The SMA anastomoses with the celiac axis via the GDA through the pancreaticoduodenal collaterals.

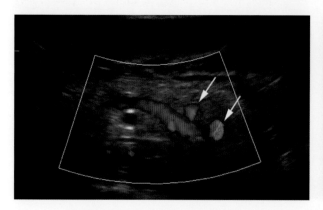

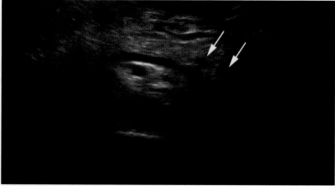

FIGURE 6–18. Transverse image of pancreatic tail. The circles (*arrows*) are the tortuous splenic artery, seen in cross section as it winds its way to the spleen from the celiac axis.

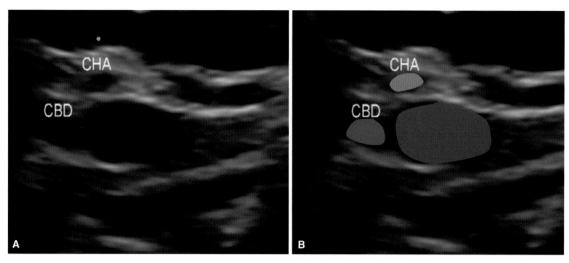

FIGURE 6–19. Portal triad. Cross-section of the portal triad at the porta hepatitis. Structures represented are common hepatic artery (CHA), common bile duct (CBD), and main portal vein (MPV).

The IMA is a small vessel, although with modern ultrasound equipment can be seen with careful scanning. The IMA typically arises from the aorta from the 1:00 position in the transverse plane, several centimeters superior to the aortic bifurcation. The IMA supplies blood to the large intestine. Figure 6–21 is a computed tomography angiogram (CTA) of the celiac axis, SMA, and IMA.

Pathology

Mesenteric Ischemia

The mesenteric (splanchnic) arteries include the celiac axis, SMA, and IMA. Stenosis or occlusion of these vessels can lead to bowel ischemia or infarction. The most common form of mesenteric ischemia in the vascular laboratory is chronic mesenteric

ischemia (CMI). CMI occurs when two of the three mesenteric vessels are occluded, causing the patient dull postprandial pain that leads to anorexia (avoidance of food) and, about 50% of the time, abdominal bruit. As a result of food avoidance, weight

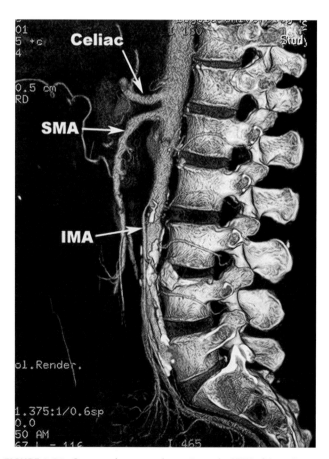

FIGURE 6–21. Computed tomography angiography (CTA) of the celiac axis, superior mesenteric artery (SMA), and inferior mesenteric artery (IMA). (Reproduced, with permission, from Brunicardi F, Andersen DK, Billiar TR, et al. *Schwartz's Principles of Surgery*, 11th ed. New York, NY; 2019; Figure 23–40. Copyright © McGraw Hill.)

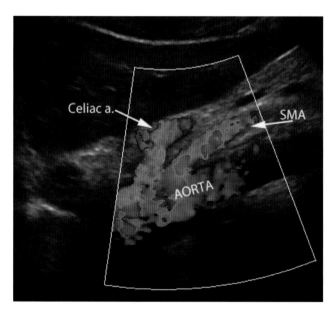

FIGURE 6–20. Sagittal image of celiac axis and superior mesenteric artery (SMA) origins.

loss is another symptom of CMI. The main cause of CMI is atherosclerosis in the mesenteric vessels. The collateral circulation present within the mesenteric vessels is the reason why two out of three vessels need to be severely stenosed or occluded before a patient will present with symptoms. The GDA and arc of Riolan are two of these collaterals.

Acute mesenteric ischemia, found more commonly in women, may be caused by arterial embolus, arterial thrombus, nonocclusive ischemia, external compression, and in rare cases venous thrombosis. These patients often present in the sixth or seventh decade with other cardiac-related medical conditions, such as atrial fibrillation, congestive heart failure, etc. Patients complain of severe abdominal pain, vomiting, and diarrhea, which may mimic other gastrointestinal (GI) diseases, such as diverticulitis or gallbladder disease, and therefore the diagnosis may be delayed. The longer the acute mesenteric ischemia diagnosis is delayed, the more bowel becomes ischemic and may infarct. Time is an issue for these patients, as acute mesenteric ischemia has a mortality rate above 60%. A serious complication of mesenteric ischemia is necrosis of the bowel wall, which is best seen with CT. Necrosis of the bowel is potentially life-threatening and is treated surgically.

Patients with acute mesenteric ischemia may be sent for computed tomography angiography (CTA) or conventional angiography instead of the vascular laboratory, as diagnosis and treatment (embolectomy and stenting) can occur in the interventional suite. Surgical treatment may be needed, such as a bypass graft. Acute mesenteric ischemia is a true medical emergency, and these patients need rapid diagnosis and treatment.

Median Arcuate Ligament Syndrome

Median arcuate ligament syndrome (MALS) is an entrapment of the CA by the median arcuate ligament of the diaphragm. Compression of the CA only occurs during exhalation, and is relieved with inspiration. Due to MALS, Doppler studies of the mesenteric vessels must include spectral Doppler waveforms of the CA in both inspiration and expiration. Figure 6–22 is an ultrasound in a patient with MALS. Note the velocity change in expiration versus inspiration.

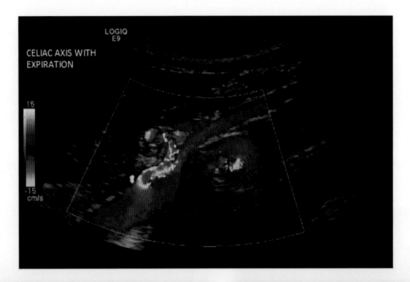

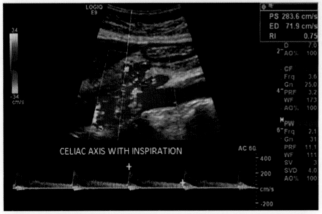

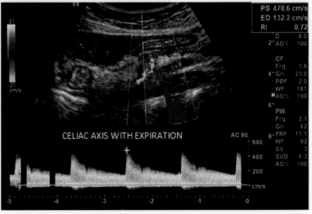

FIGURE 6–22. Ultrasound of the celiac axis in inspiration and expiration in a patient with median arcuate ligament syndrome (MALS). Notice the dramatic velocity increase in expiration. Because of MALS, the celiac axis must always be documented in both inspiration and expiration.

Aneurysm

Although aneurysms of the mesenteric vessels are rare, splenic artery aneurysms are the most common type. CT or MRI usually identifies mesenteric vessel aneurysms first, although they may be found incidentally during ultrasound examination, so it is important to know of their existence.

Scanning Protocol, Patient Assessment, and Integration of Data

Mesenteric studies are performed with a low-frequency (2-4 MHz) curvilinear transducer. The patient should fast at least 8 hours, although that number may vary laboratory to laboratory. It is helpful if the patient is able to control breathing as some images will need to be taken in deep inspiration while others in expiration. Breath holding will make for easier sampling of these small vessels, and a lot of probe pressure may be needed to move bowel gas out of the way. Mesenteric studies are performed with the patient in a fasting state in order to evaluate preprandial waveforms. For mesenteric ischemia studies, if the preprandial waveforms are normal, the study is then repeated about 30 minutes after eating a meal.

Imaging begins with grayscale images of celiac axis, SMA. The IMA is not routinely examined unless there is pathology of the celiac axis and SMA. Color and spectral Doppler should be obtained of the celiac and SMA, as well. Typically, PSV measurements are obtained at the origin of the vessels and 1-2 cm distal to the origin. Depending on the laboratory protocol, the common hepatic and splenic arteries may also be examined, and some laboratories obtain velocity waveforms of the mid and distal SMA.

In a normal fasting patient, the celiac axis, which primarily supplies blood to the liver and spleen, should have a low-resistance flow pattern due to its low-resistance distal beds. The SMA and IMA, which feed the resting bowel, exhibit a high-resistance waveform due to the constricted arterioles distally. After a meal, the intestines require blood, causing arteriolar dilatation. This normally induces a change in the feeding blood vessels, the SMA and IMA, to low-resistance flow patterns, with forward flow in all phases of the cardiac cycle. If the SMA or IMA resting flow patterns are low-resistance (monophasic) in the fasting state, then the postprandial study need not be performed because the distal arterioles are abnormally persistently dilated due to hypoxia. The diagnosis of mesenteric ischemia is not made on waveform analysis alone, but with velocities as well. Table 6–1 lists the normal and abnormal velocities for the mesenteric vessels. If celiac axis occlusion is suspected, the GDA should be imaged to evaluate for retrograde flow. The GDA becomes collateral circulation to the liver and spleen via the pancreaticoduodenal vessels from the SMA in the presence of celiac axis occlusion (Fig. 6–23).

Figure 6–24 presents normal spectral waveforms and velocities of the celiac axis and SMA. Note the low-resistance celiac axis and high-resistance SMA in this fasting patient. Figure 6–25 is a patient with celiac stenosis. In this patient's case, the celiac

TABLE 6–1 • Normal and Abnormal Values for Celiac Axis and SMA		
Vessel	**Normal**	**Abnormal (> 70% Stenosis)**
Celiac Axis	≤ 200 cm/s preprandial	> 200 cm/s
SMA	≤ 275 cm/s preprandial	> 275 cm/s
SMA	High-resistance waveform preprandial	Low-resistance waveform preprandial

velocity is abnormally elevated to 298 cm/s. Figure 6–26 is a CTA of the same patient. Figure 6–27 is a patient with a 70% SMA stenosis. Note the aliasing on the color Doppler image. This patient underwent stent placement of the SMA (Fig. 6–28).

RENAL VASCULATURE

Anatomy

The left and right renal arteries emerge from the aorta just inferior to the origin of the SMA (Fig. 6–29). Duplication of either

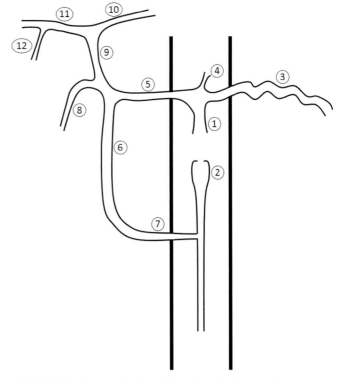

FIGURE 6–23. Diagram of celiac axis branches showing superior mesenteric artery (SMA) to celiac collaterals. (1) Celiac axis, (2) SMA, (3) splenic artery, (4) left gastric artery, (5) common hepatic artery, (6) gastroduodenal artery (GDA), (7) pancreaticoduodenal artery, (8) right gastric artery, (9) proper hepatic artery, (10) left hepatic artery, (11) right hepatic artery, and (12) cystic artery.

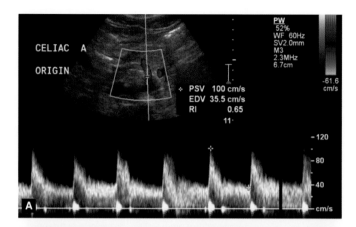

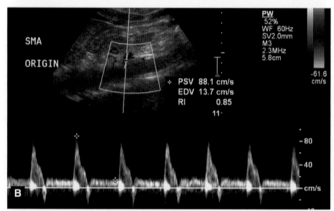

FIGURE 6–24. (A) Normal celiac axis spectral Doppler. **(B)** Normal superior mesenteric artery (SMA) spectral Doppler.

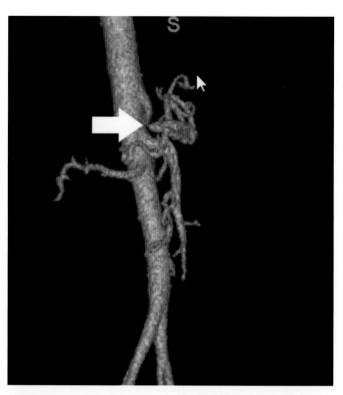

FIGURE 6–26. Computed tomography angiography (CTA) of patient with celiac stenosis. *Arrow* points to area of narrowing.

artery is common, especially the right renal artery, and there may even be more than two of each renal artery. The left renal artery, which typically emerges from the aorta at around the 3:00–4:00 position, is shorter than the right renal artery due to the aorta's location on the left side of the body. The right renal artery typically emerges from the aorta at around 10:00, travels anteriorly for about 1 cm, and then travels posteriorly toward the kidney. The right renal artery travels posterior to the inferior vena cava (IVC), and is normally the only vessel that lies posterior to the IVC. The renal arteries are depicted in color Doppler in Figure 6–30. It is not uncommon to visualize multiple renal arteries, and care should be taken to identify and document these accessory arteries (Fig. 6–31).

The left renal vein is longer than the right renal vein because the IVC is closer to the right side of the body. The left renal vein emerges from the IVC and usually travels anterior to the aorta but posterior to the SMA (Fig. 6–32). Sometimes, the left renal

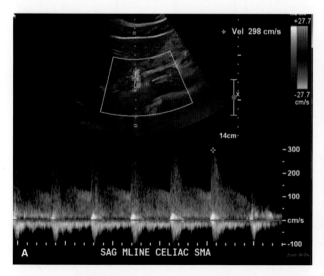

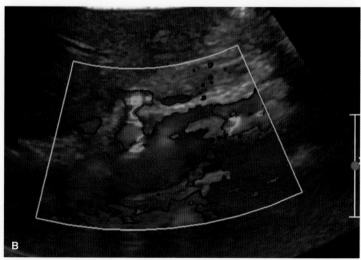

FIGURE 6–25. (A) Spectral and **(B)** color Doppler of a patient with stenosis of the celiac artery. Note the aliasing in the color Doppler image.

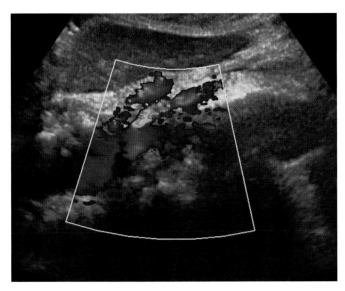

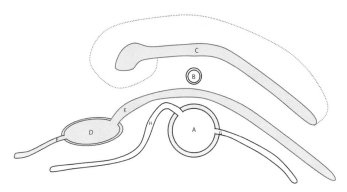

FIGURE 6–29. Diagram of the relationship of the aorta, renal arteries, renal veins, superior mesenteric artery (SMA), and splenic vein. The pancreas is represented by the dotted line **(A)** aorta, **(B)** SMA, **(C)** splenic vein, **(D)** inferior vena cava (IVC), **(E)** left renal vein, **(F)** right renal vein, **(G)** left renal artery, and **(H)** right renal artery.

FIGURE 6–27. Patient with more than 70% superior mesenteric artery (SMA) stenosis. Color Doppler image demonstrates aliasing in the region of the elevated velocities.

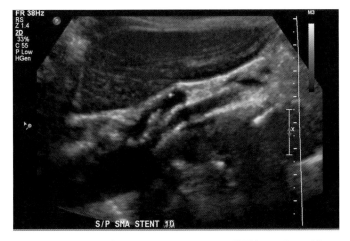

FIGURE 6–28. Stented superior mesenteric artery (SMA) in patient with history of more than 70% stenosis.

vein will travel posterior to the aorta, called a retroaortic left renal vein (Fig. 6–33). Both renal arteries lie posterior to their corresponding veins.

The main renal artery travels to the renal hilum, where it divides into the segmental arteries (Fig. 6–34). The segmental arteries, each of which correspond to a surgically resectable part of the kidney, further divide into the interlobar arteries. The interlobar arteries branch to become the curved arcuate arteries, which eventually become the terminal branches, the interlobular arteries (Fig. 6–35).

Pathology

Renal Artery Stenosis

Renal artery stenosis (RAS) is considered hemodynamically significant when there is at least a 70% reduction in lumen diameter. Stenosis or occlusion of the renal arteries can lead

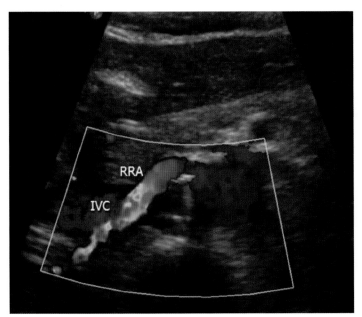

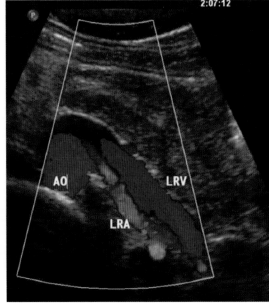

FIGURE 6–30. Right and left renal arteries. The right renal artery travels posterior to the inferior vena cava (IVC).

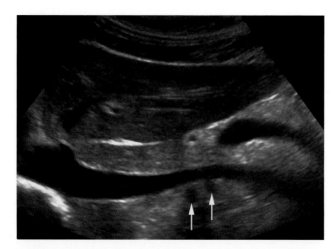

FIGURE 6–31. Sagittal grayscale image showing two right renal arteries (*arrows*) posterior to the inferior vena cava (IVC).

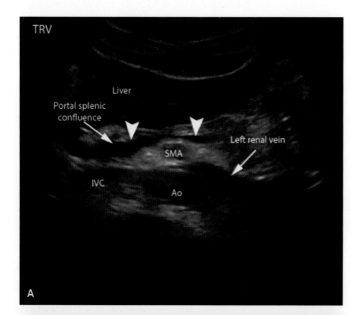

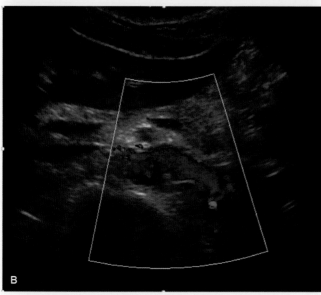

FIGURE 6–32. Transverse **(A)** grayscale (*Arrowheads* point to splenic vein) and **(B)** color Doppler of left renal vein. Note its location between the aorta and the superior mesenteric artery (SMA).

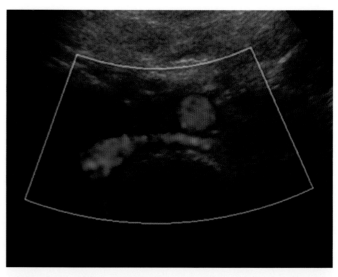

FIGURE 6–33. Power Doppler of retro-aortic left renal vein. The left renal is normally anterior to the aorta.

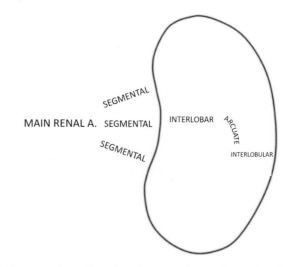

FIGURE 6–34. Arterial branches of main renal artery depicted graphically in relation to location and size in kidney.

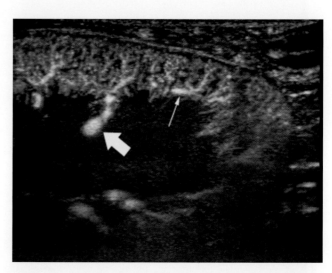

FIGURE 6–35. Microflow imaging (Toshiba America Medical Systems, Tustin, CA) of the kidney. *Large arrow*: interlobar artery; *small arrow*: arcuate artery.

to renal insufficiency, and may manifest itself as hypertension and elevated renal function tests such as blood urea nitrogen (BUN) and serum creatinine. Not all renovascular hypertension is caused by RAS. In fact, there are many disease processes that manifest as renovascular hypertension; RAS is just one of the conditions that needs to be ruled out. Many kidney diseases have no cure, and end-stage renal disease leads to the need for prolonged dialysis or kidney transplant. The diagnosis of RAS is important because it is a condition that can potentially be treated with angioplasty or stenting.

Most patients who present with hypertension have primary hypertension, formerly known as essential hypertension, which is usually idiopathic. A smaller percentage of patients will have renovascular hypertension, also called secondary hypertension, which is most commonly caused by atherosclerotic disease in patients more than 50 years old, and fibromuscular dysplasia (FMD) in patients less than 50 years old. Hypertension resulting from RAS may be a result of activation of the renin–angiotensin system, in which the kidney produces renin which is later converted to angiotensin II. This process causes vasoconstriction of the renal vasculature.

Fibromuscular Dysplasia

FMD is a segmental, nonatherosclerotic arterial disease most commonly associated with the carotid and renal arteries, although it can occur in any blood vessel. FMD occurs from abnormal cell proliferation in the arterial walls which causes abnormal architecture. Up to 90% of FMD occurs in women, typically under 50 years of age. FMD can be focal or multifocal. Focal FMD can occur in any part of the artery, while multifocal FMD usually occurs in the mid-distal segments and presents as the classic "string of beads" appearance caused by alternating areas of stenosis and dilatation (Fig. 6–36). Multifocal FMD is more common in adults, while focal FMD is more common in the pediatric population.

Renal Vein Disorders

Disorders of the renal veins include thrombus and external compression causing venous stenosis. Thrombus in the renal vein is commonly from tumor thrombus, as renal cell carcinoma and other cancers may spread into the renal vein. When this occurs on the left side in males, this may manifest itself as a severe left testicular varicocele due to the left testicular vein's insertion into the left renal vein.

"Nutcracker syndrome" may occur when the left renal vein is compressed due to its location between the SMA and the aorta, or from a retroaortic left renal vein (Fig. 6–37). A rarer version of this is a circumaortic renal vein, in which one renal vein is anterior to the aorta and another is posterior.

Renal Transplants

Although kidney transplantation is 60 years old at the time of this writing, rejection is still an issue for patients despite advances in immunosuppression and increased understanding

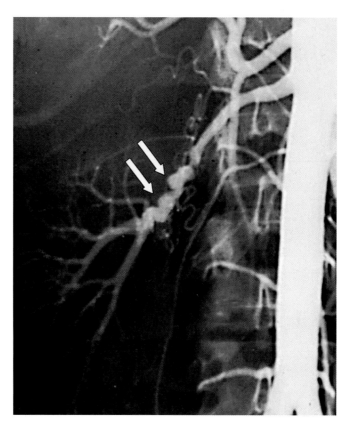

FIGURE 6–36. Angiogram of fibromuscular dysplasia (FMD). Angiogram of patient with FMD of renal artery. The renal artery (*arrows*) is very tortuous referred to as a "string of beads" appearance. (Reproduced, with permission, from Brunicardi F, Andersen DK, Billiar TR, et al. *Schwartz's Principles of Surgery,* 11th ed. New York, NY; 2019; Figure 23–44. Copyright © McGraw Hill.)

of immunology. In 2012, the survival rates for cadaver and living donor grafts were 89% and 95%, respectively. Rejection of a transplanted renal kidney is called graft rejection, or graft versus host disease. Clinicians may suspect renal transplant rejection or other problems in the presence of new hypertension, pain, anuria, rising BUN/creatinine, bruit, or abnormal kidney biopsy.

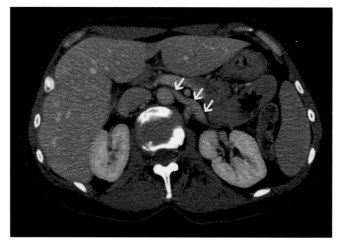

FIGURE 6–37. CT of left renal vein impingement. *Arrows* point to prominent left renal vein in patient with "nutcracker" syndrome.

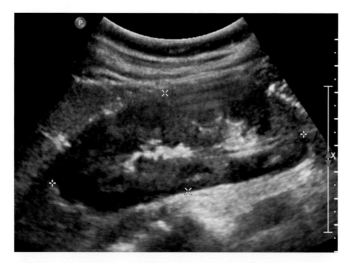

FIGURE 6–38. Kidney length and anterior–posterior (AP) measurement.

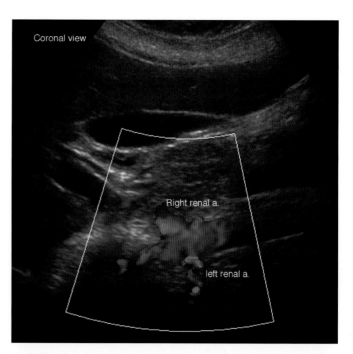

FIGURE 6–39. Coronal view of the right and left renal artery originating from the abdominal aorta. The coronal plane permits a 0-degree angle of insonation, which provides the strongest Doppler shift and therefore the best color Doppler image.

Renal artery and vein evaluation is an essential component of renal transplant follow-up. As part of the renal transplant study, the sonographer has to evaluate the new kidney for size, echogenicity, fluid collections, fistulas, and evaluate velocities and waveforms. The most common location for a transplanted kidney, called an allograft, is in the patient's right pelvis. Stenosis of the renal artery is the most common complication of renal transplants, but problems may also occur with the renal veins. Other pathologies of renal transplants include pseudoaneurysms and arteriovenous fistulas (AVFs). The patient's native kidneys are often left in situ unless infection or neoplasm is a concern.

Scanning Protocol, Patient Assessment, and Integration of Data

Renal Artery Doppler

Renal artery evaluation tends to be more technically challenging than other abdominal vascular studies due to patient body habitus issues and overlying bowel gas. A low-frequency (2-4 MHz) curvilinear transducer should be used. All renal artery evaluations should begin with evaluation of the kidneys, including a measurement of the longest axis of the kidney (Fig. 6–38). The normal adult kidney measures 9-13 cm in long axis. The renal cortex is normally isoechoic or hypoechoic to the liver, and surrounds a more echogenic hilum. A difference of more than 2 cm in length, or echogenicity greater than that of the liver, is indicative of renal disease. The optimal window for scanning renal arteries will vary from patient to patient, and an 8-12-hour fast is recommended to minimize bowel gas. The main renal arteries may be visualized either through the AP plane at the midline, or via a coronal plane by scanning parallel to the table (Fig. 6–39).

Although the exact protocol may vary from laboratory to laboratory, renal artery Doppler evaluation commonly includes the aorta, main renal arteries, segmental arteries, and, in some laboratories, parenchymal arteries as well. Angle-corrected spectral Doppler should be performed of the aorta in the region

of the renal artery origin, or ostium. Next, angle-corrected spectral Doppler waveforms of the renal artery origin should be taken bilaterally. Accessory arteries, if present, should be documented and sampled, as well (Fig. 6–40). When sampling the main renal arteries, color Doppler should be used to ensure more accurate angle correction and to look for aliasing that might signal markedly elevated velocities. Renal arterial waveforms have a compliance or early systolic peak (ESP) that may not correspond to peak systole. In making a determination between a normal arterial upstroke and a delayed upstroke, the systolic slope may be measured. This slope measurement, in which the calipers are placed along the systolic slope, is called

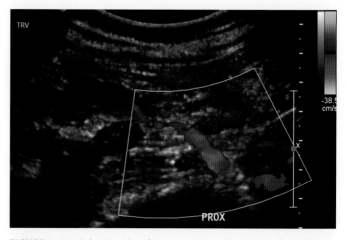

FIGURE 6–40. Color Doppler of an accessory renal artery. Accessory renal arteries should be identified and evaluated with spectral Doppler as part of a RAS study.

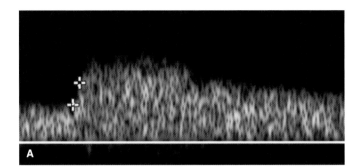

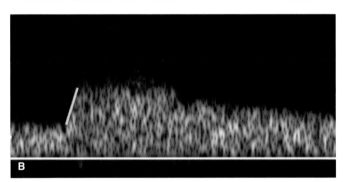

FIGURE 6-41. **(A)** Caliper placement along systolic slope to measure early systolic acceleration (ESA), also called acceleration index (AI). It is only necessary to place the calipers on the slope, not at the early systolic peak (ESP). **(B)** The *yellow line* depicts what is being measured with acceleration index—the slope of the upstroke.

early systolic acceleration (ESA) or acceleration index (AI), demonstrated in Figure 6-41.

In the main renal arteries, the waveform should be measured to obtain peak systolic and end-diastolic velocities (EDVs) (Fig. 6-42) at the origin, proximal, mid, and distal portions of the vessels. Most ultrasound machines have renal vascular calculation packages permitting measurement of AI and acceleration time (AT). AI is the time from the beginning of systolic flow to the ESP, in milliseconds. The ESP may be difficult to consistently identify, and therefore, the AT may be associated with measurement error and increased operator-to-operator variability. The normal AT is less than 0.1 second (or 100 ms). The AI, as already described, is the slope of acceleration, in cm/s^2. The AI should be greater than 300 cm/s^2. Delay in the acceleration slope is known as tardus parvus, and presents as rounding of systolic peak, versus the sharp upstroke seen in normal arteries (Fig. 6-43). Tardus parvus indicates obstruction proximal to the point of sampling.

The highest main renal artery PSV should be compared to the aortic PSV, and a renal artery-to-aorta ratio (RAR) obtained.

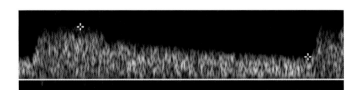

FIGURE 6-42. Measurement of peak systolic velocity (PSV) and end-diastolic velocity (EDV).

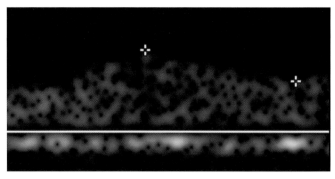

FIGURE 6-43. Tardus parvus waveform in a renal artery. Note the delayed upstroke and rounding of systole.

The RAR should be less than 3.5, and if the RAR is 3.5 or more, there is at least a 60% stenosis. Flow velocity elevation is the strongest predictor for hemodynamically significant RAS. Any areas of aliasing or color bruit should be thoroughly investigated (Fig. 6-44). Angle correction 60 degrees or less must be used any time velocities or AI are measured. In addition, any areas of spectral broadening or downstream turbulence should be documented and further evaluated. After the main renal arteries have been evaluated, the AI and/or AT is obtained in the segmental arteries at the upper, mid, and lower poles of the kidney. When sampling the parenchymal arteries (interlobar/arcuate), angle correction is not used because the vessels are too small to be visualized. The lack of angle correction means that AI and PSV cannot be obtained, but by placing the calipers at the PSV and EDV, or by tracing the waveform, the RI will be calculated. To measure the waveform components more accurately, a fast sweep speed should be used, as demonstrated in Figure 6-45. Waveform analysis is an important part of renal artery evaluation. In the presence of medical renal disease, the

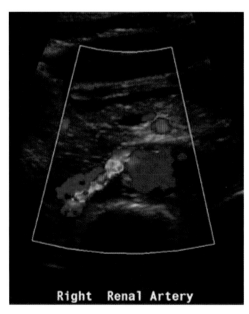

FIGURE 6-44. Color aliasing at point of stenosis in right renal artery.

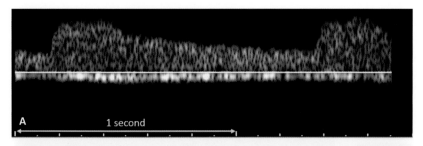

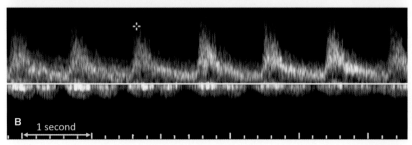

FIGURE 6–45. **(A)** Fast sweep speed used for measuring acceleration index (AI). This allows for more precise measurements of different components of the cardiac cycle. **(B)** Slower sweep speed allows for more waveforms on the screen at one time. Not optimal for measuring AI but fine for measuring peak systolic velocities (PSV).

kidney becomes more resistant, resulting in a high-resistance arterial waveform. Similarly, a proximal significant stenosis will result in downstream tardus parvus.

If the patient has a renal artery stent (Fig. 6–46), angle-corrected PSV measurements should be obtained proximal to the stent, mid-stent, and distal to the stent. Color Doppler will help visualize areas of flow abnormalities or elevated velocities. The scale/PRF may need to be adjusted for either a high-flow state, as in a stenosis, or low-flow, as in near or suspected occlusion. Be aware that velocity changes will occur as flow travels between the stent and the native vessel, each of which have different diameters. The position of the stent should also be documented with grayscale for proper placement. Normal and abnormal velocity values of the renal artery are listed in Table 6–2. There are several other published criteria used to evaluate in-stent restenosis post intervention. One of the most common suggest that a PSV 240 cm/s or more and an RAR 3.2 or more indicates a significant restenosis within the stent.

Renal Venous Disease

The two most common pathologies of the renal vein are thrombosis and tumor extension. Thrombus to the renal veins may result from IVC thrombus extension or tumor thrombus from a renal cancer, so careful evaluation using spectral and color Doppler with high-sensitivity settings is essential to evaluate for concomitant disease. Note the location and size of the left renal vein, as extrinsic compression from the SMA or an aberrant route posterior to the aorta may result in compromised flow.

Renal Transplants

Evaluation of the renal transplant should begin with a thorough grayscale evaluation of the allograft to look for seromas, hematomas, masses, and evaluate size and echogenicity. The urinary bladder should be evaluated with urine present, although not extremely full, and the presence and location of any urinary stents documented. It is best to use a 3 to 5-MHz curvilinear transducer, adjusting the frequency as necessary based on body habitus and other factors, although a linear transducer may be used for additional detail. The term "allograft" is used for the transplanted kidney when the donor is genetically nonidentical to the recipient. The transplanted kidney is typically first imaged 48 hours after transplant, and this study is used as a baseline for subsequent studies. Kidney size should be documented in three orthogonal planes. The transplanted kidney

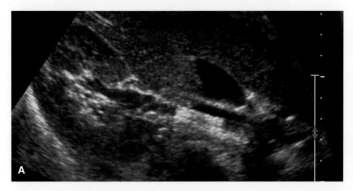

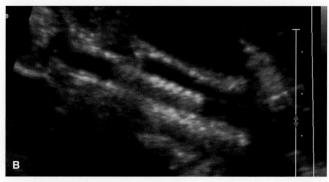

FIGURE 6–46. **(A)** Right kidney with stent visible in right renal artery. **(B)** Magnified view of renal artery stent.

TABLE 6–2 • Normal versus Abnormal Renal Artery Criteria (PST = Post-Stenotic Turbulence)		
Criteria	**Normal**	**Abnormal**
Renal Length	≥ 9 cm in adult	< 9 cm in adult or > 2 cm size discrepancy left to right
Renal Artery: Aorta Ratio (RAR)	< 3.5	≥ 3.5 (> 60% stenosis)
Peak Systolic Velocity	< 180-200 cm/s	≥ 180-200 cm/s with PST
End-Diastolic Velocity	—	> 150 cm/s (> 80% stenosis)
Early Systolic Acceleration	> 300 cm/s^2	≤ 300 cm/s^2
Acceleration Time	< 0.1 s	≥ 0.1 s

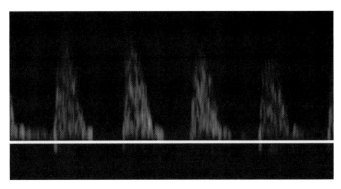

FIGURE 6–48. Six-year-old renal transplant rejection arterial waveform. Note the absence of diastolic flow.

may increase in size (up to 30%) from its initial implantation as it takes over the duty of two kidneys, known as compensatory hypertrophy. The renal arteries and veins of the transplanted kidney should be examined with color and spectral Doppler from their proximal anastomoses to the kidney, measuring PSV, AI, and resistive index RI. The use of color and power Doppler on the renal parenchyma may help visualize areas of perfusion abnormalities or other pathology. Rejection may manifest as increase in echogenicity, increase in volume, and overly prominent renal pyramids (Fig. 6–47). Other signs of rejection include changes in arterial Doppler waveforms, from the normally low-resistance arterial waveform to a high-resistance waveform that may include absent or reversal of the diastolic component (Fig. 6–48). The normal RI should be less than 0.7, but an RI of greater than or equal to 0.9 is more specific for rejection.

Stenosis of the renal artery is the most common complication of renal transplants, and other arterial complications include arterial occlusion, pseudoaneurysm, and AVF. Renal allograft arterial PSVs greater than 200 cm/s are indicative of stenosis. RIs and/or acceleration indices are usually obtained from parenchymal flow in upper, mid, and lower poles. The parenchymal RI can be predictive of successful revascularization, with patients with elevated RIs (> 0.8) having more likelihood of irreversible parenchymal damage and less chance of success.

Thrombosis of the renal vein may occur posttransplant, but is most common immediately after the transplant as opposed to being a long-term problem. Renal vein thrombus can be visualized with grayscale and color Doppler, and manifests as an enlarged kidney due to obstructed outflow. If there is occlusive renal vein thrombus, reduced outflow can lead to a high-resistance arterial waveform with reversal of diastolic flow (Fig. 6–49).

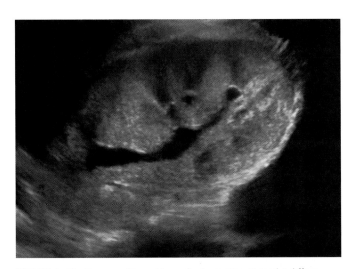

FIGURE 6–47. Six-year-old renal transplant rejection. Note the diffuse, echogenic parenchyma, and prominent renal pyramids.

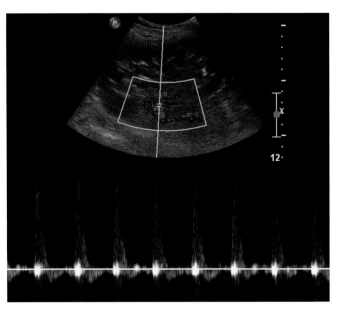

FIGURE 6–49. Reversal of flow in the renal artery due to thrombosed renal vein.

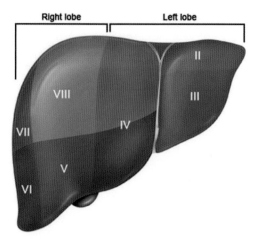
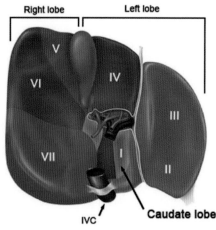

FIGURE 6–50. Couinaud's division of the liver. (Reproduced, with permission, from Brunicardi F, Andersen DK, Billiar TR, et al. *Schwartz's Principles of Surgery,* 11th ed. New York, NY; 2019; Figure 31–3. Copyright © McGraw Hill.)

THE LIVER AND PORTAL VENOUS SYSTEM

Anatomy

The liver is a large organ in the right upper quadrant (RUQ) responsible for many functions, including production of bile and detoxification of blood coming from the GI tract. The length of the liver is typically less than 15 cm. In its most basic anatomic division, the liver is made up of a right lobe and a left lobe, separated by an imaginary line between the gallbladder fossa and the IVC. Surgeons prefer Couinaud's division of the liver, which allows for resection with relation to the vascular anatomy. The liver is made up of eight segments (Fig. 6–50), with the left lobe made up of segments II, III, (the left lateral segments), and segment IV (the left medial segment). The right lobe is made up of segments V and VIII (right anterior lobe) and segments VI and VII (right posterior lobe). Segment I, the caudate lobe, is special because it receives blood from the LHA and RHA and portal veins, and drains directly into the IVC. Because of its unique blood supply, the caudate lobe is often spared in the presence of severe liver disease.

The liver receives its blood from two sources: the systemic arterial system, via the proper, or MHA, and the portal systemic circulation, via the main portal vein (MPV). Approximately 25% to 30% of the blood to the liver is from the MHA, with the remaining 70% to 75% of blood to the liver coming from the portal venous circulation. Note, however, that the oxygenated blood to the liver comes from the MHA, as the portal venous blood is mostly deoxygenated. Blood travels from the MPV to the left portal vein (LPV) and the right portal vein (RPV) branches into the liver sinusoids. After processing by the liver, blood drains into the central veins, and from there into the hepatic veins (Fig. 6–51). The left, right, and middle hepatic veins, which are part of the systemic circulation, join the IVC at the confluence in the dome of the liver, and from there the IVC drains into the right atrium of the heart (Fig. 6–52). On ultrasound, the intrahepatic portal vein tributaries have an echogenic border, which is attributed to collagen in the walls. The thin-walled hepatic veins do not have these bright walls, and are readily differentiated from the portal veins, at least in a normal appearing liver (Fig. 6–53).

The IVC is the large systemic vein that receives blood from the trunk and legs. Like all systemic veins, the IVC is thin-walled and easily compressible. The IVC is formed by the union of the left and right common iliac veins. The right gonadal veins (ovarian or testicular veins) drain into the IVC mid-abdomen. The left gonadal veins drain into the left renal vein, an important distinction. The left, middle, and right hepatic veins, which drain the liver, join the IVC at the hepatic vein confluence just inferior to the diaphragm. On ultrasound, when only the left and middle hepatic veins are visualized in the axial plane, this view was commonly called the "Playboy bunny" or "bunny" sign. However, this author prefers the term "hepatic moose" because more than two hepatic veins are routinely visualized, making them look more like antlers than ears (Fig. 6–54). There are no mesenteric veins draining into the IVC, as these vessels are part of the portal venous system. Blood flow through the IVC and hepatic veins is pulsatile due to the vessels' proximity to the right heart. The more peripheral the vein, the more this transmitted pulsatility is lost. Respiration will also affect the IVC and hepatic vein flow, with deep inspiration causing cessation of forward flow from the abdomen. For this reason, when performing spectral Doppler of the IVC and hepatic veins, shallow breathing should be used instead of sustaining a deep inspiration.

The portal venous system is a separate network of vessels designed to protect the body from ingested toxins. These toxins travel from the bowel to the liver for detoxification before being sent via the hepatic veins into the systemic circulation. In the normal adult human body, there are no natural connections between the portal venous circulation and the systemic circulation (Fig. 6–55).

The splenic vein emerges from the spleen and travels transversely across the abdomen, posterior to the pancreas from the tail of the pancreas to the pancreatic head (Fig. 6–56).

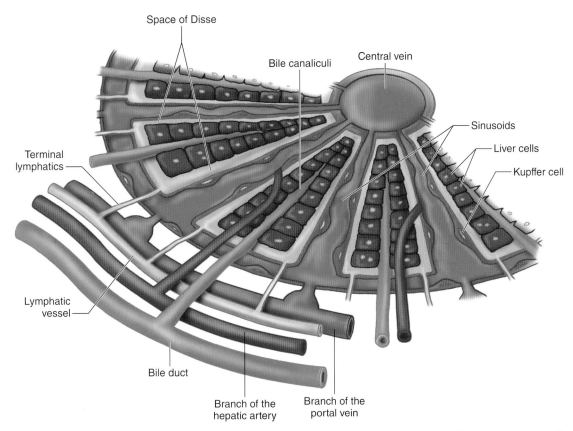

FIGURE 6–51. Detail of the liver lobule demonstrating portal triad of hepatic artery, portal vein, and bile duct. (Reproduced, with permission, from Butterworth JF IV, Mackey DC, Wasnick JD. *Morgan & Mikhail's Clinical Anesthesiology*, 5th ed. New York, NY; 2013. Figure 32–1. Copyright © McGraw Hill.)

Around mid-pancreas, the inferior mesenteric vein (IMV), which drains the large intestine, joins the splenic vein. At the head of the pancreas, the superior mesenteric vein (SMV) joins the splenic vein to form the portal splenic confluence (Fig. 6–57). The SMV predominantly drains the small intestines. The portal splenic confluence gives rise to the MPV, which enters the liver at the porta hepatis (Fig. 6–58). Inside the liver, the MPV bifurcates into LPV (Fig. 6–59) and RPV (Fig. 6–60). The LPV, which supplies the left lobe of the liver,

bifurcates into medial and lateral branches. The RPV, which supplies the right lobe of the liver, bifurcates into anterior and posterior branches. The left gastric vein, also called the coronary vein, drains the veins of the stomach into the MPV, and

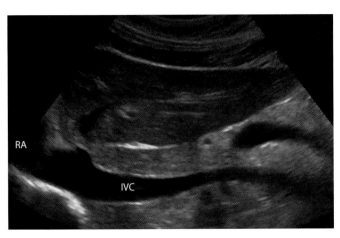

FIGURE 6–52. Sagittal grayscale image of inferior vena cava (IVC) terminating at the right atrium of the heart.

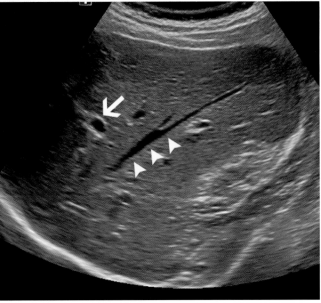

FIGURE 6–53. Grayscale differentiation of portal veins from hepatic veins. The portal veins (*thick arrow*) have thick echogenic walls while the hepatic veins (*thin arrow*) have very thin walls.

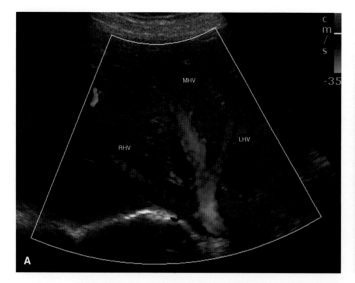 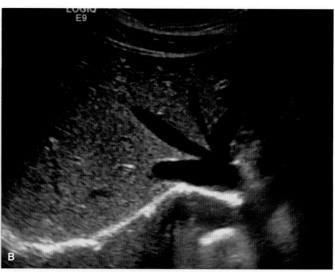

FIGURE 6–54. Transverse color Doppler and grayscale images of the hepatic vein confluence demonstrating left, middle, and right hepatic veins. **(A)** Transverse color Doppler of hepatic vein confluence with IVC. **(B)** Transverse grayscale images of the hepatic vein confluence with IVC. It's a moose, right?

has anastomoses with the esophageal veins. Figure 6–61 is an illustration of the portal venous circulation.

Blood flow through the portal veins is normally continuous with mild respiratory phasicity. Portal venous flow may be mildly pulsatile and should be hepatopetal (toward the liver).

Pathology

Portal Hypertension
The primary function of the liver is to filter the blood coming from the digestive tract. Therefore, toxins that are ingested, such as alcohol and other substances, may cause damage to

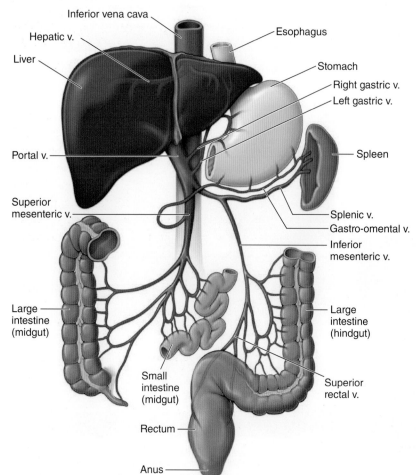

FIGURE 6–55. Illustration of liver with hepatic veins and portal veins. (Reproduced, with permission, from Morton DA, Foreman KB, Albertine KH. *The Big Picture: Gross Anatomy*, 2nd ed. New York, NY; 2011; Figure 10–4A. Copyright © McGraw Hill.)

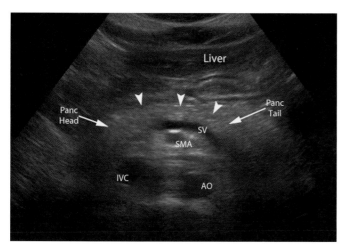

FIGURE 6–56. Transverse pancreas. The pancreas is anterior to the splenic vein. *Arrowheads* represent anterior border of body of pancreas. Only part of the pancreatic tail is visualized.

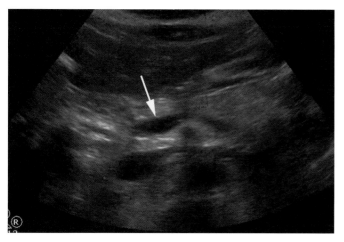

FIGURE 6–57. Transverse portal splenic confluence (*arrow*), formed by the superior mesenteric vein (SMV) and splenic vein.

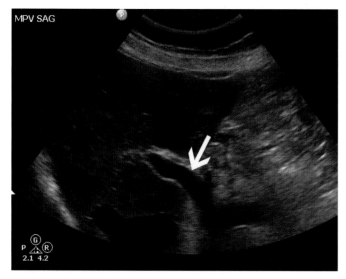

FIGURE 6–58. Oblique long-axis view of main portal vein (*arrow*) at porta hepatis.

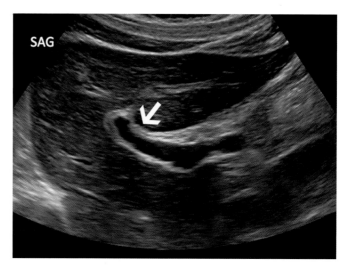

FIGURE 6–59. Sagittal and transverse views of the left portal vein (*arrows*).

the liver tissue. The liver has an amazing ability to regenerate, but damages itself in the process, causing lobulation of the liver tissue (Fig. 6–62). The liver surface should be evaluated with a 5-7 MHz frequency linear transducer to evaluate for lobulation. Normal livers are smooth while diseased livers appear "lumpy" or irregular (Fig. 6–63). End-stage liver disease is called cirrhosis, which is not specific to chronic alcohol (ETOH) abuse. Other causes of cirrhosis may be chronic hepatitis, especially hepatitis C (HCV), nonalcoholic fatty liver disease, excessive acetaminophen use, parasitic diseases such as schistosomiasis, and biliary disease. Excessive alcohol intake and HCV are the two most common causes of cirrhosis in the United States, although there is now an effective medical treatment for treatment for HCV

When disease affects the liver so that there is an increase in the pressure gradient precluding forward flow, a backup of flow termed portal hypertension (PHTN) occurs. PHTN is defined as a pressure gradient between the IVC and portal veins (hepatic venous pressure gradient, or HPVG) greater than 6 mm Hg, and may be classified as presinusoidal, sinusoidal, or postsinusoidal (Table 6–3). Clinically significant PHTN is present with a portal pressure gradient 10 mm Hg or more.

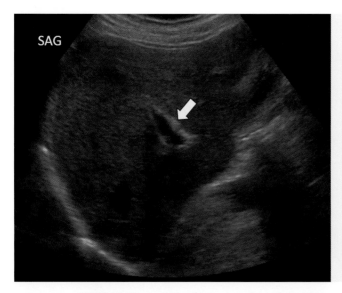
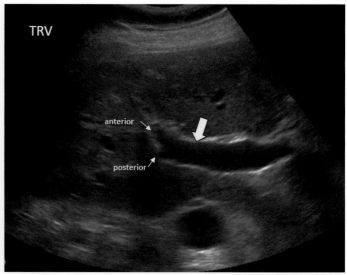

FIGURE 6–60. Sagittal and transverse views of the right portal vein (*large arrow*). The anterior and posterior branches are also identified (*small arrows*).

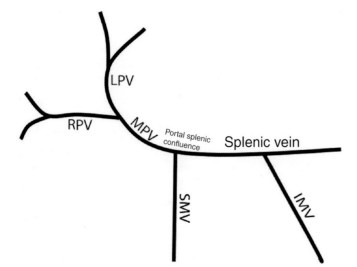

FIGURE 6–61. Illustration of the portal venous system.

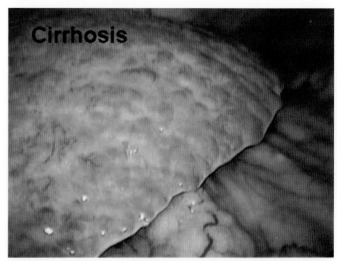

FIGURE 6–62. Surgical specimen of lobulated liver tissue. (Reproduced, with permission, from Brunicardi F, Andersen DK, Billiar TR, et al. *Schwartz's Principles of Surgery,* 11th ed. New York, NY; 2019; Figure 31–13. Copyright © McGraw Hill.)

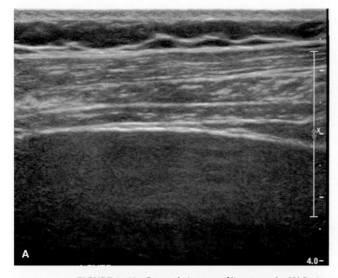
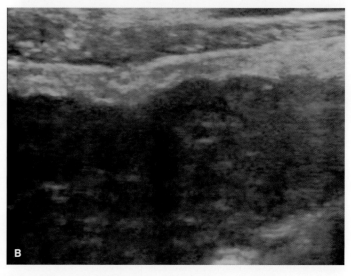

FIGURE 6–63. Grayscale images of liver capsule. **(A)** Patient with normal liver capsule. **(B)** Patient with cirrhosis demonstrating lobulated liver capsule. (Reproduced, with permission, from Doreen Kuestner, MS, RDMS, RVT.)

TABLE 6–3 • Types of Portal Hypertension

Type of Portal Hypertension	Definition
Presinusoidal	Problem with portal vein (intrinsic or extrinsic)
Sinusoidal	Problem with liver (e.g., cirrhosis)
Postsinusoidal	Problem with outflow (e.g., Budd–Chiari, thrombus in hepatic veins or IVC, right-sided heart failure)

With PHTN, as the pressure gradient increases, anastomotic channels open up that permit the flow of blood into the systemic circulation through alternate routes. Some of these pathways include recanalization of the umbilical vein (aka paraumbilical vein), splenorenal shunts, esophageal varices, and hemorrhoids via the rectal veins (Fig. 6–64). Ascites may form from PHTN or from decreased albumin levels common in severe liver disease (Fig. 6–65). Patients with ascites may need to have a procedure called a paracentesis to remove excessive fluid buildup,

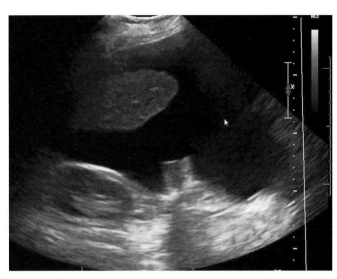

FIGURE 6–65. Ascites in the abdomen. Patient with portal hypertension and large amount of abdominal ascites.

and they will need to monitor their diet and avoid salt and certain foods.

PHTN causes many intra-abdominal changes. Splenomegaly, defined as enlargement greater than 13 cm in length (Fig. 6–66), is seen in PHTN due to reduced forward flow. In cirrhosis, the right lobe of the liver decreases in size while the caudate and left lateral lobes increase in size (Figs. 6–67 and 6–68). Abnormal flow in the portal veins may also be a result of tumor thrombus, common in hepatocellular carcinoma (HCC) (Fig. 6–69). As hepatopetal flow decreases in the portal vein, the MHA enlarges to compensate for decreased blood flow to the liver. Portal vein thrombosis may cause collateral formation around the MPV. This so-called cavernous transformation of the portal vein occurs with long-standing MPV thrombus. In cases of severe PHTN in which the MPV is thrombosed, the MHA may enlarge significantly and be mistaken for a pulsatile MPV.

A remnant of the fetal umbilical vein is found within the falciform ligament of the liver. When the pressure is increased in

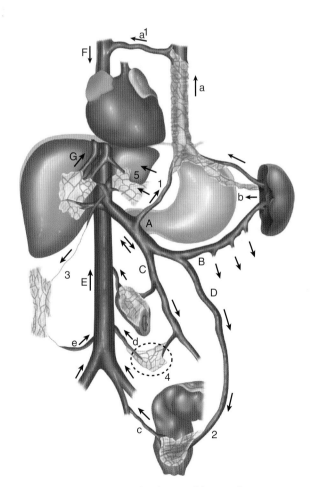

FIGURE 6–64. Potential collateral pathways of the portal venous system. (Reproduced, with permission, from Brunicardi F, Andersen DK, Billiar TR, et al. *Schwartz's Principles of Surgery,* 11th ed. New York, NY; 2019; Figure 31–14. Copyright © McGraw Hill.)

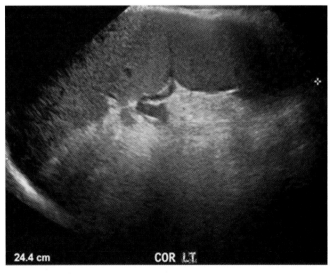

FIGURE 6–66. Sagittal spleen with splenomegaly (24.4 cm).

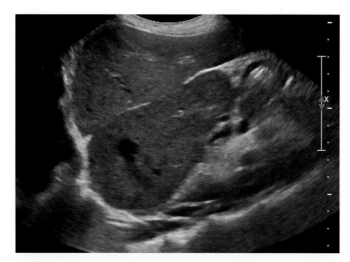

FIGURE 6–67. Sagittal caudate lobe showing enlargement.

the liver and blood can no longer easily go through the organ, the blood looks for the route with the lowest resistance (Fig. 6–70). The umbilical vein recanalizes (dilates and becomes patent), and becomes the low-resistance pathway (Figs. 6–71 and 6–72). This recanalized vein follows the falciform ligament to the anterior abdominal wall and travels inferiorly to the level of the umbilicus (Fig. 6–73). In severe cases of PHTN, the vessels form a network of what looks like red snakes on the surface of the patient's abdomen called caput medusae (Figs. 6–74 to 6–76).

The left kidney and spleen should also be evaluated to look for a splenorenal shunt. This appears as large venous varices in the splenic hilum as the splenic vein connects to the left renal vein via normally closed anastomoses (Fig. 6–77). Another vessel to examine is the left gastric vein, also called the coronary vein. Retrograde (hepatofugal) flow in the left gastric vein leads

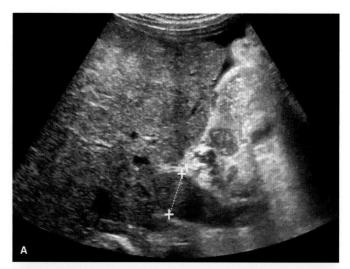

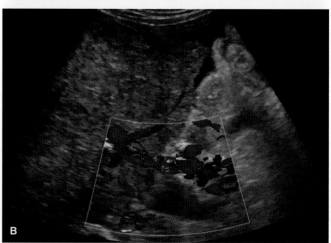

FIGURE 6–69. Portal vein with tumor thrombus. **(A)** Sagittal grayscale image of thrombosed main portal vein. **(B)** Sagittal color Doppler image of thrombosed portal vein. Note absence of flow in location of thrombus.

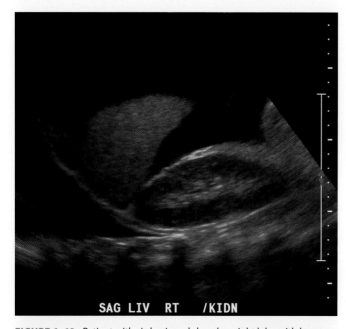

FIGURE 6–68. Patient with cirrhosis and shrunken right lobe with large amount of ascites.

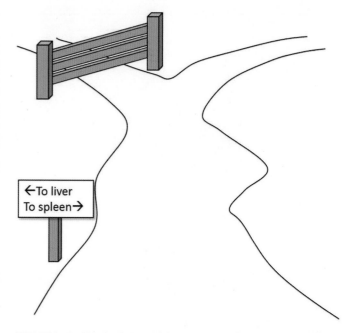

FIGURE 6–70. Blood will always follow the path of least resistance. Which way would you go?

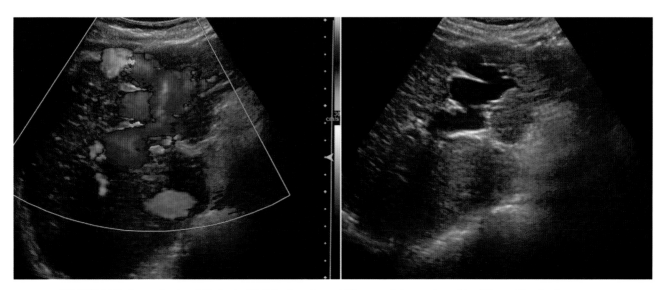

FIGURE 6–71. Recanalized umbilical vein. **(A)** Color Doppler and **(B)** grayscale image shows blood flow exiting the liver anteriorly toward the abdominal wall in a patient with severe portal hypertension. (Reproduced, with permission, from Doreen Kuestner, MS, RDMS, RVT.)

to esophageal varices, the rupture of which may lead to death (Fig. 6–78).

With chronic PHTN, in order to relieve the pressure on the portal venous system, a pathway needs to be created to bypass the liver and return portal venous flow into the systemic venous system. Normally, the portal system is completely separate from the systemic circulation, and the blood must be filtered by the liver before it is returned to the heart and distributed to the rest of the body and, most importantly, the brain. With the liver under increased pressure in end-stage disease, blood backs up, causing collaterals to open. In patients waiting for a liver transplant or patients that are not candidates for liver transplant, a transjugular intrahepatic portosystemic shunt (TIPS) can be created to bypass the liver by sending flow directly from the portal vein to the hepatic vein. Today's TIPS are a metallic stent

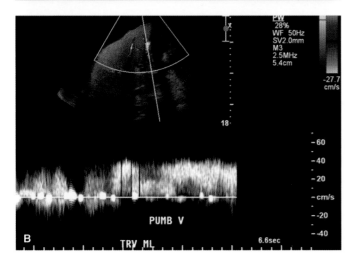

FIGURE 6–72. Color and spectral Doppler of a patient with portal hypertension and recanalization of the umbilical vein. Note the flow from the liver and toward the anterior abdominal wall.

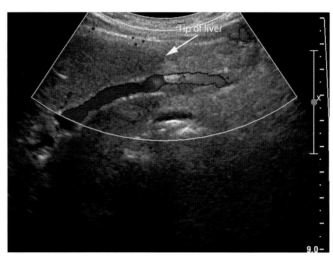

FIGURE 6–73. Recanalized umbilical vein (aka paraumbilical vein) leaving the liver and traveling along the anterior abdominal wall toward the umbilicus as a result of severe PHTN.

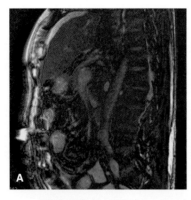
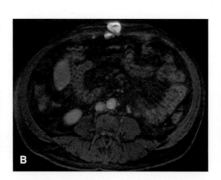
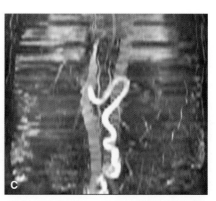

FIGURE 6–74. MRI of caput medusa. **(A)** Sagittal and **(B)** transverse views—the white structure is the dilated vein at the umbilicus. **(C)** Coronal reconstruction showing path along anterior abdominal wall.

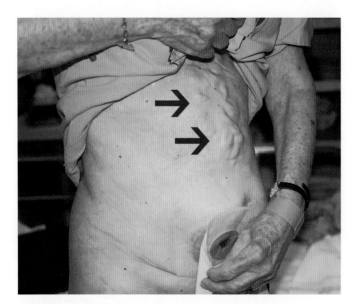

FIGURE 6–75. Ultrasound of caput medusa. Image taken at level of umbilicus showing dilated vessels as a result of portal hypertension.

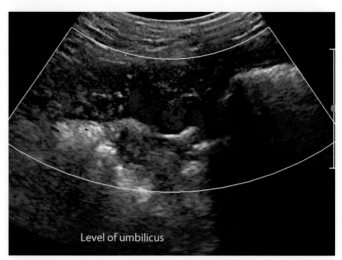

FIGURE 6–76. Caput medusa. Patient with portal hypertension and recanalization of the umbilical vein. The dilated superficial veins are visible on the surface of the patient's abdomen. (Reproduced, with permission, from Knoop KJ, Stack LB, Storrow AB, Thurman RJ. *The Atlas of Emergency Medicine*, 4th ed. New York, NY; 2016; Figure 7–43. Copyright © McGraw Hill. Photo contributor: Gary Schwartz, MD.)

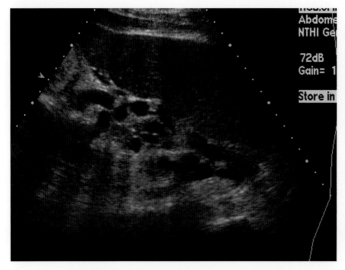
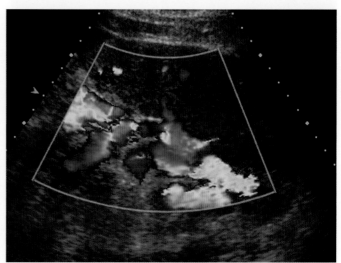

FIGURE 6–77. Images of spleen in portal hypertension. The tubular structures in the splenic hilum are splenorenal varices formed as a result of increased pressure in the liver.

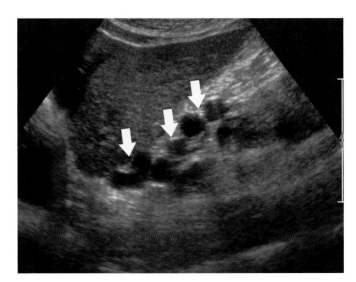

FIGURE 6–78. *Arrows* point to dilated coronary (aka left gastric) venous tributaries with esophageal varices. Image is of sagittal left lobe of liver.

covered in polytetrafluoroethylene (PTFE). Covered stents have a lower failure rate than bare metal stents. The interventional team or vascular surgeon inserts the shunt via the internal jugular vein (IJV) into the liver, connecting, in many cases, the RPV to the right hepatic vein (Figs. 6–79 and 6–80).

Hepatic Veins and IVC

Ultrasound is routinely used to evaluate the IVC and hepatic veins. Ultrasound may also be used to aid in guidance of IVC filter placement. Thrombus may occur in the IVC as a result of blood clot, usually originating from the lower extremities, or from tumor thrombus (Fig. 6–81). When deep venous thrombosis (DVT) is found and the patient is at risk for pulmonary embolism and/or cannot receive anticoagulation, an IVC filter may be placed (Figs. 6–82 and 6–83). IVC filters are inserted typically through the groin, although if the common iliac veins are clotted, they can be inserted through the IJV.

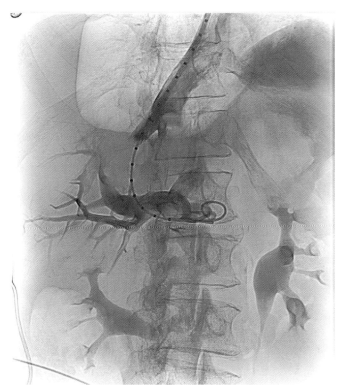

FIGURE 6–79. Angiogram of creation of transjugular intrahepatic portal systemic shunt (TIPS). There is a connection between the inferior vena cava (IVC) and the portal venous system to bypass the liver.

Occlusive hepatic vein thrombus can lead to a condition termed Budd–Chiari syndrome. The hepatic veins are responsible for draining blood from the liver, so obstruction of the outflow of the liver causes congestion of the liver and decreased inflow from the portal veins, leading to post-sinusoidal PHTN (Fig. 6–84). In studies performed for PHTN, it is important to evaluate the IVC and hepatic veins for thrombus as a cause for the PHTN. Budd–Chiari syndrome presents with the same clinical presentation as PHTN from other causes, such as abdominal

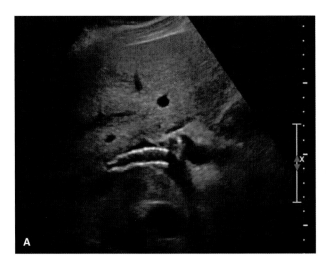

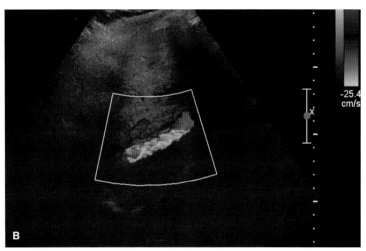

FIGURE 6–80. Ultrasound of transjugular intrahepatic portosystemic shunt (TIPS) connecting portal venous system to hepatic veins. **(A)** Grayscale of TIPS in right portal vein and **(B)** Color Doppler image of TIPS.

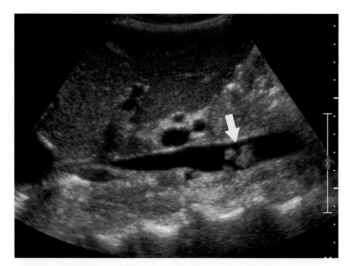

FIGURE 6–81. Sagittal image of inferior vena cava (IVC) thrombus. *Arrow* points to clot within the IVC.

fullness or pain, ascites, abnormal liver function tests (LFTs), splenomegaly, and collateral formation.

Liver Transplants

Liver transplantation has been available since the late 1960s, and ranks second in number of transplant procedures performed, after the kidney. End-stage liver disease can be caused by hepatitis C, alcoholism, biliary disease, and other disease processes. Contraindications to liver transplant include, but are not limited to, malignancy outside the liver, substance abuse, and heart or lung problems. Although partial liver transplants may come from a living donor, most come from cadavers. With a deceased donor, all or part of the liver is transplanted and placed into the RUQ after removal of the patient's diseased liver. This type of liver transplant is called an orthotopic liver transplant (OLT). Anastomoses are usually made at the IVC, extrahepatic biliary duct, MPV, and hepatic or CA. Rejection is the number one concern following transplant, followed by vascular complications. Posttransplant complications may include portal vein thrombus

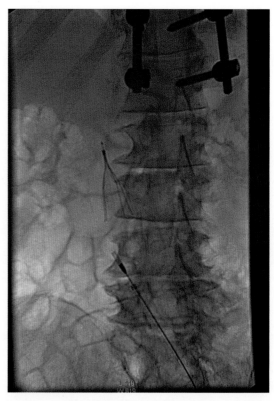

FIGURE 6–82. Angiogram of inferior vena cava (IVC) filter in place. The filter is placed at the level of the renal veins to permit blood flow to wash over any material collected in filter.

or stenosis, thrombus or stenosis of the MHA, pseudoaneurysm of the MHA, bile duct obstruction or leak, infection, and many other problems (Fig. 6–85).

Scanning Protocol, Patient Assessment, and Integration of Data

Portal Hypertension

Examination of the portal venous system normally begins with a complete grayscale evaluation of the right and left upper quadrants on a fasting patient. A curvilinear transducer in the 2 to 4-MHz range should be used, depending on patient body habitus.

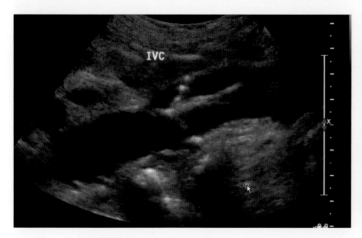

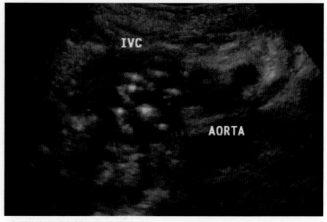

FIGURE 6–83. Sagittal and transverse grayscale images of inferior vena cava (IVC) filter in place. Note how the filter is fixed to the IVC walls to hold it in place.

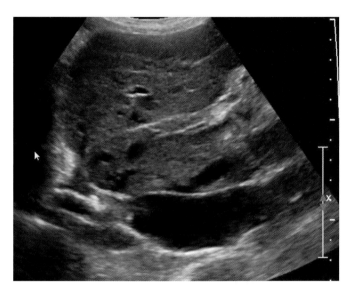

FIGURE 6–84. Enlargement of caudate lobe with dilated veins as a result of Budd–Chiari syndrome.

On patients with a fatty liver, a lower frequency may be needed even if the patient is relatively thin, due to difficulty in penetrating the liver. The liver should be evaluated for size, echogenicity, echotexture, and the presence of masses. Dedicated images of the liver surface should be undertaken with a linear transducer to evaluate for lobulation. The gallbladder, bile duct, pancreas, and kidneys are typically evaluated for pathology, as well. The spleen should be measured in its long axis, and any ascites documented.

Spectral and color Doppler should be performed in the splenic vein at the spleen, splenic vein at the pancreas, MPV, LPV, and RPV. Angle correction is not needed because velocities are not being measured, but it is critical to confirm direction of flow. Flow should be toward the liver (hepatopetal) in all of the portal system veins. In the normal portal vein, the waveform may have slight variation due to respiration or even mild pulsatility. Flow may be hepatopetal in one part of the splenic vein, but, due to collaterals may be reversed (hepatofugal) in another part of the splenic vein, so it is important to document

the splenic vein at multiple points as previously described. Memory trick: Having trouble remembering hepatopetal versus hepatofugal? Think of it like a bike: a bike moves forward when pedaled. Therefore, "hepatopetal" is toward the liver, and hepatofugal is away. If any hepatofugal flow is identified, the SMV should be documented with color and spectral Doppler to evaluate direction of flow.

If the patient has a TIPS shunt, a complete abdominal study with Doppler is performed, but the TIPS must be evaluated as well. TIPS function is determined by color Doppler and spectral Doppler velocity measurements. Unlike most venous flow studies, with a TIPS, the PSVs are measured, necessitating the use of angle correction with an angle 60 degrees or less. Angle-corrected PSV are measured in the portal vein feeding the TIPS, proximal, mid, and distal portions of the TIPS, and in the hepatic vein receiving the TIPS flow. In addition to PSV, color Doppler should be used to document the presence of thrombus and evaluate for direction of flow. TIPS stents are often evaluated shortly after placement. Similar to other grafts and covered stents placed in the body, it may not be possible to measure flow through the TIPS in the first 2-3 days after placement due to trapped air in the walls of the stent.

The pressure difference between the portal system and the systemic circulation causes flow to be pulled into the direction of the TIPS. Therefore, although the MPV should be hepatopetal, the LPV and branches of the RPVs should have hepatofugal flow as blood heads toward the path of least resistance, the TIPS (Fig. 6–86). The portal venous waveform may be more pulsatile after TIPS placement due to its direct connection with the central venous systemic circulation.

Comparison to pre-TIPS studies is helpful. Long-standing PHTN causes the MHA to dilate to increase the amount of blood going to the liver, and elevated velocities (> 130 cm/s) may be present (Fig. 6–87). Flow through the TIPS is typically 90-190 cm/s. The MPV peak velocity should be 40 cm/s or more. If the mid-TIPS velocity is less than 50 cm/s, the TIPS is stenosed. A peak velocity more than 200 cm/s within the TIPS

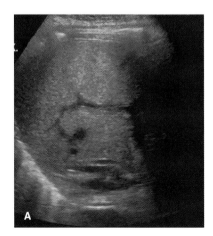 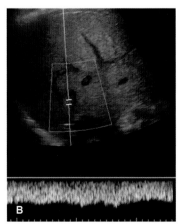 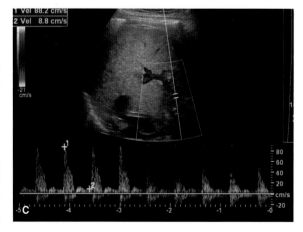

FIGURE 6–85. Rejection of liver transplant. **(A)** Liver is echogenic. **(B)** Abnormal continuous hepatic vein waveforms, suggesting edema. **(C)** The hepatic artery has an elevated resistive index (RI), suggestive of edema.

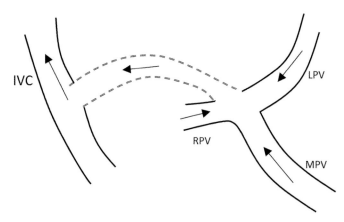

FIGURE 6–86. Illustration of blood flow in functioning transjugular intrahepatic portosystemic shunt (TIPS). Blood should be hepatopedal in main portal vein (MPV) and hepatofugal in left porteal vein (LPV) and right portal vein (RPV) as blood flows toward TIPS.

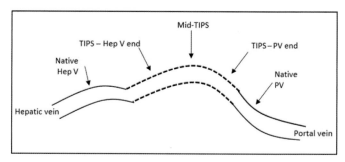

FIGURE 6–88. Transjugular intrahepatic portosystemic shunt (TIPS) evaluation and sample protocol. *Arrows* represent sampling points for TIPS. Angle-corrected velocities are obtained with angle 60 degrees or less. The recommended annotation is provided.

also indicates a TIPS stenosis, as does a velocity change of more than 50 cm/s from one location to another within the TIPS. The TIPS should not vary from one study to the next by more than 50 cm/s at each measured point. After the TIPS is placed, the patient should begin to see resolution of the PHTN symptoms. Return of those symptoms, such as ascites or esophageal varices, may indicate TIPS stenosis or occlusion. Figure 6–88 illustrates where to measure for TIPS evaluation and how to label the images. Table 6–4 presents the normal and abnormal values for TIPS. For annotation, it is best if the TIPS is labeled "portal end, mid-TIPS, hepatic end," or something similar, to avoid confusion related to where the PSV was obtained Avoid the use of the more confusing "proximal, mid, distal."

Hepatic Veins and IVC

Ultrasound of the hepatic veins and IVC uses the same scanning technique as portal venous Doppler in that a lower frequency (2-5 MHz)curvilinear probe will be used to obtain grayscale, color, and spectral Doppler images. The entire liver should be evaluated when evaluating the IVC and hepatic veins, unless the

IVC is being evaluated independently as part of a lower extremity venous ultrasound. Grayscale imaging is performed to evaluate for frank thrombus. Color Doppler permits visualization of the vessel lumen to look for markedly hypoechoic and anechoic thrombus, and spectral Doppler is used to evaluate the spectral waveforms. The spectral waveforms will vary based on the inflow and outflow of the vessels. The IVC and hepatic veins should be examined with shallow respiration. Deep inspiration and Valsalva maneuvers compress the IVC and cease forward flow, adversely affecting the waveform (Fig. 6–89). If the waveform is dampened or lacks pulsatility, there is obstruction more centrally (Fig. 6–90).

The left, right, and middle hepatic veins can be examined in the transverse plane at their confluence with the central IVC. Spectral waveforms should be obtained of each vessel to document waveform and direction of flow. Although the transverse subxiphoid plane is the best plane for the left and middle hepatic veins, in this view the right hepatic vein is angled close to 90 degrees, and therefore should be examined sagittally from the right intercostal window (Fig. 6–91).

The IVC should be evaluated in its entirety, from the confluence of the common iliac veins to its termination at the right atrium. The IVC should be evaluated for thrombus, waveform shape, and direction of flow. Thrombus usually appears as frank

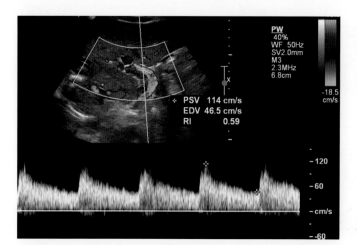

FIGURE 6–87. Dilated and low-resistance hepatic artery in presence of severe portal hypertension.

TABLE 6–4 • Abnormal TIPS Criteria
Abnormal TIPS Evaluation
Flow velocity < 50 cm/s in TIPS
Flow velocity > 200 cm/s in TIPS
Flow velocity < 30 cm/s in MPV
Presence of thrombus
Velocity difference >50 cm/s from one sampling point to another
Velocity difference >50 cm/s from prior study at same sampling point

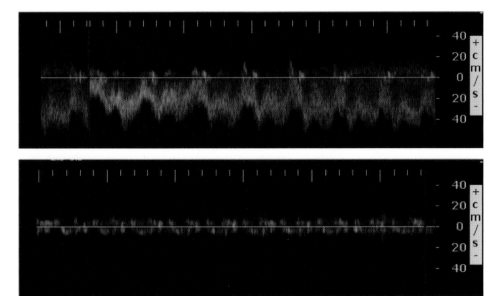

FIGURE 6–89. Inferior vena cava (IVC) waveforms with expiration **(top)** and inspiration **(bottom)**.

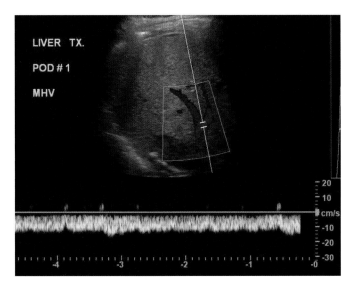

FIGURE 6–90. Dampened waveform consistent with elevated right-sided heart pressures, hepatic congestion, or central obstruction.

clot containing low-level echoes, although in some cases thrombus can be anechoic.

Liver Transplants

Preoperative evaluation of the recipient includes a complete evaluation of the abdomen with special attention to the liver. All of the portal and hepatic veins should be evaluated, as well as the biliary ducts and MHA. The liver and other abdominal organs should be evaluated for the presence of masses, which may preclude transplantation.

Posttransplant, grayscale imaging of the allograft should initially be performed in much the same way as a nontransplanted liver in that the entire liver should be evaluated and its size measured, utilizing a 2-4 MHz curvilinear transducer. Fluid collections should be sought out and documented in the subhepatic and subphrenic regions (Fig. 6–92). The extrahepatic bile duct should be measured, and any stents documented. All of the portal and hepatic vessels should be imaged with grayscale, color, and spectral Doppler. Color and spectral Doppler should

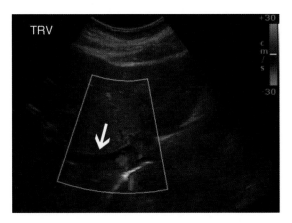
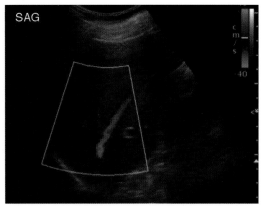

FIGURE 6–91 Doppler of right hepatic vein (RHV). In the transverse image on the left, the RHV is perpendicular to the beam, and no flow is demonstrated. The image on the right is a sagittal image taken through the intercostal window. A normal right hepatic vein is readily visualized.

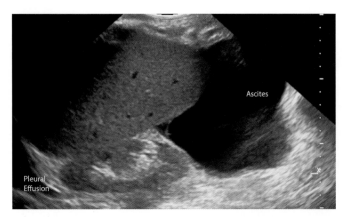

FIGURE 6–92. Liver transplant ultrasound with free fluid.

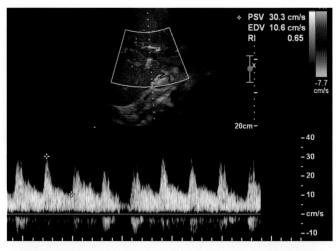

FIGURE 6–93. Spectral Doppler of normal transplanted hepatic artery.

be performed of the following blood vessels: MHA, LHA, and RHA; left, middle, and right hepatic veins; and the IVC, and LPV, RPV, and MPV. Arterial vessels should be evaluated for stenosis/occlusion, waveform morphology (tardus parvus, high resistance vs. low resistance, turbulence), velocities, and RI (Fig. 6–93). The MHA RI is typically 0.5-0.7, although there is debate in the literature regarding the prognostic value of RI in rejection of liver transplants. The portal veins should be evaluated for thrombus, direction of flow, and waveform abnormalities. The IVC and hepatic veins should similarly be evaluated for thrombus and waveform morphology. Color and spectral Doppler should be performed before, at, and distal to the anastomosis.

PELVIC VENOUS CONGESTION

Pelvic venous congestion is a cause of chronic pelvic pain that is often underdiagnosed. This disease most commonly occurs on the left side due to the aberrant insertion of the left ovarian vein into the left renal vein instead of the IVC directly. Symptoms include labial varicosities, lower extremity varicosities, pelvic pain or heaviness, and other lower extremity symptoms that

point to a more central cause of venous obstruction. Transabdominal (TA) and transvaginal ultrasound can be used to evaluate for dilated ovarian veins.

Patient preparation for TA exam begins with a full urinary bladder (from drinking water only) and an otherwise fasting patient. Transvaginal exam requires an empty urinary bladder, although a fasting patient may help reduce bowel gas. For a TA examination, the patient should be reverse Trendelenburg using a 2-5 MHz curvilinear transducer. Scan the external and internal iliac veins with B-mode, color/power, and spectral Doppler to look for dilated (> 4.0 mm) venous structures. The veins to be imaged include the IVC, left renal vein, both common/internal/external iliac veins, both ovarian/gonadal veins, and the transuterine and periuterine veins. If a dilated ovarian/gonadal vein is seen, try to elicit reflux by having the patient Valsalva during color Doppler. The veins should be measured anterior to posterior wall (Fig. 6–94). If a transvaginal ultrasound is to be performed, the patient should empty the bladder first.

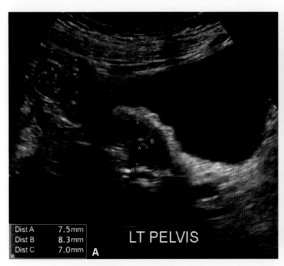

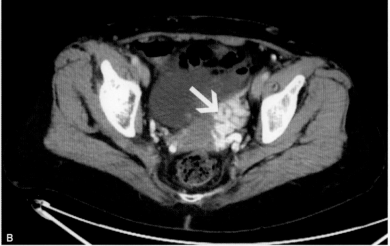

FIGURE 6–94. Ovarian vein varices. **(A)** Dilated (> 4.0 mm) ovarian veins in the left pelvis in a patient with symptoms of pelvic venous congestion. **(B)** Axial CT of same patient. Arrow points to serpiginous left ovarian vein with IV contrast.

Questions

1. What branch of the abdominal aorta sends blood to the spleen via the splenic artery?

   (A) SMA

   (B) IMA

   (C) CA

   (D) GDA

2. Which blood vessel acts as a collateral in the presence of CA obstruction?

   (A) PHA

   (B) IMA

   (C) Left gastric artery

   (D) GDA

3. The terminal branches of the renal artery are the

   (A) Interlobular arteries

   (B) Interlobar arteries

   (C) Segmental arteries

   (D) Arcuate arteries

4. The anatomic position of the left renal vein is typically anterior to the

   (A) IVC

   (B) Aorta

   (C) SMA

   (D) Right renal artery

5. Which of the following is a systemic vein?

   (A) MPV

   (B) Left hepatic vein

   (C) SMV

   (D) Splenic vein

6. Which of the following vessels follow a course that is posterior to the IVC?

   (A) The left renal vein

   (B) The right renal vein

   (C) The left renal artery

   (D) The right renal artery

7. The paraumbilical vein is a terminal branch of the

   (A) Left hepatic vein

   (B) LPV

   (C) Right hepatic vein

   (D) Cardinal vein

8. The hepatic veins terminate at the

   (A) IVC

   (B) Superior vena cava

   (C) MPV

   (D) Portal splenic confluence

9. Which blood vessel is not usually seen with ultrasound imaging?

   (A) IMA

   (B) Left gastric artery

   (C) SMV

   (D) Splenic artery

10. The portal splenic confluence is made up of the splenic vein and which portal vessel?

    (A) Splenic artery

    (B) IMV

    (C) SMV

    (D) Middle hepatic vein

11. Which mesenteric vessel originates from the anterior aorta in between the origin of the celiac axis and the origins of the renal arteries?

    (A) SMA

    (B) IMA

    (C) Left inferior phrenic artery

    (D) Right gonadal artery

12. Most of the oxygenated blood to the liver comes from the

    (A) Portal vein

    (B) IVC

    (C) SMA

    (D) Hepatic artery

13. The left gastric vein is also known as what vessel?

    (A) Cystic vein

    (B) Coronary vein

    (C) IMV

    (D) Renal vein

14. The liver receives approximately what portion of its blood from the portal vein?

    (A) 25%

    (B) 50%

    (C) 75%

    (D) 95%

15. Portal veins may be differentiated from hepatic veins by which of the following characteristics?

    (A) Hepatic veins have brighter walls

    (B) Portal veins get smaller as they exit the liver toward the right atrium

    (C) Hepatic veins originate from the portal venous system

    (D) Portal veins originate inferior to the liver

16. Which blood vessel is tortuous and lies posterosuperior to the pancreas?

    (A) Splenic artery

    (B) Splenic vein

    (C) Hepatic artery

    (D) SMV

17. What structures form the portal triad?

    (A) Portal vein, hepatic artery, splenic artery

    (B) Splenic vein, SMV, MPV

    (C) Hepatic artery, bile duct, portal vein

    (D) Hepatic vein, hepatic artery, portal vein

18. In Figure 6–95, there is a medical device placed in the patient's body. In what vessel is this device located?

    (A) IMV

    (B) MPV

    (C) Superior vena cava

    (D) IVC

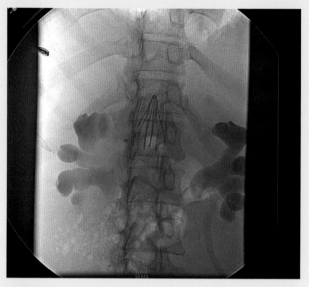

FIGURE 6–95.

19. In Figure 6–96, the arrow is pointing to which blood vessel?

    (A) Right renal artery

    (B) Left renal artery

    (C) Right renal vein

    (D) Left renal vein

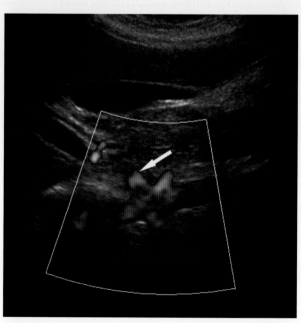

FIGURE 6–96.

20. The arrow in Figure 6–97 is pointing to which vessel?

(A) Celiac axis

(B) SMA

(C) IMA

(D) Hepatic artery

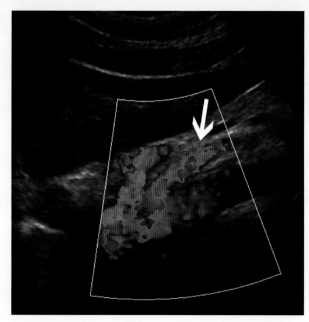

FIGURE 6–97.

21. The hepatic vein confluence is sometimes referred to as

(A) The seagull sign

(B) The ballerina

(C) The bunny sign

(D) The leaping squirrel

22. The hepatic artery branch that originates from the celiac axis is the

(A) PHA

(B) RHA

(C) LHA

(D) CHA

23. The interlobar branch of the renal artery is a direct branch off of what vessel?

(A) The segmental branch

(B) The interlobular branch

(C) The arcuate branch

(D) The main renal artery

24. Which of the following would not likely be affected in PHTN?

(A) Right renal vein

(B) Splenic vein

(C) LPV

(D) SMV

25. Which of the following is a true statement?

(A) An abdominal aorta measuring greater than 2.5 cm is always an aneurysm

(B) Saccular aneurysms are more common than fusiform

(C) An AAA measuring greater than 3 cm is a surgical emergency

(D) AAAs may present as black toes

26. "Nutcracker syndrome" may occur when

(A) The right renal artery passes posterior to the IVC

(B) The left renal vein passes posterior to the aorta

(C) The left renal vein passes anterior to the SMA

(D) The right renal vein passes anterior to the aorta

27. Which of the following is a typical measurement for the common iliac arteries?

(A) 0.25 cm

(B) 0.75 cm

(C) 1.75 cm

(D) 2.25 cm

28. What does a tardus parvus waveform in the CIA imply?

(A) This is a normal pattern in the CIA

(B) There is a more distal obstruction

(C) There is a more proximal obstruction

(D) There is a renal artery stenosis

29. From where does most of the portal venous system blood originate?

(A) The liver

(B) The IVC

(C) The lower extremities

(D) The GI tract

30. Which lobe of the liver is not usually affected in cirrhosis?

(A) Right lobe

(B) Left lobe

(C) Caudate lobe

(D) Quadrate lobe

31. In a fasting patient, which of the following waveform patterns is normal for an SMA?

    (A) Low-resistance flow
    (B) High-resistance flow
    (C) Monophasic flow with a tardus parvus pattern
    (D) To-and-fro flow

32. Which of the following is not usually seen in PHTN?

    (A) Reversal of flow in the RPV
    (B) Splenorenal varices
    (C) IVC thrombus
    (D) Hepatomegaly

33. Which of the following is synonymous with "normal flow into the liver"?

    (A) To-and-fro
    (B) Hepatopetal
    (C) Hepatofugal
    (D) Retrograde

34. Which of the waveforms would be seen distal to a hemodynamically significant stenosis of the origin of the main renal artery?

    (A) High-resistance waveform
    (B) To-and-fro flow
    (C) Multiphasic waveform
    (D) Tardus parvus waveform

35. Thrombosis of the IVC and hepatic veins is known as

    (A) Arnold–Chiari syndrome
    (B) Cavernous transformation
    (C) Vena caval thrombophlebitis
    (D) Budd–Chiari

36. Which of the following is the most common cause of cirrhosis in the United States?

    (A) Biliary tract disease
    (B) Alcohol abuse
    (C) Schistosomiasis
    (D) Hepatic artery aneurysm

37. What is the venous collateral seen in the region of the falciform ligament in the presence of PHTN?

    (A) Ductus venosus
    (B) Ductus arteriosus
    (C) Recanalized umbilical vein
    (D) Recanalized portal vein

38. Which of the following pathologies is often described as appearing like a "string of beads"?

    (A) Cavernous transformation
    (B) Thrombus
    (C) Tardus parvus
    (D) FMD

39. Hepatic veins typically exhibit what type of flow pattern?

    (A) Monophasic
    (B) Hepatopetal
    (C) Bidirectional
    (D) Unidirectional

40. Within a TIPS shunt, which of the following would be considered normal flow?

    (A) Flow toward the right atrium
    (B) Flow with a velocity more than 200 cm/s
    (C) Flow with a velocity of less than 50 cm/s
    (D) Multiphasic flow

41. Which of the following represents an abnormal RAR?

    (A) Less than 2
    (B) Less than or equal to 3
    (C) Greater than 2.5
    (D) Greater than 3.5

42. Which of the following represents normal renal lengths in an adult?

    (A) 5-7 cm
    (B) 7-10 cm
    (C) 10-12 cm
    (D) 13-15 cm

43. The normal, fasting SMA typically has PSVs less than

    (A) 50 cm/s
    (B) 175 cm/s
    (C) 275 cm/s
    (D) 300 cm/s

44. A monophasic fasting SMA is indicative of what?

    (A) A normal waveform
    (B) SMA disease
    (C) MALS
    (D) PHTN

45. **What Doppler angle should be used when obtaining the RI from the interlobular or arcuate arteries of the kidneys?**

    (A) 0 degree

    (B) 30 to 60 degrees

    (C) 60 degrees

    (D) 90 degrees

46. **How many mesenteric vessels must be abnormal in order to have mesenteric ischemia?**

    (A) None

    (B) One

    (C) Two

    (D) Three

47. **What is the most common vascular complication of renal transplant?**

    (A) Venous thrombosis

    (B) Arterial stenosis

    (C) AV fistula

    (D) Pseudoaneurysm

48. **Above what velocity is the celiac axis considered abnormal?**

    (A) 150 cm/s

    (B) 185 cm/s

    (C) 200 cm/s

    (D) 250 cm/s

49. **Which of the following is a true statement about Figure 6–98?**

    (A) The vessel is normal with a maximal AP diameter of 2.84 cm

    (B) The true lumen is 2.84 cm

    (C) The false lumen is 2.84 cm

    (D) AAA is determined solely by the length of the aneurysm

50. **A 56-year-old patient presents in the emergency department with painful black toes. Which study should be performed first?**

    (A) Lower extremity venous for DVT

    (B) Upper extremity arterial for thoracic outlet syndrome

    (C) Lower extremity plethysmography with segmental pressures

    (D) Aorta to rule out AAA

51. **This 61-year-old woman presented with hypertension and proteinuria. Figure 6–99 is an image from her right mid renal artery. The waveform represents**

    (A) Normal renal arterial flow

    (B) Delayed upstroke indicating proximal disease

    (C) High resistance indicating distal obstruction

    (D) Elevated velocities indicating stenosis at the ostium

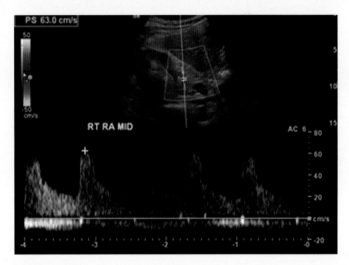

FIGURE 6–99.

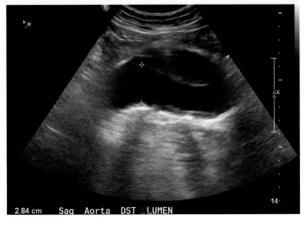

FIGURE 6–98.

52. **Figure 6–100 is a hepatic artery in a patient with postprandial pain. What does the waveform say about the patient?**

    (A) The patient most likely has IMA disease

    (B) There is renal artery stenosis

    (C) There is CA disease

    (D) The patient is without mesenteric vessel disease

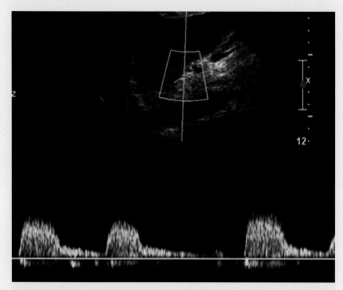

FIGURE 6–100.

53. **Figure 6–101 is a 48-year-old patient 6-month status post renal transplant. What does the spectral Doppler reveal about the transplant?**

    (A) Abnormally high-resistance flow

    (B) Normal flow pattern in segmental vessels

    (C) Proximal stenosis

    (D) Elevated velocities consistent with stricture

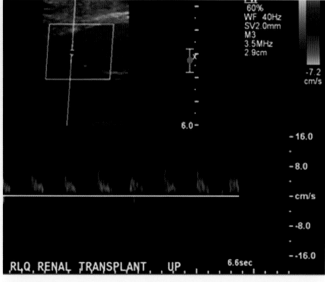

FIGURE 6–101.

54. **Figure 6–102 is that of the splenic vein and artery. Which of the following is true?**

    (A) The splenic artery is flowing in the wrong direction

    (B) The splenic vein is flowing in the wrong direction

    (C) Both vessels are flowing in the appropriate direction

    (D) It is not possible to determine direction of flow

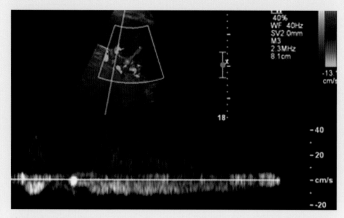

FIGURE 6–102.

55. **Which of the following is not a clinical symptom of PHTN?**

    (A) Splenomegaly

    (B) Ascites

    (C) Esophageal varices

    (D) Renal vein thrombus

56. **The normal spleen is typically**

    (A) 3-10 cm

    (B) 7-14 cm

    (C) 15-20 cm

    (D) 20 cm

57. A 62-year-old patient presents with RUQ pain and jaundice. The abdomen is distended. What does Figure 6–103 ultrasound image demonstrate?

(A) Splenomegaly

(B) Reversal of the hepatic vein flow

(C) Hepatofugal MPV flow

(D) Hepatopetal MPV flow

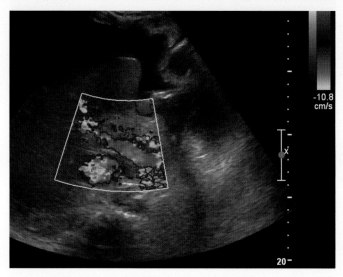

FIGURE 6–103.

58. Figure 6–104 is the left upper quadrant in a cirrhosis patient. What do the images reveal?

(A) Normal left upper quadrant

(B) Signs of collateral formation

(C) Abnormally large splenic arteries

(D) Splenic masses

59. Which collateral commonly seen in PHTN has the potential to be the most life threatening?

(A) Hemorrhoids

(B) Patent paraumbilical vein

(C) Splenorenal varices

(D) Esophageal varices

60. Impingement of the left renal vein causing hematuria and flank pain is termed

(A) Budd–Chiari syndrome

(B) Nutcracker syndrome

(C) Renovascular hypertension

(D) Nephrotic disease

61. In which portion of the aorta are most abdominal aneurysms located?

(A) Distal aorta to include CIA

(B) Proximal aorta superior to renal arteries

(C) Thoracic and proximal abdominal aorta

(D) Infrarenal aorta

62. The term "cavernous transformation" is used in which pathologic process?

(A) Thrombosis of the MPV

(B) IVC thrombus

(C) Hepatic vein and IVC thrombus

(D) Occluded hepatic artery

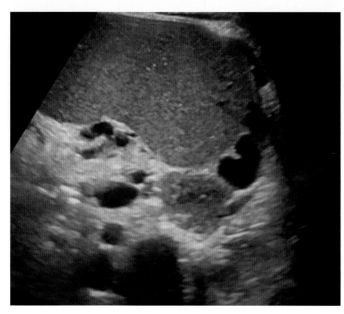

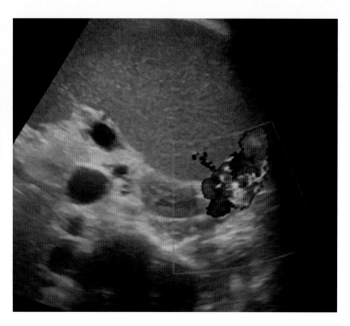

FIGURE 6–104.

63. **A TIPS shunt is placed when**

    (A) The renal arteries fail to provide sufficient flow

    (B) There is severe PHTN

    (C) There is Budd–Chiari syndrome

    (D) There is severe aortic insufficiency

64. **Which of the following is a characteristic of aortic pseudoaneurysms?**

    (A) They lack the normal layers of the vessel wall

    (B) They are very common

    (C) They have an intimal lining but no media or adventitia

    (D) They contain a neck with forward flow only into the pseudoaneurysm

65. **In a patient under 50 years of age, what is the most common cause of renovascular hypertension?**

    (A) Atherosclerotic disease

    (B) Raynaud disease

    (C) FMD

    (D) Diabetes

66. **What is the normal value for AT in the renal artery?**

    (A) Less than 100 ms

    (B) Less than 100 m/s

    (C) Less than 100 m/s^2

    (D) More than 100 m/s^2

67. **What is the name of a small, round, true aneurysm that protrudes from the aorta?**

    (A) Fusiform

    (B) Saccular

    (C) Pseudoaneurysm

    (D) False aneurysm

68. **What is the term used when aortic blood escapes the endovascular graft into the aneurysmal sac?**

    (A) Endoleak

    (B) Pseudoaneurysm

    (C) Dissection

    (D) Aortic rupture

69. **Which of the following diseases has aortic dissection as a risk factor?**

    (A) Arnold–Chiari II

    (B) Budd–Chiari

    (C) MALS

    (D) Marfan syndrome

70. **The arterial waveform in Figure 6–105 indicates what process?**

    (A) Distal occlusion

    (B) Distal stenosis

    (C) Proximal stenosis

    (D) Normal arterial waveform

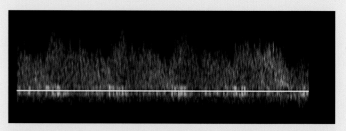

FIGURE 6–105.

71. **You are scanning a patient who is unable to provide a history and was admitted by ambulance to the emergency room (ER). On visual examination, you note the patient has jaundice and a distended abdomen. On ultrasound, there is a small liver with ascites present. In the right lobe are two parallel, echogenic lines in a superior to inferior orientation. What is the most likely reason for the right lobe structure?**

    (A) Patient has TIPS shunt

    (B) Patient had angioplasty for hepatic artery stenosis

    (C) Patient has schistosomiasis

    (D) Patient had gastric artery bypass

72. **Reversal of diastolic flow in a renal artery may be a sign of**

    (A) Proximal obstruction

    (B) Pseudoaneurysm of the renal artery

    (C) Renal vein thrombosis

    (D) Normal functioning kidney

73. **In Figure 6–106, a clot is identified in a large blood vessel. If this clot becomes an embolus, what chamber of the heart will it reach first?**

(A) Left atrium

(B) Right atrium

(C) Right ventricle

(D) Left ventricle

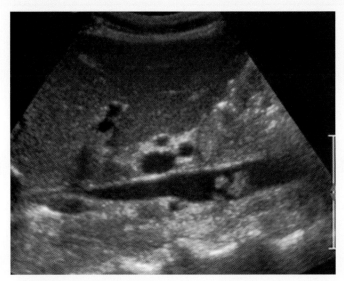

FIGURE 6–106.

74. **Central venous emboli can be potentially fatal due to what pathologic process?**

(A) Middle cerebral artery occlusion

(B) Aortic occlusion

(C) Pulmonary embolism

(D) Lower extremity emboli

75. **Figure 6–107 is of a transverse aorta. To what is the arrow pointing?**

(A) True lumen

(B) False lumen

(C) Pseudo lumen

(D) Saccular aneurysm

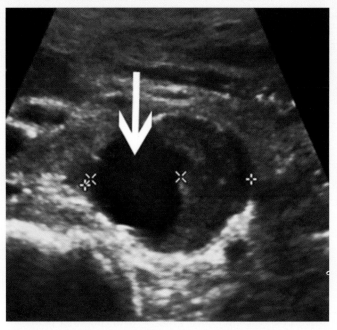

FIGURE 6–107.

76. **Which of the following is true about renal artery stenosis examinations?**

(A) Patients need not fast prior to the examination

(B) Angle-corrected Doppler of the arcuate arteries is essential

(C) The kidney length must be measured as part of the examination

(D) PSV information is not needed

77. **In MALS, which of the following is true?**

(A) The compression is relieved with inhalation

(B) The compression is relieved with deep exhale

(C) There is an increase in celiac PSV with inhalation

(D) There is an increase in SMA velocities with inhalation

78. **A Type I aortic endoleak**

(A) Is from a branch of the aorta communicating with the sac

(B) Is from a tear in the graft itself

(C) Is from a poor seal at one end of the graft

(D) Is from a nonspecified source

79. **When measuring the abdominal aorta, which of the following is true?**

(A) The most important measurement is the length of the aneurysm

(B) Only a true transverse measurement should be used

(C) Only a true AP measurement should be used

(D) The widest cross-sectional measurement should be used

80. **Which of the following would be a reason for a normal CTA of the celiac axis but an abnormal US?**

(A) CTA is less sensitive than US for CA studies

(B) CTAs are usually performed without radiopaque contrast agents

(C) CTA is typically performed with deep inspiration

(D) Unlike CT, CTA does not use ionizing radiation

81. **A 63-year-old female presents with epigastric pain after eating. She complains of weight loss without trying to lose weight. You notice occlusion of the celiac axis but you identify flow in the proper hepatic and splenic arteries. Which of the following is a likely finding?**

(A) There is a duplicated CA

(B) There is retrograde flow in the GDA

(C) There is retrograde flow in the SMA

(D) There is a high-grade stenosis in the abdominal aorta

82. **This patient (Fig. 6–108) presented with abdominal pain and leg swelling. US of the lower extremities was negative for DVT. This patient has what significant finding?**

(A) Thrombosis of the proximal aorta

(B) Left hepatic vein thrombus

(C) Central IVC thrombus

(D) Tumor thrombus of the left renal vein

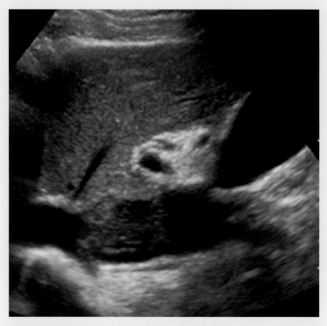

FIGURE 6–108.

83. **In Figure 6–109, in what direction is the blood flowing?**

(A) Toward the head

(B) Toward the feet

(C) Bidirectional

(D) Cannot tell from this image

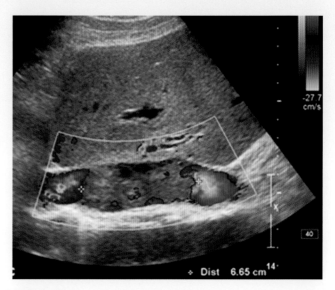

FIGURE 6–109.

84. **Blood is flowing in a hepatopetal direction in the LPV status post-TIPS placement. Which of the following is likely true?**

    (A) Patent TIPS

    (B) AVF in shunt

    (C) MPV thrombus

    (D) TIPS stenosis or failure

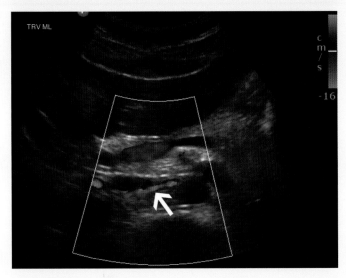

FIGURE 6–110.

85. **Why does angle correction need to be used when measuring AI in the renal artery?**

    (A) Angle corrections are not needed for AI

    (B) Because of the pulsatile nature of renal arteries

    (C) Because velocities are needed to measure AI

    (D) Because angle correction is needed for all measurements

86. **What is the maximum angle correction that may be used when measuring velocities?**

    (A) 0 degree

    (B) 45 degrees

    (C) 60 degrees

    (D) 89 degrees

87. **The main purpose of a TIPS is to**

    (A) Relieve pressure leading to esophageal varices

    (B) Increase the pressure in the MPV to force the blood through the liver

    (C) Increase flow through the paraumbilical vein

    (D) Connect the systemic arterial system to the systemic venous system

88. **What are the reasons TIPS are covered in PTFE?**

    (A) Easier to insert

    (B) Less chance of failure

    (C) Blood can travel faster

    (D) Keep it warm in winter

89. **A patient has severe abdominal pain after eating. Which vessel should be evaluated?**

    (A) SMA

    (B) MPV

    (C) Hepatic artery

    (D) Left gastric artery

90. **The renal artery**

    (A) Typically has a delayed upstroke

    (B) Is a high-resistance vessel

    (C) Has an AI more than 300 cm/s^2

    (D) Typically has reversal of diastolic flow

91. **A nonaneurysmal dilatation of the aorta less than 3 cm is called**

    (A) Ectasia

    (B) Saccular dilatation

    (C) Pseudoaneurysm

    (D) Aortic stenosis

92. **Which of the following is a prime concern in the patient with cirrhosis?**

    (A) Renal cell carcinoma

    (B) Hepatoma

    (C) Focal nodular hyperplasia

    (D) Metastasis

93. **During an abdominal ultrasound, ascites and splenomegaly are seen. Which of the following might also be seen?**

    (A) Hepatopetal flow in the MPV

    (B) Hepatofugal flow in the paraumbilical vein

    (C) Hepatofugal flow in the splenic vein

    (D) Distal IVC thrombus

94. **Which potential collateral originates from the portal vein and leads to esophageal veins?**

    (A) Rectal veins

    (B) Paraumbilical vein

    (C) Splenorenal collaterals

    (D) Coronary vein

95. **Which of the following is a criterion for TIPS failure?**

    (A) Velocity difference of 20-40 cm/s from one sampling point to another

    (B) Absence of thrombus

    (C) Flow velocity less than 50 cm/s in TIPS

    (D) Flow velocity more than 30 cm/s in MPV

96. **Normal flow through the coronary vein should be**

    (A) Toward the portal vein

    (B) Toward the esophagus

    (C) Toward the spleen

    (D) Toward the IMV

97. **In Figure 6–110, the arrow is pointing to which vessel?**

    (A) Left renal vein

    (B) Left renal artery

    (C) Right renal artery

    (D) Right renal vein

98. **In Figure 6–111, the arrow is pointing to which portal venous vessel?**

    (A) Splenic vein

    (B) SMV

    (C) IMV

    (D) Left gastric vein

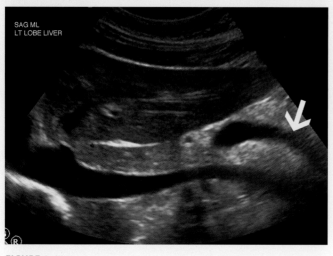

FIGURE 6–111.

99. **In Figure 6–112, the arrow is pointing to which vessel?**

    (A) Splenic vein

    (B) MPV

    (C) Superior mesenteric artery

    (D) Splenic artery

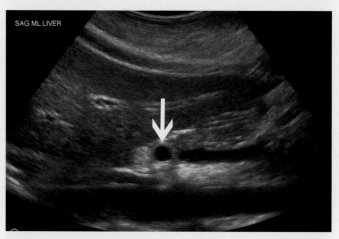

FIGURE 6–112.

100. **What is the most common type of visceral arterial aneurysm?**

    (A) Splenic artery

    (B) Renal artery

    (C) CHA

    (D) SMA

Answers and Explanations

1. **(C)** The celiac axis has three branches: the left gastric artery, not usually seen by ultrasound, the CHA, and the splenic artery.

2. **(D)** The GDA is a branch of the CHA, and connects to the SMA via collaterals. The GDA acts as a collateral in the presence of celiac axis obstruction.

3. **(A)** The interlobular branches are the most distal branches in the kidneys. They originate from the arcuate arteries.

4. **(B)** The left renal vein typically lies between the SMA and the aorta. In some patients, the left renal vein has an aberrant course posterior to the aorta, but this is not the typical presentation.

5. **(B)** The left hepatic vein is part of the systemic circulation, while the other vessels listed are part of the portal venous circulation.

6. **(D)** The right renal artery is the only major blood vessel that lies posterior to the IVC.

7. **(B)** The paraumbilical vein, also known as a recanalized umbilical vein, is a collateral that originates from the LPV. This vein is a remnant of fetal circulation, that may become patent in the presence of PHTN.

8. **(A)** The hepatic veins drain the liver and form a confluence in the superior portion of the liver that drains into the IVC.

9. **(B)** The left gastric artery, a branch of the celiac axis, is not usually visualized with ultrasound.

10. **(C)** The SMV and the splenic vein form a confluence called the portal splenic confluence. The MPV originates from this confluence.

11. **(A)** The SMA originates from the anterior aorta just inferior to the celiac axis origin and just superior to the origin of the renal arteries.

12. **(D)** The hepatic artery supplies oxygenated blood to the liver. The MPV supplies the majority of the blood to the liver, but it is poorly oxygenated.

13. **(B)** The left gastric vein, an important collateral in the presence of PHTN, is also known as the coronary vein.

14. **(C)** The liver receives approximately 75% to 80% of its blood from the portal vein. This blood is poorly oxygenated, so most of the oxygen comes via the hepatic artery.

15. **(D)** The MPV originates from the portal splenic confluence, posterior to the pancreatic head. The MPV then travels into the liver via the porta hepatis, the liver's hilum.

16. **(A)** The splenic artery, a branch of the celiac axis, is a tortuous vessel that lies posterior and superior to the pancreas.

17. **(C)** The portal triad consists of a portal vein branch, a hepatic artery branch, and a bile duct tributary.

18. **(D)** In this image, there is the presence of an IVC filter, placed because of the risk of embolization of DVT.

19. **(A)** In this coronal view of the aorta, the renal arteries are being imaged from the right side of the patient, at the top of the screen, to the left side of the patient, at the bottom of the screen. Therefore, the renal artery closest to the transducer is the right renal artery.

20. **(B)** This sagittal view of the aorta includes the celiac axis and SMA. The arrow is pointing to the SMA.

21. **(C)** The hepatic vein confluence is the region where the left, middle, and right hepatic veins terminate at the IVC. When the left and middle hepatic veins are visualized going into the IVC, it has the appearance of the iconic "bunny" sign, or as this author prefers, the "hepatic moose."

22. **(D)** The CHA originates from the celiac axis. The PHA is the branch that becomes left and right hepatic arteries.

23. **(A)** The order of renal artery branches, from central to peripheral, is segmental, interlobar, arcuate, and interlobular.

24. **(A)** The right renal vein is part of the systemic circulation. PHTN typically affects the portal venous circulation, although it eventually causes collaterals to form that bypass the liver and form an aberrant connection to the systemic circulation.

25. **(D)** AAAs may present as embolic showers to the toes, causing black toes as the presenting clinical symptom.

26. **(B)** The normal course of the left renal vein is between the SMA and the aorta. One form of "nutcracker syndrome" occurs when the left renal vein is compressed by the aorta as it passes posterior to the aorta. Another type of "nutcracker syndrome" occurs when the left renal vein is impinged by the SMA and aorta, causing backup of flow in the left renal vein.

27. **(B)** The CIA typically measure less than 1.5 cm in diameter. A measurement over 1.5 cm is considered aneurysmal.

28. **(C)** Tardus parvus waveforms imply a more proximal obstruction. In this example, the disease is most likely in the aorta.

29. **(D)** The GI tract supplies most of the blood to the portal venous system for processing by the liver.

30. **(C)** The caudate lobe is usually spared in cirrhosis due to its unique blood supply.

31. **(B)** In the normal, fasting patient, the GI tract is not working hard, so the peripheral arterioles are constricted. Therefore, the SMA will have a high-resistance flow pattern.

32. **(C)** Although it is possible to have IVC thrombus in PHTN, it is far more common for a patient to present with reversal of flow in the RPV, splenorenal varices, and hepatomegaly.

33. **(B)** Hepatopetal is the term used for forward flow into the liver. Reversal of flow, away from the liver, is termed hepatofugal.

34. **(D)** The tardus parvus waveform implies a delayed upstroke distal to a stenosis.

35. **(D)** Budd–Chiari is a syndrome characterized by thrombus in the hepatics veins and/or IVC.

36. **(B)** In the United States, alcohol abuse and hepatitis are the two most common causes of cirrhosis. Schistosomiasis is a common cause in developing nations.

37. **(C)** The recanalized umbilical vein, also known as the paraumbilical vein, is a common collateral in PHTN. It lies in the region of the falciform ligament in the liver and originates at the LPV.

38. **(D)** FMD is often characterized as appearing like a "string of beads." Although this appearance is more easily visualized on angiography, it can be seen on ultrasound, especially when it occurs in the carotid arteries.

39. **(C)** Hepatic veins tend to be bidirectional because of the influence by the right atrium.

40. **(A)** Flow within a TIPS should be in the direction toward the IVC, which leads into the right atrium. Flow should not be less than 50 cm/s or more than 200 cm/s, and it is usually a little pulsatile due to right atrial influences, but monophasic.

41. **(D)** The RAR should be less than 3.5. An elevated RAR implies a greater than 60% stenosis of the renal artery, assuming the aortic velocity is within normal limits.

42. **(C)** The normal adult kidney measures 9-13 cm. Although that exact number is not presented as a possible answer, always pick the best answer of the choices listed.

43. **(C)** SMA velocities greater than 275 cm/s in a fasting patient indicate stenosis.

44. **(B)** When there is significant disease in the mesenteric vessels, the distal arterioles dilate to permit more blood flow to the organs, even in the fasting (resting) state. This persistent dilatation causes a low-resistance bed, and the waveforms in the feeding vessels will take on a low-resistance waveform.

45. **(A)** When the vessels are too small to visualize, and only indices (not velocities) are needed, no angle correction is needed.

46. **(C)** Two mesenteric vessels need to have significant disease before there will be mesenteric ischemia.

47. **(B)** Arterial stenosis is the most common vascular complication of renal transplants, although rejection is the most common complication overall.

48. **(C)** The celiac axis should be less than or equal to 200 cm/s.

49. **(B)** The true lumen is the lumen of the vessel without thrombus. In this image, the true lumen measures 2.84 cm.

50. **(D)** AAA can be an emergency, if ruptured or leaking. Sometimes, the only symptom of AAA is embolic showers distally. Black toes are not a classic symptom of DVT, and the segmental pressure study is not an emergent examination.

51. **(A)** Even though detailed velocity information is not presented in this single image, the waveform has good diastolic flow and a sharp systolic upstroke.

52. **(C)** The hepatic artery is a tributary of the celiac axis. The waveform displays a rounded systolic upstroke with a turbulent pattern, indicative of disease more upstream, presumably from the celiac axis.

53. **(A)** There is absent diastolic flow, which is abnormal in the kidney. This pattern may be seen with transplant rejection.

54. **(C)** It is expected that the splenic artery will flow toward the spleen, while the splenic vein flows away from the spleen. The splenic artery and vein in this image are flowing in the correct directions.

55. **(D)** While renal vein thrombus may incidentally occur in a patient with PHTN, it is far more likely that PHTN will directly result in splenomegaly, esophageal varices, and ascites.

56. **(B)** The normal splenic length is less than 13 cm.

57. **(C)** This image is of the MPV. The color scale indicates that the flow in the MPV is flowing in the wrong direction, away from the liver, and therefore is hepatofugal.

58. **(B)** The "bag of worms" appearance in the splenic region is indicative of splenorenal varices as seen in PHTN.

59. **(D)** Although PHTN has many adverse consequences, the most dangerous is rupture of esophageal varices, which may lead to death.

60. **(B)** Nutcracker syndrome is a result of left renal vein impingement, which may cause flank pain and hematuria.

61. **(D)** Most AAAs are located in the infrarenal aorta.

62. **(A)** Thrombosis with subsequent collateral formation is termed cavernous transformation of the portal vein.

63. **(B)** A TIPS is placed when there is severe PHTN. The TIPS relieves pressure on the portal system by bypassing the severely diseased liver.

64. **(A)** Aortic pseudoaneurysms are rare, but all pseudoaneurysms lack the normal layers of a true vessel wall aneurysm. Pseudoaneurysms are outpouchings caused by blood leaking into the tissue adjacent to the vessel.

65. **(C)** In a patient under the age of 50, FMD is the most common cause of renovascular hypertension.

66. **(A)** Only one of the values listed is a "time." The normal AT is less than 100 ms, or less than 0.1 s.

67. **(B)** Saccular aneurysms are typically small, round, true aneurysms that protrude from the aorta. They are not as common as fusiform aneurysms, which are circumferential enlarging of the aorta.

68. **(A)** Endoleak is the term used when an EVAR leaks into the sac around the graft, potentially leading to rupture.

69. **(D)** Marfan disease is a genetic disease characterized by an increased risk of aortic dissection. Although the dissection more commonly occurs in the thoracic aorta, it may track down into the abdominal aorta and be visible to the vascular sonographer.

70. **(C)** This spectral waveform is very turbulent, indicating a more proximal stenosis. Turbulence is commonly seen downstream from a stenosis.

71. **(A)** The TIPS shunt appears as two parallel echogenic lines in the right lobe, most commonly connecting the RPV to the right hepatic vein.

72. **(C)** Reversal of diastolic flow in a renal artery may be a sign of renal vein thrombosis causing outflow obstruction.

73. **(B)** The clot is in the IVC, which drains into the right atrium. Clot in the IVC may end up as a pulmonary embolus, a potentially life-threatening condition.

74. **(C)** Pulmonary emboli are usually a result of embolic venous thrombus, most commonly from the lower extremities.

75. **(A)** The arrow is pointing to the true lumen of an AAA. The hypoechoic portion is thrombus.

76. **(C)** It is important to measure renal length during any kidney examination. In severe kidney disease, the kidney will shrink. The normal renal length is 9-13 cm.

77. **(A)** MALS is relieved with inhalation, which is why it might be missed on routine examination unless exhalation spectral Doppler waveforms are also documented.

78. **(C)** Type I EVAR endoleaks are caused by a poor seal in one or more ends of the graft.

79. **(D)** The widest measurement obtained (not length) should be used as the size of the aorta. In the transverse plane, it may not always be a "true" transverse measurement, but is the widest cross-sectional measurement.

80. **(C)** Most CTA examinations are performed with deep inspiration. The CA in MALS is normal in deep inspiration, and abnormal in expiration.

81. **(B)** The GDA is a potential collateral for the liver and spleen in the presence of CA occlusion. When CA stenosis or occlusion is suspected, the GDA should be sampled for reversal of flow.

82. **(C)** This image demonstrates thrombus in the central IVC. It may be a result of tumor thrombus or part of a Budd–Chiari complex.

83. **(A)** In the example given, red is away from the transducer, so blood is going toward the heart/head.

84. **(D)** Status post TIPS, the LPV should be hepatofugal as blood travels toward the low-pressure TIPS. If blood is traveling in a hepatopetal direction in the LPV after TIPS, the TIPS must have failed.

85. **(C)** Velocity information is needed to measure AI. Therefore, angle correction is needed. AT does not require velocity information, so no angle correction would be needed.

86. **(C)** Angle correction greater than 60 degrees should not be used because the degree of error is too high.

87. **(A)** Of the choices listed, A is the best answer because a TIPS is placed to relieve the PHTN. PHTN can lead to potentially life-threatening esophageal varices.

88. **(B)** TIPS covered in PTFE are less prone to failure than bare stents.

89. **(A)** Of the vessels listed, the SMA is the best choice. The SMA supplies part of the GI tract with blood, along with the celiac axis tributaries and IMA.

90. **(C)** The renal artery AI should be greater than 300 cm/s^2. Even if that answer was not known, the others are incorrect: renal arteries should not have a delayed upstroke, they are not high-resistance vessels, and do not normally have reversed diastolic flow.

91. **(A)** If the aorta is widened but not aneurysmal, it is called ectasia of the aorta.

92. **(B)** Hepatoma, or HCC, is a concern in the patient with chronic liver disease.

93. **(C)** The patient may have PHTN with findings of ascites and splenomegaly. Hepatofugal flow in the splenic vein would confirm this finding.

94. **(D)** The coronary vein, or left gastric vein, drains the esophageal veins. In PHTN, this flow backs up, causing esophageal varices.

95. **(C)** Flow velocities in a TIPS should be more than 50 cm/s, among other criteria.

96. **(A)** Normal flow in the coronary (left gastric) vein is from the esophageal vessels to the portal vein. Backup of flow in this vessel due to PHTN leads to esophageal varices.

97. **(C)** The arrow in this image is pointing to the right renal artery. Notice the color is away from the transducer, so

the flow is going from medial to lateral, away from the aorta. Also, the vessel is posterior to the IVC, and the right renal artery is the only vessel in this location.

98. **(B)** The arrow in this image is pointing to a large vessel that is draining into the portal splenic confluence. The view is in the sagittal plane, so it must be the SMV.

99. **(D)** This is a sagittal image of the pancreas at the level of the aorta. The circular structure superior to the pancreas is the splenic artery.

100. **(A)** Aneurysm of the splenic artery is the most common visceral arterial aneurysm.

Suggested Readings

1. AbuRhama AF, Bandyk DF. *Non-Invasive Vascular Diagnosis*. 3rd ed. London: Springer-Verlag; 2012.

2. ACR. American College of Radiology. 2014. Available online at www.acr.org. Accessed June 15, 2014.

3. ACR. ACR-AIUM-SPR-SRU Practice guideline for the performance of native renal artery duplex sonography. American College of Radiology Practice Guideline. 2013. Available online at http://www.acr.org/~/media/70460ec59008432aa63c0ee9a4960498.pdf. Accessed June 15, 2014.

4. Aichroth J, Fox T. Retroaortic left renal vein. *J Diagnostic Med Sonography*. 2012;29(1):11–14.

5. AIUM. Ultrasound examination of solid-organ transplants. American Institute of Ultrasound in Medicine. 2014. Available online at http://www.aium.org/resources/guidelines/solidOrganTransplants.pdf. Accessed June 15, 2014.

6. AIUM. Ultrasound examination of native renal artery duplex sonography. American Institute of Ultrasound in Medicine. 2014. Available online at http://www.aium.org/resources/guidelines/renalartery.pdf. Accessed June 18, 2014.

7. Aggarwal S, Qamar A, Sharma V, et al. Abdominal aortic aneurysm: A comprehensive review. *Exp Clin Cardiol*. 2011;16(1):11–15.

8. Bhatt S, Dogra VS. Catastrophes of abdominal aorta: Sonographic evaluation. *Ultrasound Clin*. 2008;3(1):93–91.

9. Bluth EI, Benson CB, Ralls PW, et al. *Ultrasound: A Practical Approach to Clinical Problems*. 2nd ed. New York, NY: Thieme; 2008.

10. Boozari B, Bahr MJ, Kubicka S, et al. Ultrasonography in patients with Budd–Chiari syndrome—Diagnostic signs and prognostic implications. *J Hepatology*. 2008;49(4):572–580.

11. Brunicardi FC, Andersen DK, Billiar TR, et al. *Schwartz's Principles of Surgery*. 11th ed. New York, NY: McGraw-Hill; 2019.

12. Colver WR, Eltahawy E, Cooper CJ. Renal artery stenosis: optimizing diagnosis and treatment. *Prog Cardiovasc Dis*. 2011;54(1):29–35.

13. Daigle R. *Techniques in Non-Invasive Vascular Diagnosis*. 4th ed. Littleton, CO: Summer Publishing; 2014.

14. Ferral H, Behrens G, Lopera J. Budd-Chiari syndrome. *Am J Roentgenol*. 2012;199(4):737–745.

15. Fidelman N, Kawn SW, LaBerge JM, et al. The transjugular intrahepatic portosystemic shunt: An update. *Am J Roentgenol*. 2012;199(4):746–755.

16. Garovic VD, Textor SC. Renovascular hypertension and ischemic nephropathy. *Circulation*. 2005;112(9):1362–1374.

17. Goel A, D'Souza D. Portal hypertension. 2014. Available online at http://radiopaedia.org/articles/portal-hypertension. Accessed June 18, 2014.

18. Goykhman Y, Ben-Haim M, Rosen G, et al. Transjugular intrahepatic portosystemic shunt: current indications, patient selection and results. *Isr Med Assoc J*. 2010;12(11):687–691.

19. Greenberger NJ, Blumberg RS, Burakoff R. *Current Diagnosis & Treatment: Gastroenterology, Hepatology, & Endoscopy*. 2nd ed. New York, NY: McGraw-Hill; 2012.

20. Heller MT. Ultrasound evaluation of the renal transplant. 2014. Available online at https://iame.com/online/ultrasound_evaluation_of_renal_transplant/content.php. Accessed June 15, 2014.

21. IAC. Intersocietal Accreditation Commission. 2019. Available online at www.intersocietal.org. Accessed November 24, 2019.

22. Kupinski AM. *Diagnostic Medical Sonography: The Vascular System*. 2nd ed. Baltimore, MD: Wolters Kluwer; 2017.

23. Lee WK, Mossop PJ, Little AF, et al. Infected (mycotic) aneurysms: spectrum of imaging appearances and management. *Radiographics*. 2008;28(7):1853–1868.

24. Butterworth JF, Mackey DC, Wasnick JD. *Morgan & Mikhail's Clinical Anesthesiology*. 5th ed. New York, NY: McGraw-Hill; 2013.

25. Morton DA, Foreman KB, Albertine KH. *The Big Picture: Gross Anatomy*. New York, NY: McGraw-Hill; 2011.

26. Mulholland MW, Lillemoe KD, Doherty GM, et al. *Greenfield's Surgery: Scientific Principles & Practice*. 6th ed. Philadelphia, PA: Lippincott Williams & Wilkins; 2016.

27. Pellerito J, Polak JF, eds. *Introduction to Vascular Ultrasonography*. 7th ed. Philadelphia, PA: Elsevier Health Sciences; 2020.

28. Rumwell C, McPharlin M. *Vascular Technology: An Illustrated Review*. 5th ed. Pasadena, CA: Davies Publishing; 2017.

29. Singh AK, Nachiappan AC, Verma HA, et al. Postoperative imaging in liver transplantation: What radiologists should know. *Radiographics*. 2010;30(2):339–351.

30. Size G, Lozanski L, Russo T. *Inside Ultrasound: Vascular Reference Guide*. In: French-Sherry E, Skelly CL, Pearce AZ, eds. Inside Ultrasound, Inc.; 2013.

31. Spyridopoulos TN, Kaziani K, Balanika AP, et al. Ultrasound as a first line screening tool for the detection of renal artery stenosis: A comprehensive review. *Med Ultrason*. 2010;12(3):228–232.

32. SVU. Renal artery duplex imaging. Society for Vascular Ultrasound. 2019. Available online at https://higherlogicdownload.s3.amazonaws.com/SVUNET/c9a8d83b-2044-4a4e-b3ec-cd4b2f542939/UploadedImages/PPG_Docs/18__Renal_Artery_Duplex_Imaging__Updated_2019_.pdf. Accessed November 20, 2019.

33. Walker DH, Dumler JS, Marrie T, et al. Rickettsial diseases. In: Jameson JL, Fauci AS, Kasper DL, et al, eds. *Harrison's Principles of Internal Medicine*. 20th ed. New York, NY: McGraw-Hill; 2019.

34. Wood MM, Romine LE, Lee YK, et al. Spectral Doppler signature waveforms in ultrasonography: A review of normal and abnormal waveforms. *Ultrasound Q*. 2010;26(2):83–99.

35. Wyers NC. Acute mesenteric ischemia: Diagnostic approach and surgical treatment. *Semin Vasc Surg*. 2010;23(1):9–20.

36. SVUnet.org. Transabdominal pelvic venous duplex evaluation practice performance guideline. Retrieved from https://higherlogicdownload.s3.amazonaws.com/SVUNET/c9a8d83b-2044-4a4e-b3ec-cd4b2f542939/UploadedImages/PPG_Docs/20__Transabdominal_Pelvic_Duplex_Evaluation__Updated_2019_.pdf. Accessed November 24, 2019.

37. Knuttinen MG, Xie K, Jani A, et al. Pelvic venous insufficiency: Imaging diagnosis, treatment approaches, and therapeutic issues. *Am J Roentgenol*. 2015;204(2):448–458.

7

Quality Assurance and Statistics

QUALITY ASSURANCE

Why Quality Assurance?

Improvement in laboratory quality has several components, including equipment maintenance, laboratory protocols and diagnostic criteria, and continuous laboratory improvement. These types of programs are sometimes referred to as quality assurance (QA) or quality control. How does a vascular laboratory know that the values used for quantification of disease (50% stenosis, 70% stenosis, etc.) are accurate when compared to a "gold standard" (GS)? A QA program with a documented quality improvement (QI) plan ensures a laboratory is producing expected results and continues to do so. If the level of quality drops off at any point, it will be easier to trace to the source if careful records are kept. Patient satisfaction is another measure of quality. Patients are more likely to return to a laboratory where they were treated well, and where they had faith that the examination was being performed correctly.

It is very important to know that the machines are calibrated and tested for reproducibility. If results vary from study to study due to equipment error, then there is an increased risk of misdiagnosis. There are certain checks that the sonographer can and should do on a routine basis. Before or after each patient, the machine should be checked. Cracked or damaged transducers should be removed from service due to risk of electrical shock as well as the degradation of image quality. Removable air filters should be vacuumed monthly to ensure free flow of air to the machine. Annually, a biomedical technician should be brought in to perform QA testing using special equipment, such as phantoms. If strip printers on the plethysmography equipment are being used, it is also important to calibrate them to ensure accurate measurements.

Continued safe operation of the equipment helps ensure good image quality. This means that it is important to ensure that staff do not run over transducer or power cords, that the machine is shut down properly each time, and the equipment is cleaned routinely. Routine cleaning of any equipment that comes in physical contact with a patient is essential to infection prevention and should be done between each patient. It is also important to always use a vendor-approved disinfectant to avoid damage to the equipment.

Phantoms

Ultrasound phantoms are calibration and testing tools of varying designs used to ensure the ultrasound machine is performing as expected. Tissue mimicking phantoms typically have pins, fake cysts, and solid mass mimickers to test for caliper accuracy, dead zone, and image quality. Modern phantoms are made of a soft-tissue mimicking material that transmits sound at 1,540 m/s and has attenuation properties similar to soft tissue. Doppler accuracy can be tested with a Doppler phantom. Doppler phantoms may have a moving string, a vibrating belt, or may be a flow phantom, which consists of a blood mimicking fluid moving through a tube via a pump. Pressure machine calibration is usually performed by a trained equipment technician and not by the sonographers. Some manufacturers have remote diagnostic capability for QA, so a biomedical engineer or technician does not have to come on site.

Calibration

Proper calibration of the equipment used for noninvasive vascular testing is critical for reproducibility. Ultrasound equipment is tested using phantoms and Doppler flow testing devices to ensure velocities are being measured accurately. Plethysmography machines are calibrated to ensure the pressure readings are accurate and the strip printer, if present, is moving at the correct rate of speed. The pressure machine cuffs are also tested to ensure they are holding the proper pressures without leaking.

QUALITY IMPROVEMENT

What Is Quality Improvement?

QI is a review process for a vascular lab to maintain high standards for quality patient care by evaluating the staff, the equipment, and the metrics used by the lab. A QI program is an ongoing process that continually evaluates the following categories:

- How appropriate the order is from the referring physician?
- Technical quality of the examination
- Quality of the interpretation by the interpreting physician
- Quality and completeness of the report and the time it took to get from dictated report to signed report to being received by the referring physician
- Level of correlation with other imaging modalities

The Intersocietal Accreditation Commission (IAC) has an online tool for vascular labs to measure QI and measures the main areas described above. The goal of QI is to improve patient safety, reduce costs, and improve patient outcomes

STATISTICS

Why Do We Have to Know Statistics?

Physicians have a lot of diagnostic tools at their disposal to diagnose vascular diseases. How does the physician know which test is best? Statistics are used to determine which test is most reliable, accurate, and has a low yield of providing false results. Many factors are taken into account when choosing a test for a patient. For example, conventional angiography has some advantages over ultrasound, but is invasive, uses ionizing radiation, and does not show the vessel walls. Carotid ultrasound is noninvasive and reproducible, but ultrasound's inability to penetrate the bone limits the extent of visualized vessels. In most labs, you will probably never need to calculate a positive predictive value (PPV) or negative predictive value (NPV), but as sonographers/vascular technologists, we should be the experts of our tests, including knowing which tests are best compared to the alternatives, and how good a job our lab is doing compared to measurable standards.

Reliability

Some tests are more reliable than others. Reliability means that if the test were repeated, the same or similar results would be achieved. Some tests are considered the "gold standard," (GS) the ideal test to be performed for that disease process. When performing statistical analysis on vascular examinations, angiography is usually considered to be the GS.

Chi Square

Chi (pronounced "kai") square is a statistical analysis tool used to compare a vascular test to the GS. The Chi square can be used to determine the PPV, NPV, sensitivity, specificity, and accuracy

FIGURE 7–1. Chi square (A) represents true positives, (B) is false positive, (C) is false negative, and (D) is true negative.

of some other imaging tests compared to the GS. The Chi square (Fig. 7–1) is a 4-box matrix consisting of a GS test on the *x*-axis, and a test being compared to the GS on the *y*-axis. Note that this may be reversed in your laboratory (or on the board examination), so it is important to determine which is on the *x*-axis and which is on the *y*-axis. It is important to remember that when comparing another test result to the result of a test considered to be the GS, the GS results are always assumed to be correct.

The Chi square is read as follows:

A: True positive: Both tests have the same positive results.

B: False positive: Your test is positive, but the GS is negative.

C: False negative: Your test is negative, but the GS is positive.

D: True negative: Both tests have the same negative results.

How well a test is able to predict a positive result is called the **PPV**. In a noninvasive vascular laboratory, PPV is determined by the number of true positives identified by the laboratory (True positives) divided by the total number identified as positive by the laboratory (True positives + False positives). PPV is determined by the following equation:

$$PPV = \frac{A}{A+B}$$

How well a test is able to predict negative results is called the **NPV**. In a noninvasive vascular laboratory, NPV is determined by the number of true negatives identified by the laboratory (True negatives) divided by the total number identified as negative by the laboratory (True negatives + False negatives). NPV is determined by the following equation:

$$NPV = \frac{D}{D+C}$$

Some tests are good at finding diseases (sensitivity), but not good at saying what the disease is (specificity). Other tests are good at saying what a disease is, but only when it eventually finds the disease.

Sensitivity is how well a test can find disease that is present. In a noninvasive vascular laboratory, the sensitivity of a test is determined by the number of true positives identified by the laboratory (True positives) divided by the total number identified as positive by the GS test (True positives + False negatives). If a test is sensitive, it means its positive findings correlate with the GS positive findings. To determine the sensitivity of a test, use the following equation:

$$\text{Sensitivity} = \frac{A}{A+C}$$

Specificity is the ability to determine which patients without disease will have a negative result. In a noninvasive vascular laboratory, the specificity of a test is determined by the number of true negatives identified by the laboratory (True negatives) divided by the total number identified as negative by the GS test (True negatives + False positives). To determine specificity, use the following equation:

$$\text{Specificity} = \frac{D}{D+B}$$

The **accuracy** of a test is how well the test provides the correct answer, positive or negative. In a noninvasive vascular laboratory, the accuracy of a test is determined by the total number identified correctly both positive and negative (True positives + True negatives) divided by the total number of tests performed (True positives + False positives + False negatives + True negatives). An important note about accuracy is that the percent accuracy falls somewhere between sensitivity and specificity as well as between PPV and NPV. To determine accuracy, use the following equation:

$$\text{Accuracy} = \frac{A+D}{A+B+C+D}$$

Memory Trick

Anyone who has studied vascular has used a memory trick of some sort to memorize all this. Visual people may do better with a graphical representation, while others may prefer rote memorization. Of course, it is always easier to remember if you have an understanding of the material and what each statistic means. Figures 7–2 to 7–6 might help as a visual aid to learn this material. The triangle is the numerator, and the sum of the contents in the box is the denominator. For example, if asked to

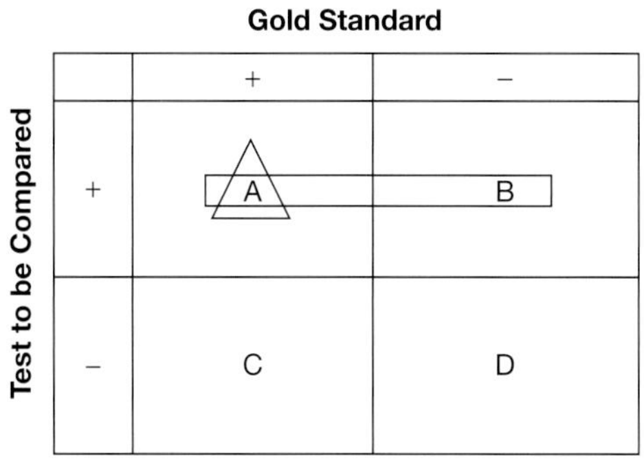

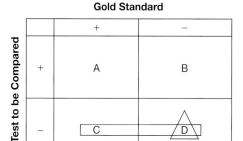

FIGURE 7–3. Negative predictive value (NPV). True negatives (D) divided by sum of true negatives and false negatives (D + C).

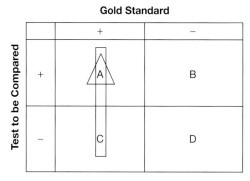

FIGURE 7–4. Sensitivity. True positives (A) divided by sum of true positives (A) and false negatives (C).

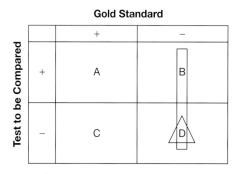

FIGURE 7–5. Specificity. True negatives (D) divided by sum of true negatives (D) and false positives (B).

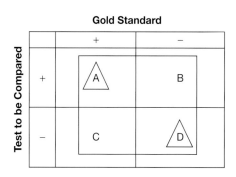

FIGURE 7–6. Accuracy. Sum of true positives (A) and true negatives (D) divided by sum of all squares (A + B + C + D).

FIGURE 7–2. Positive predictive value (PPV). True positives (A) divided by sum of true positives and false positives (A + B).

determine the specificity of a test (Fig. 7–5), the numerator, D, is in the triangle, and the denominator, D + B, is in the box.

SAMPLE PROBLEM

A new noninvasive vascular test is invented to diagnose carotid stenosis. One hundred patients were enrolled in the study to evaluate this new test. All patients had carotid angiograms, considered the "gold standard" as well as the new test. Out of the 100 patients, the angiogram reported 77 studies were positive and 23 studies were negative. Out of the 77 patients reported positive by angiogram, 71 were reported as positive by the new test, 6 were reported as negative. Out of the 23 patients reported as negative by the angiogram, 18 were reported as negative by the new test, and 5 were reported as positive. Calculate PPV, NPV, sensitivity, specificity, and accuracy of the new test.

Where to begin? First, identify the true and false positives and true and false negatives. In this example, 77 were positive according to the GS, but the new test only identified 71 positive studies. These 71 are true positives (Box A) because they matched the GS. Six of the studies were incorrectly reported as negative compared to the GS, and these are the false negatives (Box C). Now, look at the number of studies identified as negative by the GS. The GS identified 23 negatives out of the 100 studies. However, the new test only identified 18 as negative. Therefore, there are 18 true negatives (Box D) and there are 5 false positives (Box B). Add all the boxes up, and it should equal the total number of studies reviewed, which in this example is 100.

Next, draw the Chi square, and populate the true-positives, false-positives, true-negatives, and false-negatives squares with data keeping in mind that the GS test is always assumed to be the correct result. If the GS examination agreed with a positive result from the new test, it is a true-positive result. If the GS examination said the study was negative, but the new test said it was positive, that is a false-positive result. Similarly, if the GS examination agreed with a negative result from the new test, it is a true-negative result. If the GS examination said the study was positive, but the new test said it was negative, that is a false-negative result. In this example, the Chi square will look like Table 7–1.

TABLE 7–1 • Chi Square Solution for Sample Problem

		Angiogram	
		+	−
New Test	+	71 (A: True positives)	5 (B: False positives)
	−	6 (C: False negatives)	18 (D: True negatives)

Next, plug the numbers into the equations:

$$PPV = \frac{71}{71+5} = 93\%$$

$$NPV = \frac{18}{18+6} = 75\%$$

$$Sensitivity = \frac{71}{71+6} = 92\%$$

$$Specificity = \frac{18}{18+5} = 78\%$$

$$Accuracy = \frac{71+18}{71+6+5+18} = 89\%$$

The new test is able to predict about 93% of positive studies and 75% of negative studies, with an overall accuracy of 89%. The test is sensitive in that about 92% of the time, so the test can be used to find the disease. The test has lower specificity (78%), which means that although the new test is good at finding disease, it is not as good at correctly predicting a negative result.

PATIENT CARE

Vascular sonographers provide patient care in many ways. In addition to providing excellent care while in the presence of the patient, the vascular sonographer has other duties that extend beyond the actual patient visit. Before a patient is scanned, the vascular sonographer should retrieve any prior examinations for comparison. Prior studies do not have to be ultrasounds or segmental pressure studies, but may be computed tomography (CT), magnetic resonance imaging (MRI), angiography, etc. Any prior examination may be helpful to both the sonographer and the interpreting physician. In patients with grafts or fistulas, especially when multiple procedures have been performed, a "road map" of the surgery would be helpful to sort out the connections made by the vascular surgeon.

Before going to the scanning room, the vascular sonographer is responsible for retrieving the proper patient from the work list or schedule, identifying the patient with a minimum of two identifiers, and ensuring the correct study is to be performed. The sonographer should obtain a thorough and accurate medical history including but not limited to any previous related surgeries, chronic illnesses, risk factors, and signs and symptoms. Signs and symptoms are important in order to identify the proper indication for the examination. The examination should be explained to the patient, including advance warning of any discomfort the patient might experience. The sonographer must wash his/her hands before and after every examination, and whenever the gloves are removed, preferably in the presence of the patient. Patient comfort should be ensured, including protecting patient modesty whenever possible.

Room temperature should be adjusted, if possible, so it is not so cold that it may have an adverse effect on peripheral circulation. In order to ensure consistency from study to study and patient to patient, a protocol should be followed for every examination performed. The two vascular accreditation agencies, Intersocietal Accreditation Commission (IAC, http://intersocietal.org/) and American College of Radiology (ACR, www.acr.org), have protocols on their respective websites that laboratories can use. The American Institute of Ultrasound in Medicine (AIUM), Society for Vascular Ultrasound (SVU), and Society of Radiologists in Ultrasound (SRU) also list protocols and consensus statements on their websites. Membership in a professional society is one way to ensure that the sonographer stays current with terminology, technology, and protocols.

After the examination is over, the sonographer needs to write up the examination according to the institution's protocol. In some institutions, preliminary reports or examination print outs are scanned into a picture archiving and communication system (PACS), along with any images produced which are transferred digitally. One of the advantages of PACS is the ability to digitally transmit images to the vascular surgeon or other physicians. Another option is for the patient to pick up images from the institution on a CD/DVD, which are a form of optical storage.

In vascular sonography, like all areas of the medical field, critical thinking skills are very important. Not every patient conforms to what is listed in a textbook. When presented with a patient's symptoms and clinical history, the sonographer has to use that information, along with the ultrasound findings, to determine what to present to the physician. Ultrasound is not about pushing buttons on a machine but requires using knowledge and technical skills to provide the highest level of patient care.

The vascular sonographer needs to observe the Health Insurance Portability and Accountability Act (HIPAA) regulations common to all health care institutions and ensure patient privacy. The use of social media has received a lot of attention, and even if a posting does not violate HIPAA per se, it may violate the policies of the sonographer's institution. When in doubt, leave it out. Do not post it.

The key thing to remember is that everything relates to the patient. What training the sonographers have, the laboratory's QI, machine maintenance, etc., all relates to the patient and what happens to that patient next. An examination that is performed improperly may cause a patient to receive an invasive procedure or test that was not needed. For example, a patient may be unnecessarily sent for a CTA, exposing the patient to unneeded ionizing radiation; or worse, that patient has an allergic reaction to the contrast and is hospitalized. How well a sonographer performs an examination matters. How the patient is treated matters. The accuracy of the results matters. It is all about the patient.

Questions

1. If both the GS and your test produce the same positive results, this is called a

   (A) True negative
   (B) True positive
   (C) False positive
   (D) False negative

2. The PPV is used to gauge

   (A) How accurate the test is
   (B) How sensitive the test is
   (C) Ability of predicting abnormal results
   (D) Ability of predicting negative results

3. Using a standard Chi square matrix, the equation $D \div (D + C)$ is used for determining what statistic?

   (A) Accuracy
   (B) Sensitivity
   (C) PPV
   (D) NPV

4. Using a standard Chi square matrix, which of the following equations is used to determine specificity?

   (A) $A \div (A + B)$
   (B) $D \div (D + C)$
   (C) $D \div (D + B)$
   (D) $(A + D) \div (A + B + C + D)$

5. Which of the following indicates how well a test provides the correct results, regardless of whether the result is positive or negative?

   (A) Accuracy
   (B) Specificity
   (C) Sensitivity
   (D) PPV

6. What is the purpose of testing and calibrating the pressure machine on a scheduled basis?

   (A) To ensure the examination is being performed properly
   (B) The hospital's legal department requires it
   (C) To ensure the machine is performing as it is supposed to
   (D) To ensure that the sonographers are trained in calibration

7. When should ultrasound equipment be checked for defects in machine and/or transducers?

   (A) At the end of each day
   (B) During the examination
   (C) On a monthly basis, as required by the accreditation bodies
   (D) Before or after each patient

8. What is the hazard of a cracked transducer?

   (A) There is a risk that the velocities will be inaccurate
   (B) There is a risk that the machine will explode
   (C) There is a risk of electrical shock
   (D) There is no hazard. If the probe works, it is safe

9. A phantom is designed with a string that moves through a water bath. This phantom would be used to test for

   (A) Pressure cuff inflation
   (B) Doppler-based velocities
   (C) Slice thickness artifact
   (D) Contrast resolution

Five hundred patients are evaluated by conventional angiography to rule out stenosis of the internal carotid artery. You have designed a new process, called BestGuess, which you want to compare to the "gold standard" of angiography. Of the 500 patients that had angiography, 150 were positive for stenosis by angiography. Of the 150 patients who were positive by angiography, 80 were positive by BestGuess. Of the 350 patients that were negative by angiography, 180 were negative by BestGuess. Answer the following questions:

10. What is the sensitivity of the new test?

    (A) 47%
    (B) 53%
    (C) 51%
    (D) 32%

11. What is the specificity of the new test?

    (A) 47%
    (B) 53%
    (C) 51%
    (D) 32%

12. **What is the accuracy of the new test?**

    (A) 52%

    (B) 78%

    (C) 54%

    (D) Not enough information to determine

13. **What is the PPV of the new test?**

    (A) 72%

    (B) 32%

    (C) 51%

    (D) 53%

14. **What is the NPV of the new test?**

    (A) 72%

    (B) 32%

    (C) 51%

    (D) 53%

15. **A test is developed that is very good at identifying a certain disease, but it only finds the disease about half the time. This test has a low _____ and a high _____**

    (A) Sensitivity, accuracy

    (B) Specificity, sensitivity

    (C) Accuracy, specificity

    (D) Sensitivity, specificity

16. **A test is developed that is very good at determining when disease is not present. This test is said to have a high**

    (A) NPV

    (B) PPV

    (C) Accuracy

    (D) Sensitivity

17. **A test that is good at finding disease, regardless of positive or negative result, has a high**

    (A) Accuracy

    (B) Sensitivity

    (C) Specificity

    (D) NPV

18. **Which of the following is true about HIPAA?**

    (A) It is actually spelled HIPPA

    (B) It specifies criminal and civil penalties for violating patient confidentiality

    (C) It only applies to hospital employees

    (D) Celebrities are not covered under HIPAA because they are in the public eye

19. **Laboratory QI is needed because**

    (A) Vascular sonographers are very messy

    (B) Equipment is always breaking

    (C) Vascular laboratories constantly need to maintain or improve standards

    (D) You will not get paid if you do not do it

20. **Which of the following is a computer-based file storage device used by institutions to electronically store images and reports?**

    (A) Matrix camera

    (B) Kodak film

    (C) PACS

    (D) Canon scanner

21. **Who is responsible for ensuring the correct patient is being scanned, the correct study is being performed, and the correct body part is being imaged?**

    (A) The ordering physician

    (B) The nurse

    (C) The front desk clerk

    (D) The sonographer

22. **For which patients should prior examinations be reviewed?**

    (A) Patients that had studies performed within the last 12 months

    (B) Any time priors are available

    (C) When the doctor tells you to

    (D) For all portable studies

23. **Seventeen patients had a CTA performed that was positive for 70% stenosis of the ICA. Ultrasound only revealed 11 patients with similarly positive results. What is the sensitivity of the ultrasound?**

    (A) 17%

    (B) 65%

    (C) 22%

    (D) 35%

24. **Fifty patients had a negative magnetic resonance angiography (MRA) for mesenteric stenosis. Of those patients, 40 were negative by ultrasound. What is the specificity of the ultrasound?**

    (A) 80%

    (B) 90%

    (C) 50%

    (D) Not enough information to determine

25. **What is the sensitivity of your test if the true positives' number is 70 and the false negatives' number is 10?**

    (A) 70%

    (B) 88%

    (C) 12%

    (D) 0%

Answers and Explanations

1. **(B)** "True positive" is when the test you are using produces the same results as the GS.

2. **(C)** The PPV is used to describe how well a test can predict a positive, or abnormal, result.

3. **(D)** $D \div (D + C)$ is the formula for NPV, a statistic that predicts how well a test can find a negative, or normal, result. Notice all the parts of the equation are "negative." C is false negatives and D is true negatives.

4. **(C)** The equation for specificity, the statistic that states how good a test is at finding disease, is $D \div (D + B)$, where D is true negatives and B is false positives.

5. **(A)** Accuracy is how well a test provides the correct result, regardless of whether that result is positive or negative. Accuracy involves all the variables: true positives (A) + true negatives (D) divided by the sum of all the variables $(A + B + C + D)$.

6. **(C)** Ultrasound and plethysmographic equipment must have checks as part of a routine QA program. QA is required for all accredited laboratories but should be performed by nonaccredited laboratories, as well. Performing QA checks helps ensure that any error is not caused by the equipment.

7. **(D)** Before a patient is scanned, the transducer and equipment should be checked to ensure there are no cracks in the transducer or cords. After the examination, it is the responsibility of the sonographer to ensure the probe cords and power cord are not run over as part of moving the equipment, and that the machine is cleaned according to laboratory standards. Annual QA checks should be performed by a biomedical technician.

8. **(C)** Roughly 10-500 volts of electricity go through the transducer, presenting a potential shock hazard to sonographer and patient. Cracked transducers should immediately be taken out of service.

9. **(B)** There are different types of Doppler phantoms. One type uses a string in a water bath to mimic flowing blood.

For 10 through 14, the Chi square is as follows:

True positives (A): 80
False positives (B): 170
False negatives (C): 70
True negatives (D): 180

10. **(B)** Sensitivity is determined by the equation $A \div (A + C)$, where A is the true positives and C is the false negatives. The answer is $80 \div 150 = 53\%$.

11. **(C)** Specificity is determined by the equation $D \div (D + B)$, where D is the true negatives and B is the false positives. The answer is $180 \div 350 = 51\%$.

12. **(A)** Accuracy is determined by the equation $(A + D) \div (A + B + C + D)$, where A is the true positives and B is the false positives, divided by all the values in the Chi square. The answer is $250 \div 500 = 52\%$.

13. **(B)** The PPV is determined by the equation $A \div (A + B)$, where A is the true positives and B is the false positives. The answer is $80 \div 250 = 32\%$.

14. **(A)** The NPV is determined by the equation $D \div (D + C)$, where D is the true negatives and C is the false negatives. The answer is $180 \div 250 = 72\%$.

15. **(D)** The test described can identify a specific disease (high specificity), but it is not good at finding that disease (low sensitivity). An example of this type of test is anti-DNA for systemic lupus erythematosus (SLE). When the test is positive, it is very specific for SLE. However, the patient might have SLE and a negative anti-DNA because the test is not sensitive. In other words, the test may be negative even if the patient has active disease.

16. **(A)** The NPV is high when a test is good at saying that the study is normal; no disease is present.

17. **(A)** Accuracy is the ability of a test to provide a true result, regardless of positive or negative.

18. **(B)** HIPAA, the Health Insurance Portability and Accountability Act, provides for criminal and civil penalties if protected health information (PHI) is used or accessed inappropriately. Celebrities are protected by HIPAA the same as any other person. The only records the sonographer should access are those of patients with whom they have direct contact as part of their care.

19. **(C)** Continuous quality improvement is vital to ensure that patients receive the appropriate test for the clinical diagnosis, that the test is performed correctly, and that the sonographers meet the standards set forth by the laboratory and/or accreditation body.

20. **(C)** The PACS is a picture archiving and communication system that involves a computer or network that is used to store images and reports digitally. Institutions with PACS are referred to as "filmless" because hard copy film is no longer used.

21. **(D)** The sonographer is the gate keeper to ensure that the correct patient is being scanned (check for at least two identifiers), the correct study is being performed (based on a clinical history), and the correct body part is being scanned (again, based on a history). If an invasive procedure is being performed, a "time out" is required so everyone agrees on the procedure being performed.

22. **(B)** If the patient has had a study performed before, prior examination reports should be reviewed. In the presence

of pathology or complicated results, like with graft studies, the prior images should also be reviewed, if obtainable.

23. **(B)** Sensitivity is determined by true positives divided by (true positives + false negatives), or A ÷ (A + C). In this example, the results are (11) ÷ (11 + 6) = 65%.

24. **(A)** Specificity is determined by true negatives divided by (true negatives + false positives), or D ÷ (D + B). In this example, the results are 40 ÷ (40 + 10) = 80%.

25. **(B)** Sensitivity is determined by true positives divided by (true positives + false negatives), or A ÷ (A + C). In this example, the results are 70 ÷ (70 + 10) = 88%.

Suggested Readings

1. Adler AM, Carlton RR. *Radiologic Sciences and Patient Care.* 5th ed. St. Louis, MO: Elsevier; 2012.

2. Daigle R. *Techniques in Non-Invasive Vascular Diagnosis.* 4th ed. Littleton, CO: Summer Publishing; 2014.

3. Henderson MC, Tierney LM, Smetana GW. *The Patient History: An Evidence-Based Approach to Differential Diagnosis.* 2nd ed. New York, NY: McGraw-Hill; 2012.

4. Jurgen AHR. The gold standard: Not a golden standard. *BMJ.* 2005;330(7500):1121.

5. Kupinski AM. *Diagnostic Medical Sonography: The Vascular System.* 2nd ed. Baltimore, MD: Wolters Kluwer; 2017.

6. LeBlond RF, Brown DD, DeGowin RL. *DeGowin's Diagnostic Examination.* New York, NY: McGraw-Hill; 2009.

7. Penny SM, Fox TB, Godwin CH. *Examination Review for Ultrasound: Sonographic Principles & Instrumentation (SPI).* 2nd ed. Philadelphia, PA: Wolters Kluwer; 2017.

8. Weiland C, Hutchisson M. Quality assurance of the vascular laboratory. In: AbuRhama AF, Bandyk DF, eds. *Non-invasive Vascular Diagnosis.* 3rd ed. London: Springer-Verlag; 2012.

Practice Examination

Questions

1. **In this image (Fig. PT-1), the waveform indicates**

   (A) A stenosis distal to the point of sampling

   (B) A stenosis proximal to the point of sampling

   (C) A tardus parvus waveform

   (D) A normal arterial waveform

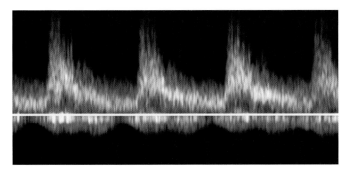

FIGURE PT-1.

2. **Which brachial artery should be used to obtain pressures in a segmental pressure study?**

   (A) The left brachial artery for left ankle-brachial index (ABI), and right brachial artery for right ABI

   (B) The lowest brachial pressure should be used

   (C) The highest brachial pressure should be used

   (D) Use the brachial artery corresponding to the leg with the most disease

3. **Esophageal varices may present intra-abdominally as**

   (A) Hepatopetal flow in the splenic vein

   (B) Retrograde flow in the coronary vein

   (C) Flow toward the liver in the superior mesenteric vein

   (D) Clot in the inferior vena cava (IVC)

4. **Tardus parvus can be described as**

   (A) Rounding of the systolic peak

   (B) Turbulence distal to a hemodynamically significant stenosis

   (C) Elevated systolic velocities in a stenosis

   (D) To-and-fro flow pattern

5. **What is the most common type of abdominal aortic aneurysm?**

   (A) Mycotic

   (B) Saccular

   (C) Pseudoaneurysm

   (D) Fusiform

6. **The portal vein in this image (Fig. PT–2) demonstrates what type of flow?**

    (A) Normal to-and-fro pattern typical of portal veins
    (B) Abnormal waveform suggestive of liver congestion
    (C) Continuous flow consistent with distal obstruction
    (D) Retrograde flow

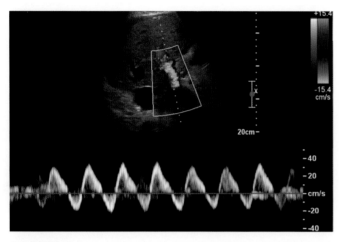

FIGURE PT–2.

7. **Assuming a nonhemodynamically significant stenosis, the lowest pressure will be found**

    (A) Immediately proximal to a stenosis
    (B) Immediately distal to a stenosis
    (C) At the level of stenosis
    (D) Downstream from a stenosis

8. **Which of the following is not typically imaged on a mesenteric arterial examination?**

    (A) The splenic vein
    (B) The superior mesenteric artery (SMA)
    (C) The celiac axis
    (D) The inferior mesenteric artery (IMA)

9. **In this image (Fig. PT–3) of the circle of Willis, what letter represents the posterior communicating artery (PCoA)?**

    (A) B
    (B) H
    (C) D
    (D) E

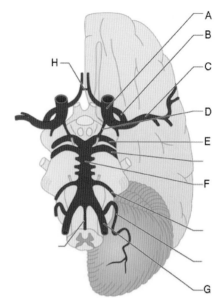

FIGURE PT–3.

10. **In this image (Fig. PT–3) of the circle of Willis, what letter represents the vessel that bifurcates into the anterior cerebral artery (ACA) and middle cerebral artery (MCA)?**

    (A) A
    (B) B
    (C) C
    (D) D

11. **The internal thoracic artery is a branch of which vessel?**

    (A) Axillary artery
    (B) External carotid artery
    (C) Vertebral artery
    (D) Subclavian artery

12. **A test is designed that has a high level of ability in predicting when there is no disease present. This test has a high**

    (A) Positive predictive value (PPV)
    (B) Negative predictive value (NPV)
    (C) Sensitivity
    (D) Specificity

13. **Peripheral resistance is determined by**

    (A) Blood pressure

    (B) Volume flow through the aorta

    (C) Arteriolar dilatation

    (D) Salt intake

14. **Normal flow in a fasting patient's SMA is typically**

    (A) High resistant

    (B) Low resistant

    (C) Monophasic

    (D) Nonpulsatile

15. **A patient complains of severe cramping in the right buttock while walking. At what level is the disease most likely located?**

    (A) Aortoiliac

    (B) Popliteal artery

    (C) Superficial femoral artery

    (D) Deep femoral artery

16. **In this image (Fig. PT–4), the waveform is consistent with**

    (A) High-resistance flow pattern

    (B) Low-resistance flow pattern

    (C) Tardus parvus flow pattern

    (D) To-and-fro flow pattern

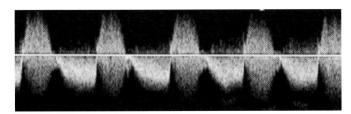

FIGURE PT–4.

17. **Conventional or digital subtraction angiography uses**

    (A) A strong magnetic field and radiofrequency signals

    (B) An arterial puncture

    (C) No contrast agent for imaging

    (D) Noninvasive imaging techniques

18. **With renal arterial stenosis**

    (A) The kidney gets larger in size

    (B) The renal artery:aorta ratio (RAR) will be more than 3.5

    (C) There will be absent venous flow

    (D) The acceleration index will be more than 300 cm/s^2

19. **A 59-year-old patient has jaundice and abdominal discomfort. He has no history of alcohol abuse, but was diagnosed with hepatitis C 15 years ago. What is the most likely diagnosis based on this image (Fig. PT–5)?**

    (A) Normal liver ultrasound

    (B) Pulmonary effusion

    (C) Portal hypertension

    (D) Hepatocellular carcinoma

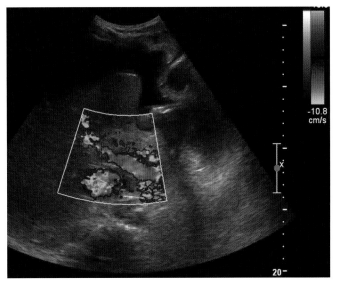

FIGURE PT–5.

20. **The sensitivity of a study is defined as which of the following?**

    (A) (True positives + true negatives) ÷ all of the values

    (B) True positives ÷ (true positives + false positives)

    (C) True positives ÷ (true positives + false negatives)

    (D) True negatives ÷ (true negatives + false positives)

21. **Which of the following techniques is the key for the diagnosis of deep venous thrombosis (DVT)?**

    (A) Color Doppler

    (B) Spectral waveforms

    (C) Augmentation

    (D) Compressions

22. **Grayscale imaging of a vessel with fibromuscular dysplasia (FMD) is often said to have the appearance of**

    (A) A seagull

    (B) A bunny rabbit

    (C) A string of beads

    (D) A keyhole

23. **The most common site of atherosclerotic disease is usually at**

    (A) The terminal end of the vessel

    (B) The origin of the vessel

    (C) In the middle of the vessel

    (D) Throughout the entirety of the vessel

24. **Median arcuate ligament syndrome (MALS) causes celiac artery stenosis**

    (A) With inspiration

    (B) With expiration

    (C) During a fatty meal

    (D) Only in the elderly

25. **Who is the most important person in the vascular laboratory?**

    (A) The vascular sonographer

    (B) The receptionist at the front desk

    (C) The nurse in the department

    (D) The patient

26. **Overmeasurement of the spectral waveform is possible if**

    (A) The Doppler gain is set too high

    (B) The Doppler gain is set too low

    (C) The frequency is too low

    (D) The pulse repetition frequency (PRF) is set too high

27. **The common femoral vein is formed by the confluence of the femoral vein and the**

    (A) Great saphenous vein

    (B) Popliteal vein

    (C) Deep femoral vein

    (D) External iliac vein

28. **Which of the following is true about a transjugular intrahepatic portosystemic shunt (TIPS) shunt?**

    (A) Flow should be from the hepatic veins toward the portal veins

    (B) Flow should be greater than 200 cm/s

    (C) Flow should be less than 50 cm/s

    (D) Flow velocity should be within 50 cm/s from sampling point to sampling point

29. **According to the segmental pressure study below (Fig. PT–6), which of the following is true?**

    (A) There is likely a right subclavian stenosis

    (B) Suprapopliteal waveforms are markedly dampened

    (C) The ankle-brachial indices are normal

    (D) There is moderate disease on the left

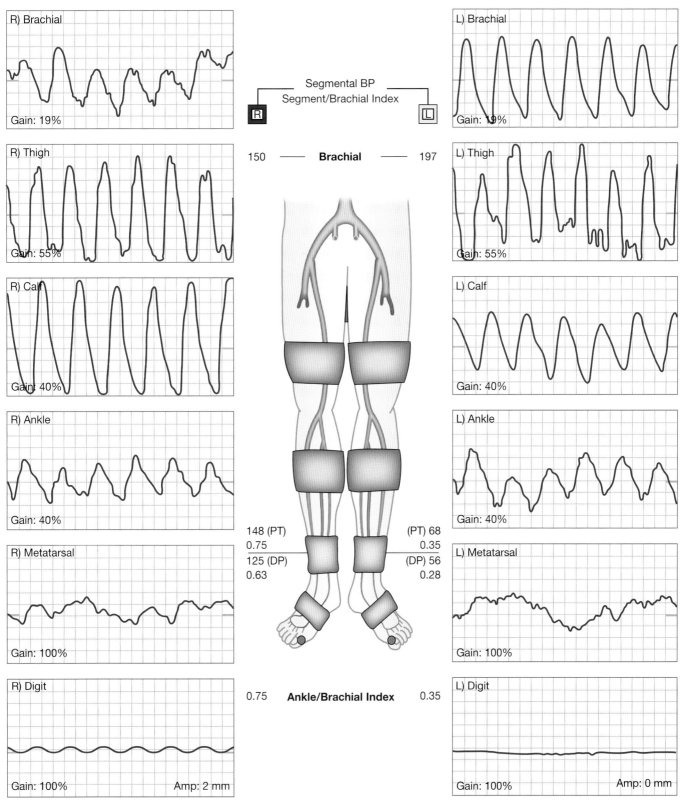

R) Brachial
Gain: 19%

R) Thigh
Gain: 55%

R) Calf
Gain: 40%

R) Ankle
Gain: 40%

R) Metatarsal
Gain: 100%

R) Digit
Gain: 100%   Amp: 2 mm

Segmental BP
Segment/Brachial Index

R   L

150 ——— **Brachial** ——— 197

L) Brachial
Gain: 19%

L) Thigh
Gain: 55%

L) Calf
Gain: 40%

L) Ankle
Gain: 40%

L) Metatarsal
Gain: 100%

L) Digit
Gain: 100%   Amp: 0 mm

148 (PT)   (PT) 68
0.75   0.35
125 (DP)   (DP) 56
0.63   0.28

0.75   **Ankle/Brachial Index**   0.35

FIGURE PT–6.

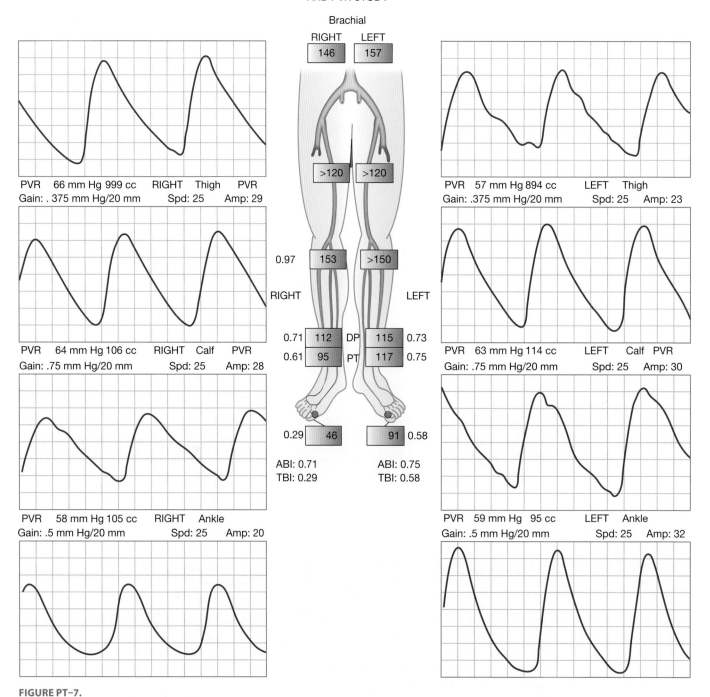

SEGMENTAL PRESSURE
AND PVR STUDY

Brachial

	RIGHT	LEFT	
	146	157	

PVR 66 mm Hg 999 cc RIGHT Thigh PVR
Gain: . 375 mm Hg/20 mm Spd: 25 Amp: 29

PVR 57 mm Hg 894 cc LEFT Thigh
Gain: .375 mm Hg/20 mm Spd: 25 Amp: 23

>120   >120

PVR 64 mm Hg 106 cc RIGHT Calf PVR
Gain: .75 mm Hg/20 mm Spd: 25 Amp: 28

0.97   153   >150

RIGHT   LEFT

PVR 63 mm Hg 114 cc LEFT Calf PVR
Gain: .75 mm Hg/20 mm Spd: 25 Amp: 30

0.71 112 DP 115 0.73
0.61 95   PT 117 0.75

PVR 58 mm Hg 105 cc RIGHT Ankle
Gain: .5 mm Hg/20 mm Spd: 25 Amp: 20

0.29 46   91 0.58

ABI: 0.71   ABI: 0.75
TBI: 0.29   TBI: 0.58

PVR 59 mm Hg 95 cc LEFT Ankle
Gain: .5 mm Hg/20 mm Spd: 25 Amp: 32

FIGURE PT–7.

30. **According to the segmental pressure study shown in Figure PT–7, what is the level of disease at the right ankle?**

    (A) Borderline

    (B) Mild to moderate

    (C) Severe

    (D) Gangrene

31. **Which of the following is true about the right internal carotid artery?**

    (A) It has extracranial branches

    (B) It supplies the facial arteries with blood

    (C) It is normally a low-resistance vessel

    (D) It originates off of the aortic arch

32. **High-resistance flow in the internal carotid artery may be indicative of what process?**

    (A) Cerebral edema

    (B) Common carotid artery (CCA) stenosis

    (C) Stenotic heart valve

    (D) Occlusion of the external carotid artery (ECA)

33. **In transcranial Doppler, the A1 portion of the ACA should have flow that is**

    (A) Bidirectional

    (B) Toward the transducer

    (C) Away from the transducer

    (D) High-resistance

34. **Assuming a suboccipital approach through the foramen magnum, in a normal transcranial Doppler (TCD) examination, the basilar artery flow is normally**

    (A) Toward the transducer

    (B) Away from the transducer

    (C) Bidirectional

    (D) Dependent on the patient position

35. **Color Doppler flash artifact is visualized in the soft tissue adjacent to the common femoral artery status post conventional angiography. Which of the following is the most likely scenario?**

    (A) Normal appearance of color Doppler

    (B) The color gain is too low

    (C) There may be an arteriovenous fistula

    (D) Deep venous thrombus may be present

36. **Budd–Chiari syndrome**

    (A) Occurs in the portal venous system

    (B) Is a result of spina bifida aperta

    (C) May occur as a result of overheparinizing the patient

    (D) Usually involves the hepatic veins and IVC

37. **Which findings are consistent with a failed TIPS?**

    (A) Hepatopetal flow in the MPV

    (B) Increasing ascites

    (C) Flow between 50 and 200 cm/s in the mid-portion of the TIPS

    (D) Flow velocity of 60 cm/s in the MPV

38. **Which of the following is expected to have a low-resistance monophasic waveform?**

    (A) The external carotid artery

    (B) The resting lower extremity artery

    (C) The renal artery

    (D) The distal aorta

39. **Which of the following is in the correct order?**

    (A) Segmental renal artery → interlobular artery → arcuate artery

    (B) Segmental renal artery → arcuate artery → interlobar artery → interlobular artery

    (C) Segmental renal artery → interlobar artery → arcuate artery → interlobular artery

    (D) Arcuate artery → segmental renal artery → interlobular artery → interlobar artery

40. **You are scanning the neck and a large, solid mass is located at the bifurcation of the internal carotid artery (ICA) and ECA. This is most likely**

    (A) A carotid body tumor

    (B) A pseudoaneurysm

    (C) A Klatskin tumor

    (D) A normal variant of the bulb

41. **Which of the following is not normally visualized on ultrasound?**

    (A) The main portal vein

    (B) The superior mesenteric vein

    (C) The left renal artery

    (D) The left gastric artery

42. **Mirror-image artifact is seen in the right subclavian vein with color Doppler. Which of the following methods may eliminate the artifact?**

    (A) Increase the color gain

    (B) Move the angle of the beam away from 90 degrees

    (C) Increase the image depth

    (D) Decrease the frequency of the transducer

43. **Esophageal varices may be formed in the presence of**

    (A) Budd–Chiari syndrome

    (B) Portal hypertension

    (C) Elevated right-sided heart pressures

    (D) Hepatopetal portal venous flow

44. **What is the consequence of using a blood pressure cuff too small for the body part?**

    (A) It is too uncomfortable for the patient

    (B) The blood pressure will be measured artificiality lower than normal

    (C) The blood pressure will be measured artificiality higher than normal

    (D) Different cuff sizes have no effect on measured blood pressure

45. **A 38-year-old woman presents to the vascular laboratory with unexplained hypertension. What is her physician's chief concern?**

    (A) Portal hypertension

    (B) Renal venous thrombosis

    (C) FMD

    (D) DVT

46. **Dilated venous structures surrounding the umbilicus in severe portal hypertension is known as**

    (A) Cavernous transformation

    (B) Splenorenal shunting

    (C) Esophageal varices

    (D) Caput medusa

47. **What is the optimal patient position for arterial segmental pressure examinations?**

    (A) Supine

    (B) Semi-Fowler's

    (C) Standing

    (D) Reverse Trendelenburg

48. **A 58-year-old patient presents 1-month status post cardiac catheterization. The venous waveforms are remarkable for high velocities and pulsatile flow, and color pixels are present within the soft tissues. What is the most likely diagnosis given the information presented?**

    (A) DVT

    (B) Arteriovenous fistula

    (C) Hematoma

    (D) Pseudoaneurysm

49. **Which of the following is the first branch of the subclavian artery?**

    (A) Thyrocervical trunk

    (B) Internal mammary artery

    (C) Superior thyroid artery

    (D) Vertebral artery

50. **Continuous flow in a peripheral leg vein may be a sign of what?**

    (A) A more peripheral obstruction

    (B) Underwear that is too tight

    (C) Portal hypertension

    (D) Arteriovenous (AV) fistula

51. **The dorsalis pedis is a terminal branch of which lower extremity vessel?**

    (A) Anterior tibial artery

    (B) Posterior tibial vein

    (C) Common femoral artery

    (D) Peroneal artery

52. **As the area of a vessel decreases, according to Bernoulli, what happens to pressure at the level of nonhemodynamically significant stenosis?**

    (A) The pressure is increased at the point of stenosis but drops distal to the stenosis

    (B) There is a pressure drop at the point of stenosis which persists distal to the stenosis

    (C) There is no change in pressure in the vessel in a nonhemodynamically significant stenosis

    (D) There is a pressure drop at the point of stenosis but normal distal to the stenosis

53. **The venous valves arise from which layer of the blood vessel?**

    (A) The tunica adventitia

    (B) The vasa vasorum

    (C) The tunica intima

    (D) The tunica media

54. **In a standing patient, where will the hydrostatic pressure be the highest?**

    (A) By the ankles

    (B) In a hand stretched over the head

    (C) At the level of the heart

    (D) In the mid-abdomen

55. **The superficial vessel that runs along the posterior calf and may be referred to as the "stocking seam" vein in the**

    (A) Great saphenous vein

    (B) Small saphenous vein

    (C) Posterior tibial vein

    (D) Dorsalis pedis

56. **A 72-year-old patient presents with amaurosis fugax that lasts almost the entire day. This patient is diagnosed with having a**

    (A) Transient ischemic attack (TIA)

    (B) Cerebrovascular accident

    (C) Myocardial infarction

    (D) Major stroke

57. **A patient's right ICA has a peak systolic velocity (PSV) of 225 cm/s and end-diastolic velocity (EDV) of 90 cm/s. The patient's category of stenosis based only on this information is**

    (A) 0% to 25% stenosis

    (B) 25% to 50% stenosis

    (C) 50% to 79% stenosis

    (D) More than 80% stenosis

58. **In the abdominal aorta, at what size (and above) will intervention usually be considered?**

    (A) 2.5 cm

    (B) 3.0 cm

    (C) 5.5 cm

    (D) 7.0 cm

59. **With subclavian steal syndrome,**

    (A) The arm with the lowest blood pressure will be contralateral to the side of stenosis

    (B) The arm with the lowest blood pressure will be ipsilateral to the side of stenosis

    (C) The blood pressures are decreased bilaterally

    (D) The blood pressures are increased bilaterally

60. **A "thumping" waveform is seen and heard**

    (A) Proximal to an occlusion

    (B) Distal to a high-grade stenosis

    (C) Distal to an occlusion

    (D) Proximal to a nonhemodynamically significant stenosis

61. **At what angle does the maximum Doppler shift occur?**

    (A) 60 degrees

    (B) 90 degrees

    (C) 45 degrees

    (D) 0 degree

62. **In this sagittal color Doppler image (Fig. PT–8) below the level of the inguinal ligament, letter "A" represents which vessel?**

    (A) Common iliac artery

    (B) Internal iliac artery

    (C) External iliac artery

    (D) Common femoral artery

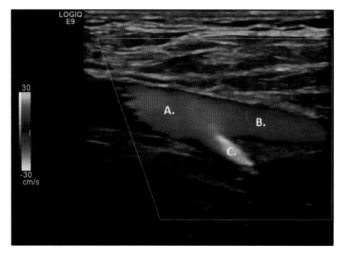

FIGURE PT–8.

63. **In this sagittal color Doppler image (Fig. PT–8) above the level of the inguinal ligament, letter "A" bifurcates into which two arteries?**

    (A) B: Internal iliac artery, C: External iliac artery

    (B) B: External iliac artery, C: Internal iliac artery

    (C) B: Superficial femoral artery, C: Profunda femoris artery

    (D) B: Profunda femoris artery, C: Superficial femoral artery

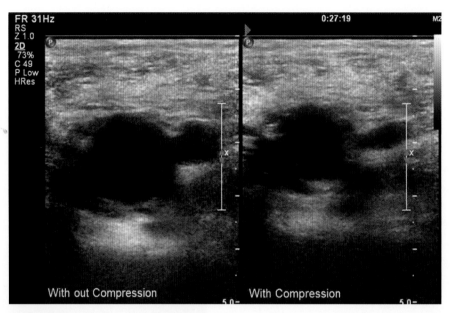

FIGURE PT–9.

64. This image (Fig. PT–9) was obtained from the left thigh just below the inguinal ligament during a venous duplex examination. What do these findings suggest?

    (A) Normal common femoral vein
    (B) Positive for chronic postthrombotic change within the common femoral vein
    (C) Positive for acute deep vein thrombosis (DVT) common femoral vein
    (D) Unable to determine without color Doppler

65. The suboccipital approach allows insonation of which vessel?

    (A) Ophthalmic artery
    (B) Posterior cerebral artery (PCA)
    (C) Extracranial internal carotid artery
    (D) Basilar artery

66. The celiac axis splits into

    (A) Splenic artery, common hepatic artery, and left gastric artery
    (B) Splenic artery, splenic vein, and SMA
    (C) Splenic artery, common hepatic artery, and gastroduodenal artery
    (D) Splenic artery, proper hepatic artery, and right renal artery

67. A patient presents to the vascular laboratory for noninvasive pressure testing. The patient describes symptoms of cramping in the calves while walking that is only relieved by rest in the absence of any other symptoms. Based on the patient's symptoms, what ABI would you expect to see on this patient?

    (A) 1.0
    (B) 0.65
    (C) 0.95
    (D) 0.25

68. A 65-year-old woman patient presents to the vascular laboratory with a suspected right ICA occlusion. During the TCD examination with the probe on the right transtemporal window, a vessel is insonated at a depth of 70 mm with flow toward the probe. What is most likely the identity of the vessel being insonated?

    (A) MCA
    (B) PCA
    (C) ACA
    (D) Terminal internal carotid artery

69. **Figure PT-10 shows an angiogram image of a lower extremity above the level of the knee. What pathology is seen on this image?**

    (A) Pseudoaneurysm

    (B) Arterial dissection

    (C) Stenosis

    (D) Occlusion

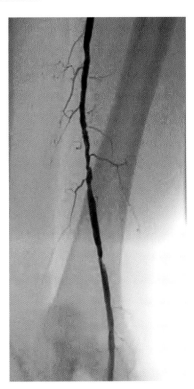

FIGURE PT-10.

70. **The vertebral artery in Figure PT-11 shows what type of flow?**

    (A) Cephalad

    (B) Caudal

    (C) Alternating

    (D) Partial occlusion

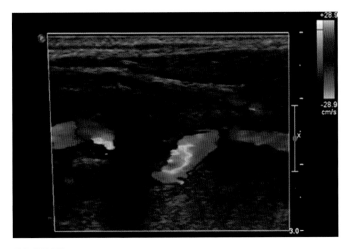

FIGURE PT-11.

71. **What condition is often referred to as the "patriotic disease" because of changes in skin color at the tips of the fingers or toes?**

    (A) Raynaud's disease

    (B) Buerger's disease

    (C) Compartment syndrome

    (D) Embolic disease

72. **A common complication associated with portal hypertension is**

    (A) Mesenteric ischemia

    (B) Varicocele

    (C) Esophageal varices

    (D) Hydronephrosis

73. **According to the North American Symptomatic Carotid Endarterectomy Trial (NASCET) criteria, what constitutes a more than 70% diameter stenosis?**

    (A) PSV more than 125 cm/s

    (B) ICA/CCA ratio more than 4.0

    (C) ICA/CCA ratio more than 2.0

    (D) EDV less than 100 cm/s

74. **Figure PT-12 shows spectral pulsed wave (PW) Doppler waveforms obtained from a patient's right cerebrovascular system. Based on these findings, what is the most likely diagnosis?**

    (A) Proximal brachiocephalic artery stenosis

    (B) Distal MCA stenosis

    (C) Proximal subclavian artery stenosis

    (D) Distal internal carotid artery occlusion

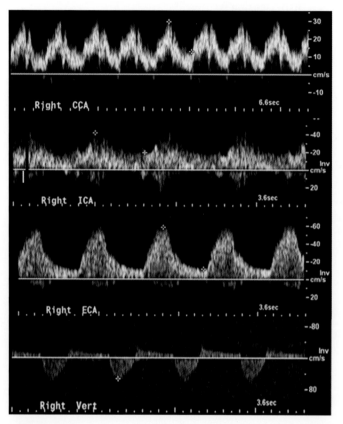

FIGURE PT-12.

75. **A patient having a renal artery duplex examination has the following findings shown in Figure PT-13. What do these findings suggest?**

    (A) Less than 60% stenosis of the left renal artery

    (B) More than 60% stenosis of the left renal artery

    (C) Velocity in aorta too low to determine

    (D) Normal study

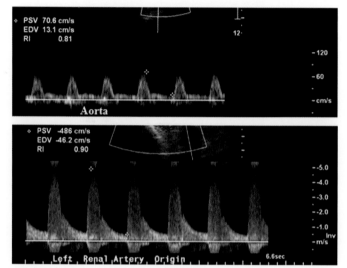

FIGURE PT-13.

76. **The type of flow pattern where the velocities increase toward the center of the vessel is known as**

    (A) Turbulent

    (B) Plug

    (C) Occluded

    (D) Laminar

77. **One hundred patients had bilateral noninvasive and invasive cerebrovascular studies. Of the 200 ICAs imaged, 80 of the ICAs showed hemodynamically significant disease in both the noninvasive and invasive studies. 100 ICAs showed no evidence of disease in both the noninvasive and invasive studies. In 18 cases, the noninvasive studies were positive but the arteriograms were negative. In 2 cases, the noninvasive studies were negative but the arteriograms were positive. How would you calculate PPV?**

    (A) 100/102

    (B) 80/98

    (C) 18/98

    (D) 100/118

78. A morbidly obese 64-year-old woman presents to the vascular laboratory for a noninvasive pressure and waveform examination. The patient has a history of hypertension and diabetes. The results of the examination show a dampened PVR waveform in the right lower extremity at the level of the calf and ankle. The ABI on the right is 1.03. What is most likely the reason for the discrepancy in these findings?

    (A) The study is within normal limits because ABIs are always more accurate than PVR waveforms

    (B) The ABIs are inaccurate as a result of technologist error

    (C) The discrepancy is most likely a malfunction of the equipment due to lack of calibration

    (D) The ABIs are falsely elevated as a result of cuff artifact and/or calcified vessels

79. The following waveform (Fig. PT–14) was obtained in the distal renal artery at the level of the renal hilum of an obese patient in which the sonographer was unable to visualize the aorta or the origin of the renal arteries. What assumption can you most likely make based on this finding?

    (A) There is normal flow within the renal artery

    (B) There is a significant proximal renal artery stenosis (RAS)

    (C) There is a significant distal RAS

    (D) There is medical renal disease present in this patient

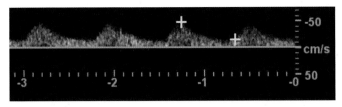

FIGURE PT–14.

80. Figure PT–15 is a transverse view of the right calf demonstrating a color Doppler image of a perforator vein. The findings in this image suggest

    (A) Normal flow from the superficial system to the deep system

    (B) Retrograde flow from the deep system to the superficial system

    (C) Normal flow from the deep system to the superficial system

    (D) Retrograde flow from the superficial system to the deep system

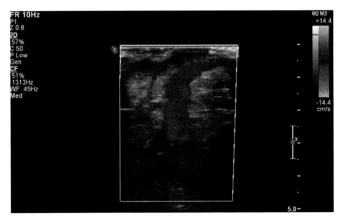

FIGURE PT–15.

81. When performing a venous insufficiency study with the patient standing, what period of reversed flow in the deep system is considered significant for venous reflux?

    (A) 0.35 s

    (B) 0.50 s

    (C) 1 s

    (D) 1.50 s

82. A 45-year-old woman with mild hypertension presents to the vascular laboratory because her primary care physician heard an asymptomatic bruit on the right side of her neck. The duplex findings reveal normal velocities within the proximal portion of the ICA and elevated velocities within the mid to distal ICA. Figure PT–16 shows a color Doppler image of the right ICA. What is most likely the cause of these findings?

(A) Atherosclerotic disease

(B) Carotid dissection

(C) FMD

(D) Carotid body tumor

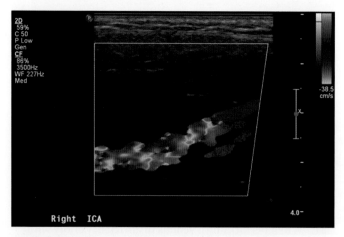

FIGURE PT–16.

83. Venous blood return from the lower extremities is greatest during which phase of respiration?

(A) Inspiration

(B) Expiration

(C) Respiration has no effect on venous flow

(D) Valsalva maneuver

84. What is the typical transducer frequency employed during a TCD examination?

(A) 1-3 MHz

(B) 3-5 MHz

(C) 5-7 MHz

(D) 10-12 MHz

85. What percent of pulmonary emboli is estimated to have originated in the lower extremities and pelvis?

(A) 30%

(B) 40%

(C) 90%

(D) 100%

86. The angle of insonance during a TCD examination is assumed to be

(A) 60 degrees

(B) 90 degrees

(C) 45 degrees

(D) 0 degree

87. What cerebral artery connects the right hemisphere circulation to the left hemisphere?

(A) PCoA

(B) Anterior communicating artery

(C) Superior cerebellar artery

(D) Anterior choroidal artery

88. A 78-year-old man patient presents to the vascular with decreased pulses in the right lower extremity 1 week following an in situ saphenous vein femoral to distal tibial artery bypass graft. The image in Figure PT–17 was obtained during a duplex examination of the lower extremity bypass graft. What is most likely the cause of these findings?

(A) Progression of atherosclerotic disease

(B) Myointimal hyperplasia

(C) Retained valve cusp

(D) Arteriovenous malformation

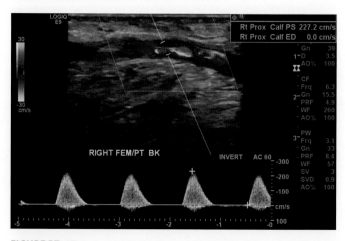

FIGURE PT–17.

89. Which of the following is not a symptom of lower extremity venous insufficiency?

(A) Skin color changes at the gaiter zone

(B) Diabetic heel ulcer

(C) Lower extremity edema

(D) Varicose veins

90. While calculating statistics for a noninvasive examination, it is determined that the sensitivity is 96% while the specificity is 85%. It is also determined that the PPV is 92% while the NPV is 83%. Based on these statistics, which of the following values is least likely to represent accuracy?

    (A) 83%

    (B) 91%

    (C) 92%

    (D) 80%

91. All of these neurological symptoms are associated with the vertebro-basilar circulation with the exception of

    (A) Amaurosis fugax

    (B) Vertigo

    (C) Diplopia

    (D) Bilateral paresthesia

92. Which of the following is not a limitation of noninvasive pressure and waveform testing?

    (A) Multiple levels of disease resulting in missing more distal disease

    (B) Cuff artifact causing falsely elevated pressure resulting in underestimation of disease

    (C) Calcified vessels causing falsely elevated pressure resulting in underestimation of disease

    (D) Pitting edema causing distortion in the shape of the pulse volume recording waveforms resulting in an overestimation of disease

93. A rare arteritis that typically affects the thoracic aortic arch and its larger branches is known as

    (A) Marfan's syndrome

    (B) Coarctation of the aorta

    (C) Takayasu's arteritis

    (D) Temporal arteritis

94. While performing a photoplethysmography (PPG) examination of the lower extremity to evaluate for venous insufficiency, a venous refill time of 6 seconds is achieved. With a tourniquet place above the knee, the test is repeated and a venous refill time of 25 seconds is achieved. What do these findings suggest?

    (A) The findings rule out the presence of venous insufficiency

    (B) There is venous insufficiency within the deep venous system

    (C) There is venous insufficiency within the small saphenous vein

    (D) There is venous insufficiency within the great saphenous vein

95. Which abdominal artery exhibits a significant increase in diastolic flow postprandial when compared to its preprandial waveform?

    (A) SMA

    (B) Celiac axis

    (C) Hepatic artery

    (D) Renal artery

96. What secondary branch of the great saphenous vein serves as a connection for several important perforators in the lower calf?

    (A) Lateral accessory saphenous vein

    (B) Posterior accessory vein

    (C) Medial accessory saphenous vein

    (D) Small saphenous vein

97. The following TCD waveforms in Figure PT–18 were obtained during an examination of a patient who is 12 days status post subarachnoid hemorrhage. What do these findings suggest?

    (A) Hyperemia

    (B) Critical stenosis

    (C) Mild vasospasm

    (D) Severe vasospasm

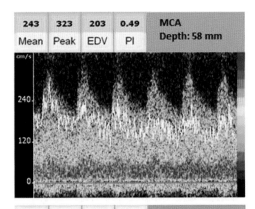

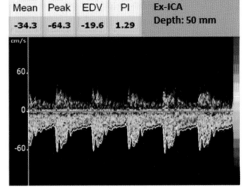

FIGURE PT–18.

98. **A phasic PW Doppler waveform obtained within the central subclavian vein suggests**

    (A) Central (proximal) obstruction
    (B) Peripheral (distal) obstruction
    (C) Increased pressure within the venous system
    (D) Normal venous hemodynamics

99. **Budd–Chiari syndrome can potentially be the cause of which type of portal hypertension?**

    (A) Presinusoidal
    (B) Sinusoidal
    (C) Postsinusoidal
    (D) Budd–Chiari syndrome and portal hypertension are unrelated

100. **Figure PT–19 is a color Doppler image obtained through the transtemporal window. Letter "A" can be identified as what vessel?**

    (A) A1 segment of the ACA
    (B) M1 segment of the MCA
    (C) PCoA
    (D) P2 segment of the PCA

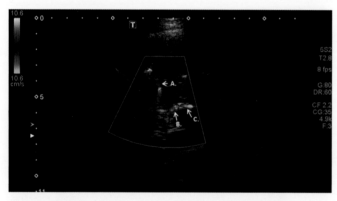

FIGURE PT–19.

101. **Figure PT–19 is a color Doppler image obtained through the transtemporal window. Letter "C" can be identified as what vessel?**

    (A) P1 segment of the PCA
    (B) M1 segment of the MCA
    (C) A2 segment of the ACA
    (D) P2 segment of the PCA

102. **Figure PT–20 is a color Doppler image above the clavicle. What do these findings suggest?**

    (A) Acute DVT subclavian vein
    (B) Chronic changes subclavian vein
    (C) Normal findings of the subclavian vein
    (D) The color scale setting is too high making it impossible for a diagnosis

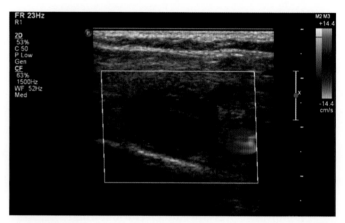

FIGURE PT–20.

103. **Figure PT–21 is a color Doppler image at the distal anastomosis of a lower extremity bypass graft. The flow represented as blue on this image is consistent with which finding?**

    (A) Normal retrograde flow found proximal to the distal anastomosis
    (B) Retrograde flow suggesting a distal occlusion
    (C) Retrograde flow suggesting impending bypass graft failure
    (D) Retrograde flow suggesting stenosis of the distal anastomosis

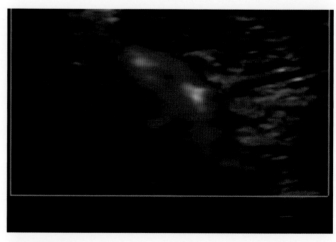

FIGURE PT–21.

104. **The spectral PW Doppler waveforms in Figure PT–22 were obtained during a venous duplex examination of the lower extremities on a patient with extreme bilateral leg edema. What do these findings most likely suggest?**

    (A) Proximal obstruction of the left common iliac vein

    (B) Proximal obstruction of the right common iliac vein

    (C) Proximal obstruction of the IVC

    (D) The bilateral common femoral waveforms suggest normal venous hemodynamics

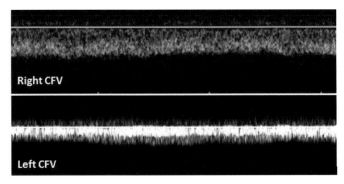

FIGURE PT–22.

105. **The plaque seen in Figure PT–23 can be characterized as all of the following EXCEPT**

    (A) Low level echogenicity

    (B) Calcified

    (C) Soft plaque

    (D) Homogeneous

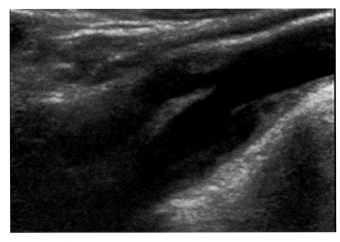

FIGURE PT–23.

106. **Which vessels make up the classic arterial trifurcation below the knee?**

    (A) Anterior tibial artery, posterior tibial artery, peroneal artery

    (B) Popliteal artery, peroneal artery, anterior tibial artery

    (C) Anterior tibial artery, dorsalis pedis artery, posterior tibial artery

    (D) Tibioperoneal trunk, posterior tibial artery, peroneal artery

107. **Classic rest pain is always associated with what degree of peripheral arterial disease?**

    (A) Mild

    (B) Moderate

    (C) Severe

    (D) Unrelated to vascular disease

108. **The following two waveforms in Figure PT–24 were obtained from the celiac axis at different phases of respiration. What is most likely the diagnosis?**

    (A) Acute occlusion

    (B) MALS

    (C) Normal celiac artery

    (D) Postprandial changes

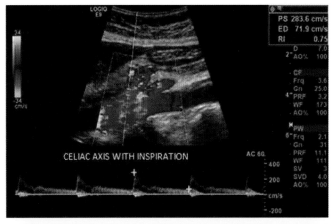

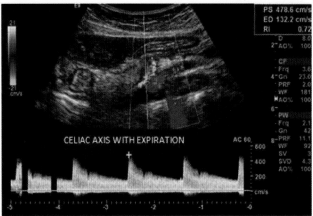

FIGURE PT–24.

109. Which of the following is NOT true regarding the typical course of the left renal vein?

    (A) It courses posterior to the SMA

    (B) It courses posterior to the left renal artery

    (C) It courses anterior to the aorta

    (D) It enters the left lateral portion of the IVC

110. Figure PT–25 demonstrates the duplex findings in a patient with right-sided hemiparalysis. What is most likely the cause of the patient's symptoms?

    (A) These findings are consistent with a critical stenosis of the left ICA which would cause symptoms on the contralateral side

    (B) These findings are consistent with a critical stenosis of the left ICA which would cause symptoms on the ipsilateral side

    (C) These findings are consistent with normal ICA flow and do not explain the patient's symptoms

    (D) These findings are unrelated to the patient's symptoms

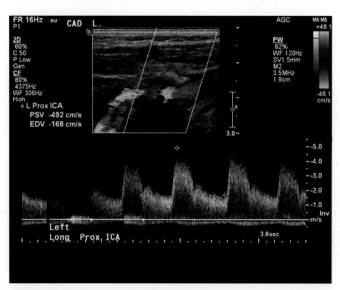

FIGURE PT–25.

111. Figure PT–26 shows a spectral PW Doppler waveform obtained from the transtemporal window. What vessel is being insonated?

    (A) Internal carotid artery

    (B) MCA

    (C) PCA

    (D) ACA

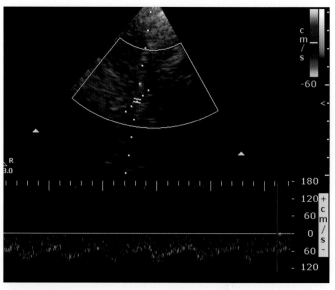

FIGURE PT–26.

112. The following TCD waveform (Fig. PT–27) was obtained from the left transorbital approach in a patient with a left extracranial internal carotid artery occlusion. What do these findings suggest?

    (A) Normal hemodynamics within the ophthalmic artery

    (B) Normal hemodynamics within the carotid siphon

    (C) Collateral flow through the ophthalmic artery via the ECA branches

    (D) Hemodynamically significant stenosis within the carotid siphon

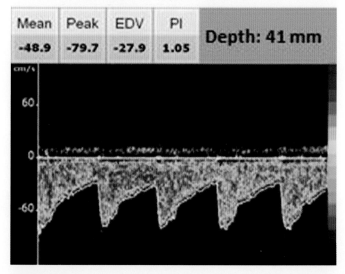

FIGURE PT–27.

113. All of the following are characteristics in determining ICA from ECA during a carotid duplex examination EXCEPT

(A) That the ICA has a lower resistant signal compared to the ECA

(B) That the ICA is typically smaller in caliber compared to the ECA

(C) That the ICA is typically located more laterally that the ECA

(D) That the ICA does not have extracranial branches while the ECA does

114. The gastrocnemius veins drain blood from the upper calf muscle and can be visualized during a venous duplex examination, where they connect to which lower extremity vein?

(A) Posterior tibial vein

(B) Peroneal vein

(C) Anterior tibial vein

(D) Popliteal vein

115. What is the most common cause of venous insufficiency in the lower extremities?

(A) Congenital defects to the venous valves

(B) Genetics

(C) Inactivity

(D) Postthrombotic syndrome

116. A 67-year-old patient presents to the vascular laboratory for a postoperative carotid duplex examination the year following his right carotid endarterectomy surgery. The findings of the duplex reveal a hemodynamically significant stenosis at the origin of the right ICA. What is most likely the cause of the restenosis?

(A) Progression of atherosclerosis

(B) Neointimal hyperplasia

(C) Clamp injury from the surgery

(D) FMD

117. Figure PT–28 is a transverse view of the common femoral vein with and without compression. What do these findings suggest?

(A) Findings are consistent with a normal common femoral vein

(B) Findings are consistent with acute DVT of the common femoral vein

(C) Findings are consistent with chronic postthrombotic change of the common femoral vein

(D) Findings are consistent with subacute DVT of the common femoral vein

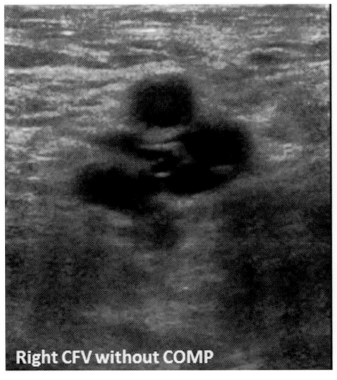
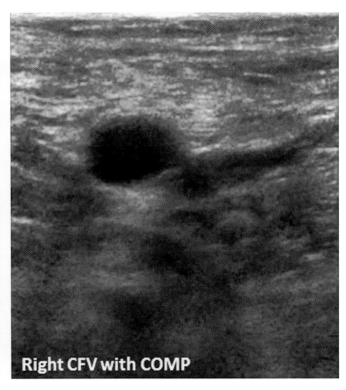

FIGURE PT–28.

118. **The condition involving an outflow obstruction of the venous system that presents with extreme swelling, cyanosis, and reduced arterial inflow is known as**

    (A) Dependent rubor
    (B) Venous insufficiency
    (C) Phlegmasia alba dolens
    (D) Phlegmasia cerulea dolens

119. **What is the most reliable parameter in determining vasospasm versus hyperemia in a patient with a subarachnoid hemorrhage?**

    (A) MCA/ICA ratio
    (B) Mean flow velocity
    (C) Peak systolic velocity
    (D) EDV

120. **All of the following increase your risk of developing DVT EXCEPT**

    (A) Immobility
    (B) Trauma
    (C) Hypertension
    (D) Postoperative

Answers and Explanations

1. **(B)** This waveform is characteristic of turbulence, which may be seen distal to a stenosis.

2. **(C)** Unless a blood pressure cannot be taken due to a contraindication, the highest pressure between the two arms is always used for all indices.

3. **(B)** The coronary vein, or left gastric vein, normally drains the esophagus. Portal hypertension may cause esophageal varices, presenting as reversal of flow in a dilated coronary vein.

4. **(A)** Tardus parvus is a delay in the systolic upstroke, and looks like a rounding of the systolic peak, unlike its normal appearance of a sharp upstroke.

5. **(D)** Fusiform aneurysms are more common than saccular or mycotic. Pseudoaneurysms are not true aneurysms, and are not common in the aorta.

6. **(B)** This waveform is a to-and-fro pattern, not normal in the portal vein. The normal portal vein is mildly pulsatile. This waveform suggests a problem distally.

7. **(C)** According to Bernoulli's principle, the lowest pressure will be at the region of the highest velocity. The continuity equation (Q = VA) states that in a nonhemodynamically significant stenosis, where the area is the smallest, the velocity is the highest. Thus, this is the region where the pressure is the lowest.

8. **(A)** The splenic vein is part of the portal venous system and is not examined routinely as part of a mesenteric arterial study.

9. **(C)** The letter "D" represents the posterior communicating artery.

10. **(A)** The letter "A" represents the terminal ICA, which bifurcates into MCA and ACA.

11. **(D)** The internal thoracic, or mammary artery, is a branch of the subclavian artery.

12. **(B)** A test with a high NPV is good at predicating a negative or normal study.

13. **(C)** It is dilatation of the peripheral arterioles that determines distal resistance. According to Poiseuille's law, radius is the most significant factor in determining resistance, and therefore, flow. The arterioles' muscular layer expands or contracts, which determines resistance.

14. **(A)** The SMA and IMA are normally high resistant in a fasting patient.

15. **(A)** Aortoiliac disease usually presents as buttock pain. Since the pain in this example is unilateral, disease is probably located in the right common iliac artery.

16. **(D)** This waveform is a classic to-and-fro waveform, as commonly seen in the neck of a pseudoaneurysm.

17. **(B)** Conventional or digital subtraction angiography uses a needle inserted into the common femoral artery, a contrast agent, and ionizing radiation to produce images of the blood vessels.

18. **(B)** RAS of more than 60% presents with an RAR greater than 3.5.

19. **(C)** According to the color flow, there is reversal of flow in the main portal vein, consistent with portal hypertension. Ascites is also present, another finding of portal hypertension.

20. **(C)** Sensitivity is defined as the number of true positives divided by the number of true positives + the number of false negatives.

21. **(D)** The diagnosis of DVT is made by compressions. Color and spectral Doppler may add additional information, but the ability of vein walls to completely coapt makes the diagnosis.

22. **(C)** The "string of beads" appearance is characteristic of FMD. This sign may be better seen on angiography than ultrasound.

23. **(B)** Disease usually occurs at bifurcations, so is more likely to occur at the origin of vessels.

24. **(B)** MALS is diagnosed when the patient has normal celiac arterial signals on inspiration but abnormal signals on expiration.

25. **(D)** The most important person in the vascular laboratory is the patient. Without the patient, there would be no need for physicians, sonographers, or nurses. Patient care is not just about performing a diagnostic examination, but also how the patient is treated by everyone.

26. **(A)** Overgaining the spectral signal will cause overmeasurement of the velocities.

27. **(C)** The common femoral vein is formed by the confluence of the femoral vein and the deep femoral vein (aka profunda femoris vein).

28. **(D)** Flow in a TIPS should be from portal veins to hepatic veins. Flow velocities should not change more than 50 cm/s from sampling point to sampling point within the TIPS.

29. **(A)** There is a more than 20 mm Hg difference in pressures between the right and left brachial arteries. The blood pressure will be lower on the side ipsilateral to the subclavian stenosis.

30. **(B)** According to criteria, ABIs of 0.41-0.90 falls in the mild to moderate range.

31. **(C)** The internal carotid artery feeds the brain, a normally low-resistance vascular bed. Therefore, ICA waveforms should be low resistant.

32. **(A)** In the presence of cerebral edema, the brain becomes a high-resistance pathway. Therefore, the ICA, which supplies this bed, becomes high resistant. In cases of severe cerebral edema or brain death, the ICA may become to-and-fro as flow ceases to move forward through systole and diastole.

33. **(C)** From a transtemporal window, the A1 portion of the ipsilateral ACA should have flow away from the transducer.

34. **(B)** From the suboccipital window via the foramen magnum, the basilar artery has flow in a direction away from the transducer.

35. **(C)** Color pixels seen in soft tissue may be a color bruit, which is a tissue vibration causing a Doppler shift outside of the blood vessels. This may be a sign of a stenosis within a vessel, a pseudoaneurysm, or arteriovenous fistula.

36. **(D)** Budd–Chiari syndrome is obstruction of the IVC and/or hepatic veins. Budd–Chiari syndrome may lead to postsinusoidal portal hypertension.

37. **(B)** The return of symptoms associated with portal hypertension is an indication of a failed TIPS. Examples include hepatopetal flow in the left or right portal vein branches, ascites, and splenomegaly.

38. **(C)** The kidney is a low-resistant vascular bed, and therefore its feeding vessels and the renal arteries, will exhibit a low-resistance monophasic waveform.

39. **(C)** The renal arteries are, in the order, main renal artery; segmental renal artery; interlobar artery, arcuate artery, interlobular artery.

40. **(A)** A carotid body tumor is (usually) a benign, vascular mass (paraganglioma) that occurs extrinsic to the carotid in the region of the carotid bifurcation.

41. **(D)** The left gastric artery, a branch off of the celiac axis, is usually not seen by ultrasound.

42. **(B)** Mirror-image artifact most commonly occurs under two conditions: angle to flow of 90 degrees or excessive gain. Fixing one or both of these problems will usually eliminate the artifact.

43. **(B)** Portal hypertension has several clinical findings, but one of the most severe is esophageal varices. Ruptured esophageal varices may cause rapid death from exsanguination.

44. **(C)** Cuff artifact can occur when the blood pressure is taken with a cuff that is too small for the area being sampled.

45. **(C)** Young females with hypertension should be screened for renal FMD.

46. **(D)** Caput medusae refer to the snake-like vessels that form around the umbilicus as a result of severe portal hypertension recanalizing the umbilical vein.

47. **(A)** Due to the effects of hydrostatic pressure, the most accurate readings will come from a patient that is supine.

48. **(B)** Given the history of recent invasive procedure, iatrogenic injury must be considered. High-velocity, pulsatile waveforms in the venous system are indicative of an AV fistula.

49. **(D)** The first branch of the subclavian artery bilaterally is the vertebral artery.

50. **(B)** Any central compression may cause continuous flow peripherally. Common causes are constrictive clothing, intrinsic clot, and extrinsic compression (e.g., from a tumor).

51. **(A)** The dorsalis pedis artery is a terminal branch of the anterior tibial artery.

52. **(D)** In a nonhemodynamically significant stenosis, the pressure drops at the area of narrowing but resumes to a normal pressure distal to the narrowing.

53. **(C)** Valves arise from the intimal layer of the vessel.

54. **(A)** In an erect patient, the farther from the heart (i.e., the closer to the ground), the higher the hydrostatic pressure.

55. **(B)** The small saphenous vein is a superficial vessel that runs down the back of the calf.

56. **(A)** TIAs, also called "mini-strokes," last less than 24 hours.

57. **(C)** PSV equal to or above 125 cm/s signify at least a 50% stenosis, regardless of EDV. Because the EDV in this example is less than 140 cm/s, the stenosis is graded at 50% to 79%, based on the limited information provided.

58. **(C)** Abdominal aortic aneurysms above 5.5 cm are usually considered for intervention.

59. **(B)** In a vertebral steal, the affected (ipsilateral) side will have the lowest blood pressure.

60. **(A)** The "thumping" sound is heard when blood smacks up against an obstruction. In other words, proximal to an occlusion.

61. **(D)** When flow is toward the transducer at a 0 degree, the Doppler shift is the greatest. The Doppler shift decreases progressively at higher angles, with no Doppler shift occurring at 90 degrees.

62. **(D)** Common femoral artery. The external iliac artery becomes the common femoral artery below the level of the inguinal ligament.

63. **(C)** The common femoral artery bifurcates into the superficial femoral artery (B) and the profunda femoris (C).

64. **(C)** The findings of a noncompressible but deformable common femoral vein with low level echogenicity are consistent with acute DVT.

65. (D) The suboccipital window is used to insonate the vertebral and basilar arteries.

66. (A) The celiac axis splits into the left gastric, splenic, and common hepatic arteries.

67. (B) An ABI of 0.65 is consistent with symptoms of claudication. An ABI above 0.90 is considered normal or borderline. An ABI 0.25 or less is associated with ischemia.

68. (C) With an extracranial internal carotid artery occlusion, it is common to find reversed flow within the ACA on the ipsilateral side of the disease suggesting collateral "crossover" flow through the anterior communicating artery.

69. (C) Figure PT–10 shows a filling defect within the distal superficial femoral artery consistent with a stenosis.

70. (A) Figure PT–11 shows a tortuous vertebral artery with normal cephalic flow toward the head.

71. (A) Raynaud's disease is often referred to as the "patriotic disease" because the tips of the patients digits initially turn white followed by blue and then eventually turn red during the rewarming period.

72. (C) Esophageal varices are a serious complication of portal hypertension caused by increased pressure in the portal system resulting in retrograde (hepatofugal) flow in the left gastric (coronary) vein.

73. (B) While some criteria use PSV and EDV to determine percent stenosis, the NASCET criteria uses an ICA/CCA ratio more than 4.0 for determining a more than 70% stenosis.

74. (A) The waveforms obtained within the CCA, ICA, and ECA all have a delay to peak systolic (tardus parvus) suggesting a proximal stenosis. The vertebral artery waveform demonstrates alternating flow suggesting the presence of proximal disease as well. Because the brachiocephalic artery gives rise to both the common carotid artery and the right subclavian, a significant stenosis would affect both vessels in this way.

75. (B) There is an elevated PSV (> 200 cm/s) in the main real artery resulting in an abnormal renal aortic ratio (RAR) of 6.9. An RAR that is greater than 3.5 is consistent with a more than 60% stenosis of the main renal artery.

76. (D) Laminar flow has a parabolic velocity profile when the velocity of flow increases toward the center of the blood vessel and decreases toward the vessel walls.

77. (B) PPV is calculated by taking the true positives (80) and dividing that by the true positive (80) + False positives (18). Thus, PPV = 80/98.

78. (D) Two main causes for falsely elevated pressure readings during a noninvasive arterial examination are cuff artifact and calcified vessels, which are common problems with obese (cuff artifact) and diabetic (calcified vessels) patients. Pulse volume recording waveforms are typically more accurate than systolic segment pressures as they are not affected by these two issues.

79. (B) The waveform displayed in Figure PT–14 of the distal renal artery is a tardus parvus waveform suggesting significant proximal disease.

80. (B) Normal flow within a perforating vein is from the superficial system to the deep. The flow within this perforator is going toward the probe from the deep system to the superficial system in an abnormal retrograde fashion.

81. (C) When performing a venous insufficiency study on a patient in a standing position, a reflux time for the deep venous system more than 1.0 s is positive for reflux.

82. (C) Atherosclerosis typically occurs within the proximal internal carotid artery and is relatively rare in the mid to distal segments. FMD is a nonatherosclerotic disease that usually occurs within the mid to distal segments.

83. (B) As a person exhales, the diaphragm rises decreasing the intra-abdominal pressure resulting in venous return from the lower extremities increasing. During inspiration, the diaphragm lowers resulting in an increase in intra-abdominal pressure as well as a decrease in thoracic pressure resulting in venous return from the upper extremities increasing.

84. (A) The typical transducer frequency for both TCD and transcranial Doppler imaging (TCDI) examinations is in between 1 and 3 MHz.

85. (C) It is estimated that the majority (90%) of pulmonary emboli are the result of DVT in the lower extremities.

86. (D) The angle of insonance during a TCD examination is assumed to be 0 degree.

87. (B) The anterior communicating artery connects the right hemisphere circulation to the left hemisphere and can be a source of collateral flow in the presence of extracranial carotid disease.

88. (C) The findings of an elevated PSV with turbulent flow seen on color Doppler are consistent with a hemodynamically significant stenosis. The most common cause of a lower extremity bypass graft stenosis is typically myointimal hyperplasia. Myointimal hyperplasia typically occurs within the first 2 years; however, with a stenosis occurring within a week of the surgery is more likely to be the result of techniques such as a retained valve.

89. (B) Skin changes in the gaiter zone, edema, and varicose veins are all findings consistent with venous insufficiency. Diabetic heel ulcers are often related to arterial insufficiency.

90. (D) Accuracy falls somewhere in between sensitivity and specificity as well as between PPV and NPV.

91. (A) Amaurosis fugax is caused by emboli that travel through the internal carotid artery to the ophthalmic artery and is not related to the posterior circulation.

92. **(D)** Pitting edema may result in a decrease in amplitude of a PVR waveform; however, the shape of the PVR waveform will not be affected. Cuff artifact and calcified vessels are two of the most common limitations of pressure testing as well as multiple levels of disease which results in the more distal disease going undiagnosed due to poor inflow.

93. **(C)** Takayasu's arteritis is a rare arteritis that typically affects the aortic arch and its larger branches.

94. **(D)** A venous refill time less than 20 seconds during a PPG examination for venous insufficiency indicates significant reflux. When the results of a PPG examination demonstrate reflux without the tourniquet and change to negative with the tourniquet at the level of the great saphenous vein, it proves that the great saphenous vein is the cause of the insufficiency.

95. **(A)** The SMA normally has a high-resistance type waveform in a fasting patient (preprandial). When the patient eats a meal (postprandial), the distal arteriole beds in the intestines dilate, increasing the diastolic flow in the SMA.

96. **(B)** The posterior accessory vein is a secondary branch of the great saphenous vein and serves as a connection for the posterior tibial perforators.

97. **(D)** Vasospasm is a multistage process causing narrowing of the cerebral arteries in the presence of a subarachnoid hemorrhage. The TCD findings suggesting severe vasospasm are a mean velocity more than 200 cm/s with a MCA/ICA ratio more than 6. The maximum degree of vasospasm typically occurs between 7 and 14 days following the bleed.

98. **(A)** The normal flow in the central veins closest to the heart should have a pulsatile component. The absence of the pulsatile component suggests a central obstruction to flow and should always be compared to the contralateral side.

99. **(C)** Postsinusoidal portal hypertension is caused by an obstruction in the outflow of the liver. Budd–Chiari syndrome refers to the thrombosis of the hepatic veins that normally drain blood from the liver back to the IVC.

100. **(B)** M1 segment of the MCA with flow toward the transducer.

101. **(D)** P2 segment of the PCA with flow away from the transducer.

102. **(A)** The absence of color Doppler flow in a dilated subclavian vein with low level echoes within the lumen is consistent with acute DVT.

103. **(A)** It is common to have retrograde flow proximal to the distal anastomosis and can often be a source of perfusion to the diseased limb and beneficial to the patient.

104. **(C)** A continuous venous waveform suggests the presence of a proximal obstruction. Bilateral continuous waveforms within the common femoral veins most likely indicate an obstruction of the IVC.

105. **(B)** Calcified plaque would be accompanied with distal shadowing. The plaque seen in Figure PT–23 has uniform low level echoes without the presence of calcifications.

106. **(A)** The trifurcation is made up of the anterior tibial, posterior tibial, and peroneal arteries.

107. **(C)** Rest pain is pain in the distal portion of the limb (feet) that occurs when the legs are elevated at or above the level of the heart and is always associated with severe peripheral arterial disease.

108. **(B)** MALS is compression of the celiac axis resulting in an increase in velocity that occurs during expiration.

109. **(B)** The left renal vein courses from the hilum of the left kidney, anterior to the left renal artery, between the SMA and the aorta to enter the left lateral side of the IVC.

110. **(A)** There is a critical stenosis of this left ICA, which would cause problems with the left side of the brain. Because the left brain controls the right side of the body, there are symptoms on the right side.

111. **(D)** The reversed flow at the location presented is indicative of normal flow within the A1 segment of the ACA.

112. **(C)** This image is representative of reversal of flow as well as a change in resistance in the ophthalmic artery, consistent with ECA collateralization due to ICA occlusion.

113. **(B)** The ICA is usually lateral to the ECA, usually has a lower-resistant waveform, does not have extracranial branches, and is typically larger than the ECA.

114. **(D)** The gastrocnemius veins typically terminate in the popliteal vein.

115. **(D)** Postthrombotic syndrome, which occurs after DVT, is the most common cause of lower extremity venous insufficiency.

116. **(B)** Neointimal hyperplasia is the most common cause of restenosis within the first 2 years after carotid endarterectomy surgery.

117. **(C)** The image to the left without compression shows hyperechoic material within the lumen of the vein which is commonly termed "synechiae." The image with compression shows compression of the vein around the echogenic material. These findings are consistent with chronic postthrombotic change in the common femoral vein.

118. **(D)** Severe venous obstructive disease may cause inflow obstruction because the blood has no way out of the leg. Phlegmasia cerulea dolens ("painful blue leg") is severe obstruction with swelling and cyanosis.

119. **(A)** The MCA/ICA ratio is the most reliable parameter when determining vasospasm versus hyperemia.

120. **(C)** Hypertension is more commonly associated with arterial disease, not venous disease. Immobility, trauma, and postoperative stasis are risk factors for DVT.

Index

Note: Page number followed by f and t indicates figure and table respectively.